TALKING BACK TO RITALIN

What Doctors Aren't Telling You About Stimulants and ADHD

REVISED EDITION

Peter R. Breggin, M.D.

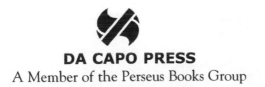

DA CAPO PRESS

A Member of the Perseus Books Group

Library of Congress Cataloging-in-Publication Data
Breggin, Peter Roger, 1936–
Talking back to Ritalin :
what doctors aren't telling you about stimulants for children/
Peter R. Breggin—Rev.ed.
p. cm.
Includes bibliographical references and index.
ISBN 1-56751-213-5 (cloth)—ISBN 0-7382-0544-3 (pbk.)
1. Attention-deficit hyperactivity disorder—Treatment. 2. Methylphenidate
hydrochloride—Side effects. 3. Attention-deficit hyperactivity disorder—
Alternative treatment. I.Title

RJ506.H9 B74 2000
618.92'858906—dc21   00-064521

Da Capo Press is a member of the Perseus Books Group.

Find us on the World Wide Web at
http://www.dacapopress.com

Da Capo Press books are available for special discounts for bulk purchases in the
U.S. by corporations, institutions, and other organizations. For more information,
please contact the Special Markets Department at the Perseus Books Group, 11
Cambridge Center, Cambridge, MA 02142, or call 1-617-252-5298.

10 9 8 7 6 5 4 3 2

For my wife, Ginger, and for her parents, Jean and Phil,
with gratitude for their love

A CAUTION TO THE READER

*T*alking Back to Ritalin is a critique of the use of stimulant drugs such as Ritalin, Concerta, Metadate ER, Dexedrine, and Adderall for the behavioral control of children. There are dozens of books on the market which take a more positive view of these medications but this is the only book that examines their mechanism of action and their adverse effects in depth and detail. Much of the material in this book has not been previously available even to physicians and other health professionals. This revised edition has been bolstered with breaking news events and additional scientific data.

Psychiatric drugs are not only dangerous to take, they are dangerous to *stop* taking as well. When stopping stimulant medications, the child's original symptoms may grow worse or new symptoms may develop. Withdrawal can cause "crashing" with lethargy, fatigue, depression and suicidal feelings. Severe "hyperactivity" and psychosis can develop. Therefore, withdrawal from stimulants should usually be done slowly, with experienced clinical supervision and careful attention to the child's needs and feelings of comfort.

This book is not a treatment guide. No book can substitute for a clinical evaluation.

CONTENTS

Part Three

The Politics of the ADHD/Ritalin Lobby

Part Four

How We Can Help Our Children

ACKNOWLEDGMENTS

Many individuals read the first edition of this book in manuscript form and made useful suggestions and editorial comments. They include Kevin McCready, Brian Kean, David Cohen, Ron David, Steve Baldwin, Doug Smith, and Ginger Ross Breggin. A number of others read portions, including John Friedberg, James O'Donnell, Sharon Collins, Jean Ross, Jim Tucker, Eileen Walkenstein, and Fred Baughman. Nelia Butler and Keith Hoeller contributed valuable comments and copy-editing. Thank you also to the many families who spoke with me or with Ginger about their personal experiences.

I take sole responsibility for any errors that may have slipped through the editing process while I wish to share responsibility with others for many of its good points.

Many people continue to send me items of various kinds that ended up in this book or otherwise proved useful. I apologize for the dozens of people inadvertently left out of the following list. Please keep sending me stuff even if you're not on the list: Tom Mabee, Bob Jacobs, David and Sandra Jacobs, Peter Oas, Sue and Michael Parry, Connie Schuster, Louise Armstrong, Howard Blevins, Ty C. Colbert, Susan Dekking, Victor Sanua, Michael Valentine, John George, Don Weitz, Judi Chamberlin, Kate Clarke, Leighton Whitaker, Mimi Noorani, Dave Dauer, Sharon Collins, Judi Striano, Val Levin, Robert Morgan, Robert Foltz, Richard Horobin, Fred Bemak, Gerald Coles, Chappell Dew, Al Siebert, Samella Abdullah, Victor Sanua, Joseph Tarantolo, David Oaks, and Thomas Greening.

I want to thank our interns who contributed enormously to this book with their research efforts and their ideas: Kristen Vaccaro, Berlos Davis, and Vance A. Hartke. Each of them initially interned when the book was nothing more than a concept, each helped to gather the mass of research papers, each made valuable suggestions. My very special thanks to the three of you and to your professor, Bill Bruck, for making it possible for you to be with us. I also want to thank Alex Laris who joined our internship program in time to provide editorial assistance. Kathy McCain worked ably and hard as a part-time assistant throughout much of this time.

For the new edition of the book, I have been assisted extensively by Ian Goddard in library research and by Linda Linson in the office. They both helped with the editing as well and made my work much more efficient. More recently, Janet Bleck has helped to polish the new chapters.

My agent, Andrew Blauner, continues to be a pleasure to work with.

My wife, Ginger Ross Breggin, was made Executive Director of the International Center for the Study of Psychiatry and Psychology shortly before the first edition of this book came out. The board appointed her by acclamation and then officially voted her into the position at the annual meeting. She earned the volunteer (unpaid) job by setting up the web site, getting the newsletters into production, creating a communications system for the advisory council and board of directors, sending out information packages, staying in touch with board and advisory council, organizing the annual meeting, and myriad other accomplishments. At the same time, Ginger handles many other tasks in our shared lives, making it possible for me to focus on projects such as this book.

In the two years since the first edition, Ginger has further expanded her extraordinary contributions. Most remarkable, perhaps, she originated the idea for the creation of the Center's new peer-review journal, *Ethical Human Sciences and Services*, and was then drafted as its volunteer managing editor. Because of her, the first issues of the journal have come out in a timely fashion with a plethora of good articles.

Ginger also played the key role in the National Institutes of Health (NIH) inviting me to be the scientific presenter on psychiatric drugs for children at the Consensus Conference on ADHD and its treatment in November 1998. She also enabled me to allocate innumerable hours to developing the research for my presentation.

Ginger is in many ways the co-author of everything I do. I cannot separate my accomplishments from Ginger's knowledge, insights, and wisdom. After seventeen years together, I continue to marvel at the richness of her intellect and spirit. Each day, like the rising of the sun, I am once again inspired by her presence.

Peter R. Breggin, M.D.
Bethesda, Maryland
May 2001

FOREWORD

When I made the decision to declare war in the courtroom against Big Tobacco, I was especially outraged that these corporations knowingly promoted their addictive, deadly products to children. We all remember the Joe Camel advertisements that were tailored to appeal to pre-teens. Some of us remember how eagerly the tobacco companies "donated" cigarettes to the Red Cross and other agencies for distribution to the young boys risking their lives in defense of the nation.

Why were the tobacco companies so vigorous in their efforts to sell their products to children and youth? It was not merely to profit from the young people themselves. They wanted to hook the children for the rest of their lives. The companies knew that addicting a child to cigarettes almost guaranteed a lifetime consumer—however shortened that life might be.

After the war with Big Tobacco, I along with a number of other attorneys began to focus on where we should next direct our experience and resources. My concern for the health of Americans persisted. As part of that concern, I initiated litigation against HMOs who exist in an arena where profits come before the health of human beings, especially children.

Then I became aware of the work of Peter Breggin in raising serious questions about many practices of the mental health industry. In reading his book, *Talking Back to Ritalin*, I began to ask myself if there could be significant similarities between the conduct of the pharmaceutical industry and the tobacco industry. I asked myself if the large sums of money earned by the pharmaceutical industry could corrupt their research in the same way as in the tobacco industry. Much as the tobacco industry promoted and marketed its products with children in mind, I began to wonder if our vulnerable children were again being targeted for corporate profit.

Here, the marketing of stimulants to children is even more insidious—and ultimately more shrewd and effective—than the marketing of cigarettes. The stimulants are disguised as "medicines." Their imposition on children is called "treatment." A "disorder" has been manipulated to justify their use.

Cigarettes of course cause cancer. But as this book confirms, stimulants can cause many different kinds of physical harm to children. Forcing diagnoses and drugs on children also assaults their self-confidence and esteem, making them feel unable to take charge of their lives.

Ultimately, stimulants steal childhood. They make children more manageable at the cost of their spirit. They substitute for what's really needed—

a national consensus to improve our schools, our family life, and all our public and private commitments to children.

Our consortium of attorneys is bringing a series of class action suits against Novartis (the manufacturers of Ritalin), CHADD (the parents' group that promotes drugs on behalf of the industry), and the American Psychiatric Association (who benefits from drug company largesse). Dr. Breggin tells me that he is proud of his role in raising serious questions in the minds of those pursuing this litigation.

I am happy to recognize the valuable contribution Dr. Breggin has made in alerting many to the controversies surrounding the use of drugs such as Ritalin and how he has raised important questions about psychiatric diagnoses. While some may disagree with Dr. Breggin, everyone will find this a thought-provoking book.

Dick Scruggs
Pascagoula, Mississippi

Introduction

THE IMPACT OF THE FIRST EDITION

The original publication of *Talking Back to Ritalin* in 1998 helped to raise public awareness about the escalating use of stimulant drugs like Ritalin and Adderall to control the behavior of children. It became a source book for parents, professionals, media representatives, and attorneys who became involved in the growing controversy. It led the National Institutes of Health (NIH) to appoint me as the scientific presenter on the adverse effects of psychiatric drugs, including stimulants, at the November 1998 Consensus Development Conference on "The Diagnosis and Treatment of Attention Deficit Hyperactivity Disorder." The book, as well as my presentations, helped to provide much-needed balance and thwarted an otherwise guaranteed victory for the Ritalin/ADHD lobby.

Most dramatically, detailed information in *Talking Back to Ritalin* inspired some of the nation's most experienced and resourceful attorneys to bring class action and fraud suits against Novartis, the manufacturer of Ritalin, for the over-promotion of ADHD and Ritalin. As a result, I was able to work as a medical consultant on the formulation of the initial suit. The class action lawsuits also name the American Psychiatric Association and CHADD, a parents' group, as co-conspirators.

Many parents have told me how the first edition of this book helped them to respond to their children's family and educational needs without resort to medications. Many others made up their minds to take their children off medication, and found much more successful parenting and educational alternatives.

Despite these successes, the overall situation has worsened. Studies have shown that 7-10% or more of America's school children are on stimulant drugs prescribed for ADHD. School systems and the courts have increased their efforts to force parents to give stimulant drugs to their children. The International Center for the Study of Psychiatry and Psychology (ICSPP) has received hundreds of communications from parents who feel pressured by teachers and even threatened with child protective service interventions if they do not drug their children (see Appendix B for more information on ICSPP). In the extreme, voices like psychiatrist Peter Jensen have advocated for a virtual psychiatric police state in which parents are forced to put their children on drugs that blunt their spirit while subduing their behavior (chapter 1).

Drug companies and the government have worked together to expand the child drug market. Two long-acting preparations of methylphenidate (Ritalin) have been developed. Named Concerta and Metadate ER, they will make it even easier to drug children throughout the school day. Furthermore, the long-acting preparations will be more dangerous. Because each dose will remain for a longer period of time in the body, any adverse drug reactions will also be prolonged.

To keep up with these rapidly unfolding events, *Talking Back to Ritalin* has been extensively revised and augmented with new information. Chapter 1 is entirely new and focuses on the scientific and political controversy that has flared up over the past two years. Chapter 8, which is also new, provides a scientific critique of badly flawed government studies used to justify the drugging of children. Chapters 2, 3, and 4 have been extensively updated with new scientific data about the dangers of stimulant drugs. To make room for the new materials, two chapters have been cut from the book and several others have been tightened up.

Overall, five chapters in addition to this introduction are new or substantially transformed to provide a considerable amount of useful material even for those who have read the original 1998 edition. In addition, four new tables have been added. They not only provide an overview of harmful drug effects, they summarize findings from dozens of scientific studies.

I hope this new edition will inspire even greater numbers of people to stand up against the psychopharmaceutical threat to our children and to advocate for their genuine needs in our families, schools, and communities.

PART ONE

RITALIN, DEXEDRINE, ADDERALL, CONCERTA, METADATE ER AND OTHER STIMULANT DRUGS

Chapter 1

THE TIDE IS SHIFTING

Events Since the First Edition of
Talking Back To Ritalin

Except for a minority of cases involving distinct medical problems such as hyperthyroidism and explicit brain injuries, most youngsters diagnosed with [Attention Deficit Hyperactivity Disorder] ADHD may simply be normal, highly playful children who have difficulty adjusting to certain institutional expectations... [P]erhaps society should try to nurture this type of human variability or to adjust to it, rather than seeking to pathologize it and eliminate it with attention-focusing psychostimulants. It is certainly more rational to try to solve social problems with social solutions than with drugs, especially when the drugs are so similar to the ones we are trying to purge from our society.

—Jaak Panksepp (1998)

America's children are being deluged by psychiatric drugs, especially stimulants like Ritalin and Adderall that are used to control hyperactive, impulsive, or inattentive behavior.

Recent studies have shown that 7–10% or more of America's school-age children are being prescribed stimulant drugs to control their behavior, and the actual figures may be higher. The percentage of boys being drugged is disproportionately large and probably reaches or exceeds 15–20%. One recent survey of two Virginia school districts found that 20% of fifth grade boys were being administered stimulant drugs during the hours they were actually in school.[1]

There has been a tenfold increase in the production of methylphenidate (Ritalin) in the United States in the last decade, and the rates are probably rising.[2] While there are no comprehensive statistics concerning the total number of children taking stimulants, it probably is reaching 4–5 million (almost 10% of school children) and may grow much greater. As we shall document in this chapter, some drug advocates believe that 8 million of America's children should be taking some kind of psychiatric medication.

Meanwhile, the 53 million children enrolled in the nation's schools will confront increased overcrowding and teacher shortages.[3] These stressful conditions will motivate teachers and schools to put additional pressure on parents to medicate their children. Parents who find their children doing poorly in these schools may themselves choose to drug their children to make them adapt to these circumstances. Many medical doctors will continue to prescribe drugs in a knee-jerk fashion to any parent who describes a child as hyperactive, impulsive or inattentive at home or school.

The Controversy Grows

Inspired in part by the publication of the first edition of *Talking Back to Ritalin* in 1998, the controversy surrounding the medicating of America's children has grown at a rapid rate. Many more people now understand that something is wrong when society finds it expedient to give psychoactive chemicals to millions of children. They suspect that the diagnosis of Attention Deficit Hyperactivity Disorder (ADHD) may be little more than an excuse for giving drugs to control children instead of meeting their genuine needs. They believe that our children require improved family, school, and community life rather than psychiatric diagnoses and psychoactive drugs.

On September 29, 2000 the U.S. House of Representatives Committee on Education and the Workforce held hearings on the over-use of psychiatric medication for children and focused on the trend for schools to coerce parents into putting their children on stimulants. Representative Bob Schaffer of Colorado sponsored the hearing at which I testified, and he created a tenor that was wholly critical of using drugs to substitute for improved education in the schools.[4]

Concerns about the over-prescription of stimulants and collusion among the interested parties recently culminated in a series of class action lawsuits brought against the manufacturer of Ritalin, Novartis, as well as against the American Psychiatric Association, and CHADD, a parents' group that takes money from drug companies. As we shall see, some of the nation's most respected and powerful attorneys are involved in the suits.

International agencies concerned with drug abuse and addiction have become increasingly worried about the widespread prescription of stimulants to children. The U.S. Drug Enforcement Administration (DEA)[5] warned about a record sixfold increase in Ritalin production between 1990 and 1995. In 1995, the International Narcotics Control Board (INCB), a agency of the World Health Organization, deplored that "10 to 12 percent of all boys between the ages 6 and 14 in the United States have been diagnosed as having ADD and are being treated with methylphenidate [Ritalin]." In March 1997, the agency declared, "The therapeutic use of methylphenidate is now under scrutiny by the American medical community; the INCB welcomes this." It warned:

However, concerns have been raised that doctors are resorting to methylphenidate as an "easy" solution for behavioral problems which may have complex causes. Critics warn that parents' and teachers' assessment of what constitutes "inattention" and "impulsivity" are highly subjective and that doctors' prescribing practices for methylphenidate are far from uniform. ... Since the drug is touted as "accepted medication" for children, abusers are unaware of its health hazards, which include addiction and a range of stimulant-abuse problems.... In its current report, the Board reiterates its request to all governments to exercise the utmost care to prevent overdiagnosing of ADD in children and medically unjustified treatment.

In 1999, the INCB continued to show concerns about the over-prescription of stimulants to children. It observed, "In the Americas, particularly in the United States, performance enhancing drugs are being given to children to boost school performance or to help them conform to the demands of school life." It noted that in some individual American schools, 30–40% of children are diagnosed and treated with stimulants without sufficient regard for the abuse and dependency potential of these drugs. The international drug regulatory agency was critical of "aggressive advertising by certain pharmaceutical firms" and reported rising rates of prescriptions in Australia, Canada, and "several European countries."

A large, ever-increasing segment of America's children are being subjected to drugs to control their minds and behavior. No such experiment in mass drugging has ever before been attempted in the history of any society or nation. Never before have so many parents been told that their children need psychiatric drug treatment for difficulties at school and in the home. This unprecedented situation is not the result of some inexplicable increase in "mental illness." It is, instead, the result of an increasing failure to identify and to meet the needs of children in our homes, schools, and communities, as well as a growing tendency to seek quick and seemingly easy medical cures to difficult individual and social problems. .

Marketing "Speed" in New Forms

In the face of recent opposition, advocates of psychiatric drugs have escalated their efforts to push their chemical wares on children. The marketing of older drugs in a new package is one method of promoting the stimulant drugs.

In the mid-1950s, Ritalin (methylphenidate) and Dexedrine (dextroamphetamine) became the first two stimulants approved for the control of behavior in children. Later Desoxyn and Gradumet (both forms of methamphetamine) were approved. Amid a great deal of marketing promotion, Adderall has recently been added to the market. Despite the hype about its newness, Adderall is a mixture of four closely related forms of old-fashioned amphetamines and differs little from Dexedrine. Most recently, Metadate and Concerta have been approved. They are longer-acting preparations of Ritalin (methylphenidate).

All of these drugs are amphetamine-like (Ritalin, Metadate, and Concerta) or they are outright amphetamines (Adderall, Dexedrine, Desoxyn, Gradumet). For most purposes, they can be considered as one class of drug with a similar adverse reaction profile, including a high potential for addiction and abuse. For example, each of them has been placed in Schedule II of the Drug Enforcement Administration (DEA). Schedule II—which also includes cocaine, opium, morphine, and the most dangerous barbiturates—is intended for drugs with the most extreme abuse and addiction potential. On this basis alone, stimulant drugs should never be considered benign.

Another stimulant, Cylert (pemoline), is not as addictive or prone to abuse, but has unique dangers, including fatal liver toxicity.

Growing More Aggressive
in the Promotion of Stimulants for Children

The government has joined forces with the pharmaceutical industry in trying to convince the professions and the public that stimulants are safe and effective. As this chapter will describe, the National Institute of Mental Health (NIMH) held a conference in November 1998 that was calculated to promote the medicating of children. And as chapter 8 will detail, NIMH also funded and then used the media to tout a greatly flawed study to vindicate Ritalin as an effective treatment for Attention Deficit Hyperactivity Disorder (ADHD).

Making Parents Drug Their Children

Two recent opinion pieces in *USA Today* highlight the escalating controversy.[6] On August 8, 2000, the newspaper published a report about mothers and fathers being pressured to medicate their children against their parental wishes.[7] In one case, a court threatened parents with being forced to medicate their child with stimulants, and the parents gave in. In the other, allegations of medical neglect were brought against parents who refused to drug their child.

On August 15, 2000, *USA Today* responded with an editorial that warned, "no arm of the state should be ramming the drug treatment down parents'— or children's—throats."

Psychiatrist Peter Jensen wrote an opposing view. While at NIMH, Jensen organized the government's promotion of Ritalin and now at Columbia University he continues in the same role.[8] To justify coercing parents into drugging their children, Jensen pointed out that "society requires that children's caretakers see that children get immunized, fed and clothed and receive treatments for other disorders such as asthma and diabetes." In these remarks, Jensen confuses the use of drugs for social control—for drugging children into conformity and submission—with genuine public health measures, medical treatment, and food and shelter.

When Jensen endorsed the use of police powers to make parents drug their children, he raised biopsychiatric oppression to a new level. For two hundred years, society has accepted the involuntary hospitalization of individuals labeled "mentally ill." In the last few years, organized psychiatry has successfully pushed for the right to force individual adult patients to take their medication even while they live at home. Most states now empower mental health authorities to come to the home to forcibly administer medication. But the call to force parents to drug their children will hopefully meet much greater public resistance.

Doctors Turn to Massive Over-Drugging

Despite public criticism, the prescription practices of many doctors throughout the nation have grown more aggressive and dangerous. In my private practice of psychiatry, where I work with adults and children, desperate parents often bring their children to me as a last resort. Their pediatrician, family doctor, or psychiatrist has suggested the addition of a fourth or fifth mind-altering drug to their child's treatment regimen. By this time, the child is being bounced around on an emotional roller coaster ride by the multiple medications.

Here is a pattern I have seen repeated a number of times in recent months. First the child is put on Ritalin or Adderall for minor school or family problems. When the stimulant causes insomnia, a sedating drug like Klonopin (clonazepam) or clonidine is added at night. When the drug combination makes the child depressed, an antidepressant like Prozac or Paxil is added. When the three drugs impair the child's emotional stability, making him aggressive and unpredictable for the first time, the parents are told that their child's "bipolar" or "manic-depressive" disorder has "emerged." Now lithium or Depakote is added as a "mood stabilizer." When this medically negligent over-dosing with four drugs leads to bizarre behavior, the child is put on an "antipsychotic" such as Risperdal or Zyprexa.

Of all the drugs that this child was prescribed, only the stimulants were FDA-approved for children. Although the parents were not told, four out of five of the drugs were "off label" and the combination was wholly unjustified on any clinical or scientific grounds. The "cocktail" of medications was guaranteed to ruin the child's mental life and eventually to leave lasting harmful effects. Yet this "polypharmacy" approach has become too commonplace.

I briefly described this typical case of the psychiatric abuse of children when I testified before Congress on September 29, 2000. The very next day,

yet another child, Raymond, was brought to my office on a similar combination of drugs, including the antipsychotic agent, Zyprexa. On examination, I
found that Raymond had abnormal tongue movements, telltale early signs of
drug-induced tardive dyskinesia. He also reported twitches of his arms. The
combination of abnormal tongue movements and twitches is diagnostic of
tardive dyskinesia, a neurological disorder caused by antipsychotic (neuroleptic) drugs like Risperdal and Zyprexa. It can result in a lifetime of
untreatable disfiguring twitches and spasms.[9] In severe cases, tardive dyskinesia can disable children, making it difficult for them to stand or to walk.
Raymond was nine years old and in danger of becoming permanently neurologically disfigured and physically impaired.

During two and one-half hours with Raymond, his father, and several
members of his extended family, I could find nothing whatsoever wrong with
the child, other than the adverse drug effects. He was bright, intelligent,
cooperative, playful, and charming. His father's family confirmed that he was
always this way with them. Even on the daylong car ride to get to my office,
Raymond had caused no trouble at all.

What had brought the full force of biopsychiatry upon Raymond? His
father and mother were divorced, and his mother had custody. Raymond had
been caught in escalating personal conflicts with his mother and she had
taken him to doctors who immediately began to treat Raymond with drugs.
Although only nine years old and weighing little more than seventy pounds,
Raymond was now taking large doses of four psychoactive drugs, only one of
them even approved for the psychiatric treatment of children.

Fortunately, when parents are devoted to their children and willing to
learn new approaches to helping them at home or in school, an experienced
doctor can gradually withdraw a child like Raymond from all psychiatric
drugs over several months or less. Frequently drug withdrawal can be
accomplished over the summer vacation. To their joy, the parents will see
their offspring's spirit re-emerge, and they will exclaim, "We have our child
back."

When parents are given proper guidance in how to relate to their children, they will quickly discover that the drugs were doing more harm than
good. With the removal of each medication, their child looks and acts better. When the child's real needs at home and at school are simultaneously
addressed, the parents and child can learn to resolve their worst conflicts,
vastly improving the child's home and school life.

While responsible parents often blame themselves for having allowed the
drug treatment go so overboard, it is the physicians who are responsible for
bamboozling them into focusing their efforts on their child's brain rather
than their child's life. The physicians should be faulted for conducting what
amounts to dangerous and destructive experimentation on children under
the guise of legitimate medical treatment.

Legal Opposition to the Widespread Drugging of Children

Meanwhile, efforts to promote psychiatric drugs for children are running into increasing professional, public, and legal opposition. A series of class action lawsuits have been filed against Novartis (Ciba Geigy), the manufacturer of Ritalin, accusing the giant pharmaceutical company of fraud in over-promoting its stimulant drug, Ritalin, as well as the ADHD diagnosis. The suits also charge the American Psychiatric Association and the parents' group CHADD of conspiring with the drug company to promote sales of the drug.

The Ritalin class action suits build on experience gained by attorneys who have brought similar legal actions against companies that manufacture and sell lethal substances such as asbestos and tobacco. When used as insulation in factories, homes, and schools, asbestos dust was inhaled by workers, families, and school children, causing cancer and respiratory disorders. Corporations were successfully sued for covering up the dangers of asbestos while continuing to expose the public to the hazardous material. Tobacco companies sold cigarettes to hundreds of millions of adults and children around the world, causing untold numbers to become addicted and to die from illnesses such as cancer, emphysema, and heart disease. The companies not only knew about the dangers of cigarettes, they denied and withheld the data, at the same time promoting cigarettes to children.

Asbestos and tobacco class action suits have demonstrated the efficacy of civil litigation to protect consumers and enforce ethical standards of corporate conduct. They have also provided attorneys with the know-how and the funds to bring other legal actions on behalf of consumers beleaguered or defrauded by giant corporations.

In early 2000, former asbestos attorney C. Andrew Waters of Dallas, Texas, began to read *Talking Back to Ritalin*. Soon after he asked to meet with me to talk about a possible class action suit related to the over-prescription of Ritalin to millions of children. Waters and his associates in Texas then hired me as their medical consultant to help formulate the original national class action suit filed in Brownsville, Texas, on May 1, 2000.[10] Dick Scruggs, who wrote the forward to this book, has now become the lead attorney for the many similar Ritalin class actions that have been brought around the nation.

The Ritalin class action suit alleges "fraud" and "conspiracy" in over-promoting both the diagnosis of Attention Deficit Hyperactivity Disorder (ADHD) and its treatment with the stimulant medication Ritalin. Three national organizations are named as defendants: (1) Novartis (formerly Ciba Geigy), the manufacturer of Ritalin, (2) CHADD (Children and Adults with Attention Deficit/Hyperactivity Disorder), a parents' organization that is partially funded by drug companies, and (3) the American Psychiatric Association, the nation's largest and most powerful psychiatric organization.

The class action suit alleges that Novartis "deliberately, intentionally, and negligently promoted the diagnosis of ADD/ADHD and sales of Ritalin through its promotional literature and its training of sales representatives." It contends that the defendants "willfully failed to address or provide adequate information to consumers, doctors, and/or schools concerning many significant hazards of methylphenidate..."

The suit also charges Novartis with "Actively supporting groups such as Defendant CHADD, both financially and with other means, so that such organizations would promote and support (as a supposed neutral party) the ever-increasing implementation of the ADD/ADHD diagnosis as well as directly increasing Ritalin sales." It further claims that "Defendant American Psychiatric Association (APA) conspired, colluded and cooperated with the other Defendants" while taking "financial contributions from Ciba [Novartis] as well as other members of the pharmaceutical industry..."

Although the Ritalin class action suit was motivated by concern about the over-medicating of America's children, it is not restricted to children. Adults who have purchased Ritalin for children or for themselves are potentially eligible to participate in the suit. The suit seeks compensation for those who paid for Ritalin, regardless of whether or not the medication caused any harm or damage. Waters and Kraus anticipate bringing additional suits over specific individual damages.

Not long after Mr. Waters contacted me, several other nationally known attorneys asked my opinion on similar class action suits against Novartis, including Richard Scruggs of Pascagoula, Mississippi, who played a prominent role in the tobacco suits. I referred them to Mr. Waters, and soon a coalition of attorneys evolved with the addition of John P. Coale of Washington, DC and Donald F. Hildre of San Diego, California. In September 2000 this group of powerful, knowledgeable lawyers brought several more suits aimed at stopping the massive drugging of America's children with Ritalin.

Don Hildre filed two civil actions against Novartis for fraud and conspiracy against the citizens of California. Mr. Hildre declared, "The turning point in the tobacco litigation was when we showed the tobacco companies were targeting children. And I believe that is going to be the turning point here."[11]

Increasing Media Concern and Objectivity

At the same time, greater numbers of major print and television representatives began showing interest in the suit and sought my opinion about the high-pressure marketing of psychiatric drugs. *The Wall Street Journal, The New York Times*, and *USA Today* carried objective news reports on the class action suits.[12] These reports signal that the media and the public are becoming aware that psychiatric drugs, and especially stimulants for children, are grossly oversold. With growing public sophistication about the dangers of psychiatric drugs and about the role of high power marketing in selling them, the future may witness a wave of class action lawsuits and media investigations related to the over-promotion of psychiatric drugs in our society.

In an effort to counter the early signs of a future ground swell of public and professional criticism, NIMH in the mid-1990s began to plan a national conference that it hoped would lay to rest all the controversy surrounding the diagnosis and treatment of ADHD.

Scenes from a Gathering of Experts

The office of the director of the National Institutes of Health (NIH) invited me to be the scientific presenter on adverse drug effects in children at the NIH Consensus Development Conference on "The Diagnosis and Treatment of Attention Deficit Hyperactivity Disorder" that took place in November 1998. It was unusual for the government to invite a well-known critic of biological psychiatric treatment to participate in this kind of conference.

At a government consensus conference, scientists present and interpret data to a panel, which then issues a report which attempts to reflect a consensus. The viewpoints of people selected for the panel will, of course, tend to predetermine the panel's conclusions. For example, if the panel is comprised of "middle of the road" professionals who fear "making any waves," then the panel is likely to develop a conventional consensus that does not offend the medical establishment, the drug companies, or the government. Similarly, the biases or viewpoints of the scientific presenters will also tend to influence the outcome.

Stacking the Conference

Planning for the ADHD/Ritalin consensus conference was led by child psychiatrist Peter Jensen who was, at the time, on the staff of National Institute of Mental Health (NIMH). Jensen tried to ensure a consensus in favor of medicating children. For example, as the chairman of the supposedly objective consensus panel, NIMH chose David Kupfer, M.D. Kupfer is chairman of the Department of Psychiatry at the University of Pittsburgh, a medical center that has received particularly extensive funding from NIMH for research based on the supposed validity of the ADHD diagnosis and stimulant treatment. A panel chaired by such a devoted establishment psychiatrist was bound to support the diagnosis of ADHD and its treatment with drugs. Furthermore, NIMH initially failed to invite any critics of the medication to speak at the conference and planned no specific presentation on adverse drug effects.

Although NIMH was running this particular conference, the larger umbrella organization, the National Institutes of Health (NIH), retains ultimate responsibility for monitoring the quality and fairness of all consensus conferences. As director of the International Center for the Study of Psychiatry and Psychology, I appealed to NIH to create more balance in the conference by adding several scientists with more critical views of ADHD and stimulants. Fortunately, the office of the director of NIH seemed to agree that the conference format was biased. After members of the staff read some of my publications, including the first edition of this book, NIH required the conference planners to designate me as the scientific presenter on the over-all subject of adverse drug effects in children. By inviting me, the National Institutes of Health (NIH) sent a message to its member institute, NIMH, that NIH would not tolerate a completely lopsided conference devoted wholly to celebrating the medicating of children. Unfortunately, no additional critics other than myself were added to the list of scientific presenters, and so the group of designated conference scientists remained heavily loaded in favor of diagnosing and drugging children.

At the conference, most of the thirty scientific presenters repeated the same old unfounded claims about the validity of the ADHD diagnosis and the value of stimulants. Four panelists, including myself, presented important new research that raised questions about the ADHD diagnosis and/or the safety of medications.

Ritalin as a Gateway Drug

Nadine Lambert, Ph.D., Professor and Director of the School Psychology Program at the University of California, Berkeley, reported on her continuing study of adults who have been prescribed stimulants in childhood. Lambert found that childhood treatment with stimulant medication is "significantly and pervasively implicated in the uptake of regular smoking, in daily smoking in adulthood, in cocaine dependence, and in lifetime use of cocaine and stimulants."[13] She attributed the increased risk of cocaine abuse to sensitization of the brain during childhood use of pre-scribed stimulants. This sensitization predisposed the young adults to cocaine abuse.

It may seem a stretch to think that using a stimulant in childhood would lead to cocaine addiction in young adulthood. But think about the familiar example of tobacco. Children who smoke cigarettes are of course more likely to become addicted to nicotine as young adults. Clinical experience indicates that they may end up with more severe nicotine addictions than those who begin smoking at a later date.

The childhood use of stimulants or nicotine encourages lifelong dependence by several means. First, children who smoke tobacco or who are prescribed stimulants develop the habit of using these drugs to deal with painful emotions or out-of-control behavior. When the habit develops early, it has a greater tendency to become a lifelong pattern. Second, the nicotine or stimulants will change the child's developing brain, making it dependent on these substances, encouraging further use later on in life. Third, in regard to stimulants, children diagnosed with ADHD have been told that they have a medical need for stimulants. Sometimes, they are misled into believing that they have a biochemical imbalance that requires Ritalin. When they discover that cocaine is simply a more potent stimulant, they are primed to use it habitually in young adulthood.

Creating a Wave of Ritalin Abuse

Gretchen Feussner (1998), a pharmacologist on the staff of the Drug Enforcement Administration (DEA), warned the conference about the increasing danger of Ritalin addiction and abuse among children. She confirmed that the United States still uses 90% of the world's production of methylphenidate and described an eight-fold increase in domestic U.S. production from 1,768 kilograms in 1990 to 14,442 kilograms in 1998.

Feussner reminded the conference that animals and humans react in similar ways to Ritalin, amphetamine, and cocaine: "In clinical studies, MPH [Ritalin] produces behavioral, psychological, subjective, and reinforcing effects similar to d-amphetamine and cocaine."[14] She noted that "Psychotic episodes, paranoid delusions, hallucinations, and bizarre behavioral characteristics similar to amphetamine-like toxic effects have been associated with MPH [Ritalin] abuse."[15]

The DEA official warned about sloppy methods on the part of schools in dispensing Ritalin to students. She observed, "It is important to note that many schools have more MPH [Ritalin] stored for student daytime dosing than is available in some pharmacies." She explained that "While State and Federal laws require accountability of controlled substances by licensed handlers, no such regulations are imposed at this level" in the schools.

Feussner cited evidence that students are giving or selling their Ritalin to other students "who frequently crush the tablets and snort the power like cocaine."[16] She reported data about increased numbers of emergency room visits associated with Ritalin use and abuse in children and teenagers (ages 10 to 17). She concluded by warning that a large amount of prescribed Ritalin is being diverted to nonprescription use and that a growing number of adolescents are using Ritalin illicitly.

Drugging Normal Children

William Carey, a professor of pediatrics at the University of Pennsylvania, went to the heart of the matter, entitling his consensus conference presentation, "Is ADHD a valid diagnosis?" He concluded that the behaviors associated with the diagnosis reflect a continuum or spectrum of normal temperaments rather than a disorder. He declared that ADHD "appears to be a set of normal behavioral variations" that lead to "dissonant environmental interactions."[17] That is, when the varied but normal temperaments of children bring them into conflict with parents and teachers, the adults try to end the conflicts by diagnosing the children with ADHD.

Killing Brain Cells

In my scientific presentation at the Consensus Conference, I summarized dozens of controlled clinical trials and numerous reviews that describe a wide variety of harmful stimulant effects on children, including drug-induced depression, lethargy, robotic behavior, obsessive-compulsive behavior, tics, heart disorders, and psychosis. The stunting of growth, I pointed out, is caused not only by appetite suppression but also by drug-induced disruptions of growth hormone production, thus afflicting the growth of the entire body and all its organs, including the brain.

I also debunked attempts by one of the other scientific presenters who claimed that stimulants do not stunt growth.[18] I had studied his flawed report and was easily able to refute it. Among other gross methodical problems, it used only one height and weight measurement, rather than several over a period of time, in order to reach its conclusions. I also confronted another presenter who claimed that there were few cases of psychoses reported to the FDA. I had hand counted the data from reports to the FDA between 1985 and March 3, 1997. The reports included psychosis (38 total), psychotic depression (11 total), and hallucinations (43 total) (see chapter 2). While significant in themselves, these numbers reflect on the tip of a much larger iceberg. Only a tiny fraction of adverse reactions get reported to the FDA. Furthermore, when a drug has been in use for decades like Ritalin, even fewer reports will be made to the FDA.

Perhaps most distressing, I described animal research demonstrating that in short-term, relatively low doses, amphetamines, such as Adderall and Dexedrine, kill brain cells. The research also found that Ritalin causes long-term brain changes. (See chapters 2 and 3 for a more complete analysis of stimulant adverse effects.)

Suppressing the Spirit of Children

In my presentation to the Consensus Conference, I documented how harmful stimulant effects are almost always mistaken for improvement in the child's behavior. Basically, stimulants suppress all spontaneous behavior and mental life, and enforce obsessive-compulsive behaviors, such as focusing on something boring to the exclusion of all else, or repeating a boring task over and over again. When the child becomes more subdued and more obsessive in behavior, over-stressed parents and teachers are likely to see it as an improvement rather than as a negative drug effect. Chapter 4 will discuss in detail how stimulants work by impairing the functions of the brain and mind.

The Brain Scan Scam

The task of proving that ADHD has a biological basis rested on the shoulders of James Swanson, Ph.D., Professor of Pediatrics at the University of California, Irvine. Swanson's slide presentation at the consensus conference included multiple photographs of brain scans supposedly showing that children with ADHD have different brains than ordinary children. For much of the audience, it must have looked totally convincing. Then a child neurologist in the audience raised a telling point.[19] He noted that psychiatric drugs are potentially very toxic to a child's brain. Then he asked Swanson, in effect, "How many of the children with supposedly abnormal brains had been previously exposed to psychiatric drugs?" Swanson was forced to admit that all the children with "different" or "abnormal" brains in all the studies had been previously exposed to psychiatric drugs. The meaning was clear: Abnormalities that had been passed off as evidence of ADHD weren't necessarily connected to ADHD in any way, shape, or form. They were much more likely caused by exposure to psychiatric drugs.

Then came the devastating follow-up question: "How could you withhold such vital information from your presentation?" Swanson made no direct reply.

Swanson's failure to mention the children's prior exposure to psychiatric drugs was no mere oversight. It is part of a propaganda campaign aimed at the public and professionals, an effort I have labeled the Brain Scan Scam. Swanson's written report for the conference also failed to mention anything about the role of psychiatric drugs in modifying or damaging the brains of children.[20] Instead, he speculated about a possible abnormality in dopamine neurotransmission in association with ADHD. However, the stimulant drugs, and even the Prozac-like antidepressants, negatively impact on dopamine. These brain-disabling agents are much more likely culprits than "ADHD" in causing dysfunction and damage in that neurotransmitter system (see chapters 2 and 3). I urged the panel to add Swanson's testimony to my own as further evidence of the damaging effects of psychiatric drugs.

The Panel Refuses to Knuckle Under to NIMH

The panel sifted through the predominantly pro-medication testimony, compared it to the few critical presentations, and arrived at conclusions that disappointed and even shocked the conference organizers. The panel raised many questions about the validity of the diagnosis of ADHD, as well as the benefits and risks of stimulant drugs. Most disappointing to the medication advocates, the panel cast reasonable doubt on the validity of the ADHD diagnosis. It also concluded that there were *no* "data to indicate that ADHD is due to a brain malfunction. Further research to establish the validity of the disorder continues to be a problem."

The rejection of a biological basis for ADHD appeared in the final consensus draft distributed to the press and the public at the end of the conference. However, that conclusion was so embarrassing to the pro-medication organizers of the conference, led by Peter Jensen, that they edited it out of the final statement. Instead, they crafted a carefully worded substitute that read, "Although research has suggested a central nervous system basis for ADHD, further research is necessary to firmly establish ADHD as a brain disorder. This is not unique to ADHD, but applies as well to most psychiatric disorders, including disabling diseases such as schizophrenia." Thus the myth that ADHD exists as a biological or medical entity was resurrected by rewriting the consensus panel's original conclusion.

Jensen had to admit that the consensus conference found no proof that "ADHD reflects a disordered biological state."[21] In trying to dance around this lack of evidence for a biological basis for ADHD, Jensen (2000) observed that ADHD has a "central nervous basis (as do all normal and abnormal behaviors, thoughts and emotions)." In other words, ADHD behaviors, like any and all behaviors, have something to do with the brain. This, of course, is a meaningless statement that in no way supports the concept of a brain disorder in children diagnosed with ADHD. Unfortunately, the public and many professionals have been misled into believing that there's a lot more substance to the supposed biological basis of ADHD.

The panel also went further than expected in warning about cardiac and neurological problems associated with stimulants.

Overall, a few critical voices among the thirty presenters undermined the intended celebration of stimulant treatment and brought about a more skeptical report than desired and expected by the government, Novartis, and drug advocates.

Members of the press told me that it was the most confusing consensus conference report they'd ever seen; it seemed to come to no definitive conclusions. That, to me, was good news. NIMH had hoped the consensus statement would provide a total vindication of ADHD and stimulant drugs.

The consensus conference panel raised so many doubts about the concept of ADHD and its treatment with drugs the conference planners had to rewrite much of it themselves after the panel had gone home. This, of course, was highly misleading and unethical. The consensus statement that has been published and that appears on NIMH's web site is a gross distortion of the actual conclusions of the panel at the conference. But the rewrite still falls far short of the kind of ringing endorsement NIMH had hoped for.

Later, Jensen subtitled his commentary on the conference in ambivalent terms, "Win, Lose, or Draw?"[22] Clearly, he had hoped for an uncontested "win," meaning an enthusiastic endorsement of the ADHD diagnosis and the use of drugs. He not only rewrote the original consensus conclusions of the panel, he left out all the critics—Lambert, Feussner, Carey, and Breggin—

from his own published discussion of the conference and from his bibliography.

Recently when asked by a reporter to name critics of ADHD and Ritalin, Jensen explained there weren't any. He has apparently expunged all the critics from his verbal communications as well as his writing. But I do not wish to focus criticism on Jensen as a person. He is but an illustration of the attitudes displayed by most advocates of ADHD and stimulant drugs. No amount of rational scientific criticism, or public outrage, will in itself stop them from pushing drugs on children. That is why legal strategies, such as the Ritalin class action suits, are needed to protect America's children.

Novartis, the drug company that manufactures and distributes Ritalin, had also anticipated a complete victory for its product at the consensus conference. Ahead of time, the public relations department told the media that the conference would finally put to rest any controversy surrounding ADHD and stimulant drugs. Afterward, the drug company wasn't bragging.

NIMH Continues Pushing Drugs for Children

There have been few scientifically sound long-term studies of the positive or negative effects of Ritalin. At the consensus conference, Peter Jensen and other participants made numerous claims that they were gathering data from an as yet unpublished study that proved the efficacy and safety of stimulant drugs for children over a fourteen-month period. The study, conducted at six medical centers, was funded by NIMH. Only the advocates themselves were privy to the details of that research.

At the Consensus Conference I took a strong stand against the panel relying on biased hearsay statements about a study that was unpublished and therefore not subject to independent evaluation. Despite my warnings, the panel briefly referred to the research in confirming the value of stimulants. Jensen then added the supposed findings of the study to the consensus report after the conference was over. It became part of the cosmetic re-write.

When finally published, the giant NIMH research project turned out to be a scientific runt. It violated the most essential scientific canons for clinical trials. For example, the stimulant drug studies lacked a placebo (sugar pill) control group. Furthermore, the research was not double-blind, enabling the biased raters to know which children were taking the drugs. Overall, NIMH was so desperate to promote drugs, that it wasted millions on a scientifically worthless study. Because it provides a model for drug marketing posing as genuine science, I will examine the study in greater detail in chapter 8.

Peter Jensen, meanwhile, has left NIMH to become a professor at Columbia University and the New York Psychiatric Institute. Is it a coincidence that this is one of the six medical centers that received funds from the NIMH Ritalin project when Jensen was holding the purse strings? Members of the drug establishment often move freely about among each other's institutions, enjoying the benefits of the Psychopharmaceutical Complex.[23]

The White House Intervenes

In June 1999—shortly after the school shootings in Colorado and Georgia—the Clintons and the Gores held the first ever White House Conference on Mental Health.[24] The conference featured President Bill Clinton and Hillary Clinton and Vice-President Al Gore and Tipper Gore. Taking advantage of the nation's concern about school shootings, the conference leadership pushed for more psychiatric interventions into the schools and touted psychoactive drug treatment for children. It was never mentioned that some of the shooters had been receiving psychiatric medications.

T. J. Solomon, the shooter at Heritage High School in Conyers, Georgia was taking Ritalin and Eric Harris from Columbine High School in Littleton, Colorado was taking a Prozac knock-off called Luvox. As I have already documented in *Reclaiming Our Children*, and will further elaborate in this book, stimulant drugs such as Ritalin and antidepressant drugs such as Prozac and Luvox can cause paranoid thinking, aggression, and in the extreme, psychotic mania. Mania can involve elaborate, bizarre planning and spawn potentially violent actions. Children are especially susceptible to developing abnormal behavioral reactions to these drugs. There are indications that some of the other school shooters may have also been taking stimulants.[25]

Because of the pro-drug agenda at the White House Conference, there was no mention of any association between psychiatric drug intake and violence. Tipper Gore had recently disclosed that she had taken antidepressants and been appointed as the Mental Health Advisor to the President. Hillary Clinton also advocated biological psychiatry and drugs. She introduced New York University psychiatrist Harold Koplewicz, one of the most radical advocates of psychiatric drugs for children. Koplewicz told the White House Conference that "absent fathers, working mothers, over-permissive parents" do not and cannot cause mental disturbances in children. He said that not even "bad childhood traumas" can cause emotional disturbances in children. Instead, mental disorders in children and young people are caused exclusively by genetic and biological defects in their brains. The number of these children and teenagers, in his opinion, is 8 million or "12% of the population under age eighteen."

Koplewicz means what he says. He has previously written that even the sexual abuse of children will not cause mental disorders unless the children are already suffering from pre-existing biological brain diseases. Specifically, Koplewicz wrote that "sexual abuse" and "traumatic experiences—abuse, divorce, the death of a loved one," as well as being "abandoned or beaten," will not in themselves cause a psychiatric disorder in children.[26] This, of course, goes against common sense, clinical experience, and a mountain of research about the harmful effects of child abuse on later adult life.[27]

In response to Koplewicz's presentation, Mrs. Clinton declared that children and young people must receive psychiatric treatment "whether or not they want it or are willing to accept it."

The director of the National Institute of Mental Health (NIMH), Steven Hyman, was the other star psychiatric apologist at the conference. Hyman displayed brain scans comparing depressed and non-depressed patients, as if he could demonstrate a biological difference between the brains. In reality, there is no way to diagnose or identify any mental disorder using a brain scan. It's all smoke and mirrors for public relations purposes.

In a critical analysis of the White House Conference in the June 12, 2000 issue of *Insight*, Kelly O'Meara revealed that Hyman himself was already on record as stating, "Magnetic Resonance Imaging, or MRIs, produce scientifically meaningless pretty pictures which are reminiscent of phrenology." Phrenology, of course, attempted to plumb an individual's psychological and moral qualities by examining the shape of the skull and bumps on the head.

As the concluding speaker on the opening day, President Clinton announced plans for a nationwide educational program to push for mental health interventions in the schools. Through video satellite, the President explained, a program encouraging mental health interventions in the school would be broadcast to 1,000 schools. Ultimately, he anticipated, it would be broadcast to every school in the nation.

The proposed program has been delayed in its implementation, and was not ready for its starting date in the fall of 1999. As the Clinton presidency came to an end, it was apparently still in development. I've also been informed that it may not be as radically biological as Hillary and Tipper were advocating. Unfortunately, even if the program turns out to be more reserved about promoting drugs than the conference itself, it will still encourage teachers to think like front-line mental health workers with a duty to recruit more children into the mental health system. In the current psychiatric climate, most of those children will end up being drugged.

The Surgeon General's Report on Mental Health came out shortly after the conference.[28] Another "first" inspired by Tipper Gore, the report turned out to be more moderate than the White House Conference. It recognized that stress and trauma are harmful to children. But it gave unhesitant support for the concept of ADHD and stimulant medication in a nation that has already gone over the edge in drugging its children.

I was so concerned and even outraged by the White House Conference that I wrote a chapter about it in my book *Reclaiming Our Children*. Although my book's official publication date was February 2000, it hit the book stores early in December 1999. Based on the media surrounding publication of the book, I was able to conduct a national campaign to expose the Clinton/Gore program for increasing psychiatric interventions in the nation's schools. I criticized the conference and its leaders on dozens of radio and television shows, and wrote an Op Ed piece about it in *USA Today*.[29] But I was unprepared for the next political move by the White House.

The AMA's Journal Warns Against the Drugging of Small Children

In February 2000, a research study and an editorial published in *The Journal of the American Medical Association (JAMA)* alerted the nation to the dangers of drugging very young children. The report by Maryland researchers led by Julie Zito examined prescription rates for psychiatric drugs for two to four year old toddlers. The researchers found an average three-fold increase in prescriptions of stimulant drugs, especially Ritalin, for these tiny tots from 1990 to 1995. Prescriptions for Prozac-like antidepressants were also escalating. The data collection did not go beyond 1995, but in the current pro-drug environment, it has almost certainly continued to escalate.

Ritalin is not FDA-approved for children under the age of six, and antidepressants are not approved for children or youth of any age. Giving these psychiatric medications to such young children is not approved by the FDA and is not supported by research or clinical experience. Instead, studies show that stimulants cause especially severe adverse reactions in young children, and that antidepressants can produce very dangerous effects in children of all ages.[30] As Zito and her colleagues correctly observed, the adverse effects of Ritalin and Prozac-like drugs "for preschool children are more pronounced than for older youths."[31]

The Zito study also found that these small children were being given the anti-hypertension agent, clonidine, in order to quiet them through its sedative effects. Clonidine was also being given to the children to counteract the stimulation of Ritalin. As the researchers observed, clonidine, especially in combination with stimulants, can cause potentially fatal heart problems. Rapid withdrawal from clonidine can also cause hypertensive crises.

The report in JAMA was accompanied by a remarkable editorial written by Harvard Medical School psychiatrist Joseph T. Coyle. Coyle expressed concern that "1% to 1.5% of all children 2 to 4 years old enrolled in these programs currently are receiving stimulants, antidepressants, or antipsychotic medication."[32]

Three out of four of the child populations studied were on Medicaid, leading Dr. Coyle to voice concern that children in poverty are being especially exposed to the escalation in drugging. Populations of poor children are likely to include disproportionately large numbers of children from minority groups, such as African-Americans, Hispanics, and Native Americans.

Dr. Coyle challenged the validity and reliability of psychiatric diagnoses in such small children. He personally surveyed a group of well-respected physicians and most reported that they rarely or never prescribed these psychiatric drugs for such young children.

In his editorial, Dr. Coyle went on to make a point that I have emphasized for years—that psychiatric drugs bathe the brains of children with agents that interfere with the normal development of the brain. Dr. Coyle declared, "Given that there is no empirical evidence to support psychotropic drug treatment in very young children and that there are valid concerns that such treatment could have deleterious effects on the developing brain, the reasons for these troubling changes in practice need to be identified."[33] He also criticized "quick and inexpensive pharmacological fixes" and called them "disturbing prescription practices" that reflect "a growing crisis in mental health services to children."

Young children are not the only ones with growing, vulnerable brains. New research confirms that the teen and young adult brain continues to grow as well. According to Jay Giedd of the National Institute of Mental Health, "Maturation [of the brain] does not stop at age 10, but continues into the teen years and even the 20's. What is most interesting is that you get a second wave of overproduction of gray matter, something that was thought to happen only in the first 18 months of life." [34]

The continued growth of the teenager's brain is good news. It is never too late to help young men and women to make major, lasting improvements in their ability to master their lives. Parents, teachers, and counselors should never give up on the young people in their care. But the continued growth of the teenage and young adult brain should also raise warning flags. We should be as concerned about drugging the brains of teenagers as we are about drugging the brains of toddlers.

Damage Control at the White House

The Zito report and the editorial in the *Journal of the American Medical Association* aroused "immense public concern" about the psychiatric drugging of very young children.[35] In one day I was interviewed by all three major TV networks concerning my reactions to the report, and this overall media interest continued for several weeks before slacking off.

Mrs. Clinton was actively involved in her political campaign for U. S. Senator from New York State, and she now seemed to perform a 180 degree turnabout from her previous advocacy of psychiatric drugs for children. After the Zito report, she received positive publicity for raising concerns about the drugging of preschool children. (Unfortunately, she continued to call stimulants a "God-send" for many children.) She claimed to have held a conference of professionals concerned about the issue. In fact, it was a damage control meeting of the relevant Clinton appointees, including NIMH director Steven Hyman, Surgeon General David Satcher, and commissioner of the Food and Drug Administration (FDA), Jane Henney, as well as the President of the

American Psychiatric Association, Allan Tasman.[36] It was a rogue's gallery of professionals wedded to biological psychiatry and drug interventions.

In response to Hillary Clinton's "concerns," NIMH announced plans for massive experimentation on preschoolers. NIMH director Hyman said his institute would spend $5 million over the next five years to study whether Ritalin is safe and effective in treating *preschoolers*. Hyman said that *hundreds* of boys and girls at research centers around the country would receive stimulants, behavior therapy or some combination of the two.[37] This sounds exactly like the badly flawed NIMH study of older children which lacked both a double blind and placebo controls (see chapter 8 for an analysis).

Hillary Clinton's endorsement of the new research on children was greeted by many as a positive advance. After all, she was encouraging "science" and "research." In fact, Mrs. Clinton had enabled the government to carry out unethical, scientifically unjustified research on the very young.

Previous to Mrs. Clinton's encouragement, NIMH would have been afraid of media and public outrage over plans to expose *hundreds of preschool children* to psychiatric drugs. The endorsement of this project by the First Lady put an aura of sanctity around this new expression of technological child abuse.

According to child psychiatrist and drug advocate Laurence Greenhill, government plans for clinical trials on toddlers were already underway before Hillary Clinton's public endorsement. Greenhill observed, "The media made it look like a knee-jerk that came out of thin air, but we've been working on putting together a Ritalin study for more than two years."[38] But they had been doing so under the cover of silence until Mrs. Clinton's endorsement. Hillary Clinton's call for more "research" did not promote the interests of America's children. Instead, it ennobled plans already in the works by the nation's most avid drug advocates.

An Assault on the Youngest of Young Children

The government should be stopped from going ahead with psychiatric drug trials involving toddlers. First, there is already sufficient research on the effects of psychiatric drugs on the very young to know that the children will be harmed. Second, we can be almost certain that NIMH, as it did with its study of stimulants for older children (chapter 8), will skew the research to come out in favor of drugging children of any age. Third, the FDA will feel encouraged by the White House and NIMH to allow and even to encourage similar drug company research on small children. Ever eager to expand their markets, pharmaceutical companies will very likely seize the opportunity to begin testing their products on preschoolers.

The FDA Drug Modernization Act of 1997 will require drug companies to test their products on children starting in the year 2002. This legislation was another Clinton political maneuver that was touted as beneficial to America's children. The argument went this way: Since many psychiatric drugs are prescribed for children without proper testing or FDA approval, a benevolent government should force all the drug companies to test their new drugs on children to see if they are safe and effective.

In reality, this legislation encouraged the future drugging of children by requiring drug companies to test their products on children. Since it's almost always possible to rig drugs trials to come out favorably for the sponsoring drug companies, many additional psychiatric drugs will end up approved for children. And since the research was mandated by legislation, it may make it easier for the drug companies to defend themselves in court if the research causes harm. With the additional Clinton initiative for testing on toddlers, the FDA and the drug companies will be able to target, and eventually market to even the youngest of the young children.

Stopping NIMH's proposed drug research on preschoolers should be one of the top priorities of all individuals and organizations concerned about the rights and well-being of children in America. If unopposed, it will not only damage the hundreds of children in the actual clinical trials, inevitably it will also lead to a further escalation of drugging toddlers and preschoolers throughout the nation.

The American Academy of Pediatrics Weighs In

Medical organizations such as the American Psychiatric Association and the American Medical Association rarely if ever criticize any treatment that is widely used by their professional constituents. Instead, the American Psychiatric Association has sponsored reports for the purpose of endorsing controversial, harmful treatments, such as lobotomy and electroshock. So, it is no surprise that the association has made no criticism of drugging small children.

If a medical organization such as the American Psychiatric Association were to criticize a commonly used treatment or method of practice, it would expose its professional members to censure and even to malpractice suits. It would also threaten to undermine government and foundation support for researchers in related fields. Most painful for these professional organizations, their criticism of medication practices would almost surely drive away financial support from the affected drug companies.

Any criticism of the widespread medicating of children would prove very costly to individual practitioners. The psychiatric medicating of children is now a significant source of income, identity, and authority in the field of pediatrics, family practice, neurology, and psychiatry.

With so many vested interests involved, it was no surprise when the American Academy of Pediatrics in May 2000 issued a set of guidelines for the diagnosis of ADHD by pediatricians and family practitioners. The guidelines, which followed those already described in the American Psychiatric Association's 1994 diagnostic manual, purposefully empowered pediatricians and family doctors to take an even larger role in diagnosing and treating children diagnosed with ADHD.

While a later academy guideline will deal with treatment, the diagnostic guidelines nonetheless opened the way to a further escalation of medicating children by estimating that ADHD may affect up to 12% of school age children. That's a lot of business for pediatricians and family physicians.

Despite its endorsement of the ADHD diagnosis, the American Academy of Pediatrics, like the NIH consensus development panel, found no convincing evidence that ADHD is biological in origin. The academy concluded that brain scans and similar studies "do not show reliable differences between children with ADHD and controls" and that they "do not discriminate reliably between children with and without this condition."

The public and the health profession have been inundated with multicolor photographs of brain scans that supposedly show something abnormal or different in the brains of children diagnosed with ADHD. Hopefully this scientific farce will be brought to an end by the rejection of these claims by the November 1998 Consensus Development Conference and the May 2000 report by the American Academy of Pediatrics.

However, given the power and the persistence of the ADHD/Ritalin lobby, the Brain Scan Scam has a lot of life left in it. Even the official press release of the American Academy of Pediatrics (2000a) continued to call ADHD a "neurobehavioral disorder." The prefix, "neuro-," means "pertaining to the nervous system." Nonetheless, the academy in fact found no evidence of a defect in the nervous system of children labeled ADHD.

More Scrutiny of Heart Failure Caused by Ritalin

On March 21, 2000, fourteen-year-old Matthew Smith collapsed while skateboarding and died shortly afterward.[39] Ljubisa Dragovic, chief medical examiner for Oakland County, Pontiac, Michigan, performed the autopsy. He found fibrosis and narrowing of the vessel walls of the heart and attributed the child's death to heart disease caused by ten years of exposure to Ritalin. In a telephone interview with me in early June 2000, Dr. Dragovic explained that he commonly has found similar and more extensive cardiac pathology in stimulant addicts. He was trying, without much success, to interest the FDA in investigating the cardiac risk for children taking stimulants.

Recently a case has been filed against the manufacturer, Novartis, by the parents of a child who died of a heart arrhythmia after an increased dose of Ritalin. Michael Mosher of Paris, Texas, is the attorney and I am a medical expert in the case.

Educational and Political Backlash Against ADHD and Ritalin

The Board of Education of the State of Colorado became the first to raise concerns about teachers and schools recommending or encouraging Ritalin.

In a non-binding resolution, it urged school districts to help children through educational rather than medical means.[41]

The school board's decision came days after a number of experts, including myself, testified before a committee of the Colorado State Legislature on November 9, 1999 concerning the adverse effects of psychiatric drugs on children.[42] The hearing was inspired and chaired by Representative Penn Pfiffner. I specifically addressed the fact that Colorado school shooter Eric Harris was taking Luvox (fluvoxamine), a Prozac knock-off known to cause mania in children. The FDA-approved label for Luvox notes that manic reactions developed in 4% of the children in brief controlled clinical trials. The percentages will be even higher in actual clinical practice where drugs are given for much longer periods of time with much less medical supervision. As a result, thousands of children are literally being driven mad by the drug.

More recently, on May 3, 2000 I testified on similar issues in Little Rock before a committee of the Arkansas State Legislature. The hearings were held in association with Arkansas State Representative Randy Minton's proposal to study the relationship between school violence and the use of prescribed drugs. One of the legislators challenged me, "I don't believe a drug can make anybody do anything." I pointed out that the scientific data proves otherwise. Time and again in controlled clinical trials, people become irrational and crazy in reaction to psychiatric drugs while they do not as commonly act abnormally in response to the placebo or sugar pill.

I also reminded the legislator that we are talking about children taking drugs that have been prescribed to them. We might not want to exonerate an adult for misbehaving on a drug such as alcohol. After all, the adult willingly imbibed the alcohol with full knowledge that the drug can impair judgment and self-control. The adult is therefore responsible for any irresponsible actions on alcohol. But the child taking psychiatric drugs is not fully mature. Furthermore, the child has not been forewarned about the dangers. The child thinks the drug is supposed to help, thereby adding to his or her confusion when the drug ends up making the child angry or insane.

Coercing Parents to Drug Their Children

Many parents are being indirectly and even directly coerced into giving psychiatric drugs to their children. In an "Orwellian" case reported in the media, school administrators in Albany called the county child protective services alleging child abuse against the parents because they wanted to take their child off Ritalin.[43] The child was suffering from typical adverse effects of stimulants, including insomnia and extreme loss of appetite. The family was justifiably concerned. Fortunately, the parents have not been prosecuted. However, the parents have been stigmatized by the charges and by a record of being investigated for child abuse. In early 2000, the Boston Globe found other cases of school systems coercing parents to drug their children.[44]

In March 2000 Patricia Weathers brought her son Michael's situation to media attention, including syndicated columnist Arianna Huffington, who has led the way in alerting the public to the dangers of drugging children. As a medical consultant in the case, I was able to ascertain that nine-year-old Michael had been driven into a disturbed mental state by the Prozac-like antidepressant, Paxil (paroxetine). The drug caused hallucinations and angry outbursts, as well as feelings of despair in the fourth grader. Scoffing at the idea that Paxil made the child mentally disturbed, school authorities reported the parents to a child protective agency to force them to continue drugging their child. Michael fortunately recovered over several weeks after being withdrawn from Paxil, and when interviewed by me, was entirely normal. The child abuse investigation has been dropped and Michael is now doing well in a private school. Pat Weathers testified effectively at the recent hearings held by the House of Representatives (2000).

In more subtle cases, many of which have come to my attention, teachers and school officials are coercing parents to have their child medically examined for prescription drugs. Even when unspoken, there is an underlying threat of serious repercussions, such as removal of the children from mainstream classrooms, if the parents fail to comply.

In cases in my clinical practice, parents have been pushed to medicate their children because the youngsters were "daydreaming in class" or "failing to fulfill their potential," i.e., not getting the highest possible grades. Throughout the nation, teachers themselves are being pressured to make their students perform better, especially on standardized achievement tests. Regardless of what we think of these tests, we should never drug our children in the hope of getting them to perform better on them. First, as chapter 4 will document, stimulant drugs do not improve learning or academic performance. Second, even if they did help children achieve higher test scores, it wouldn't be worth the risk of long-term damage to the brain.

Caught in the Crossfire

I am also familiar with a number of heartbreaking situations in which divorced parents have clashed over the medicating of their child. Often one parent feels easily able to handle the child without resorting to drugs while the other parent feels there is an absolute necessity for medication to keep the child in line. In the family situations I have observed, the parent desiring to drug the child has been less able to implement rational, consistent discipline, or has been less available to the child. In court cases, I have seen parents lose custody of their children because of their refusal to drug them.[45] This trend appears to have grown worse in the last year or two. It is ironic that parents are losing their parental rights for refusing to give stimulants to their children while other adults are going to jail for selling the very same drugs to children on the street.

While there is an encouraging trend to question the widespread psychiatric medicating of America's children, this has not yet resulted in any decline in the practice. When it comes to abusive practices involving psychiatric drugs, the medical profession has often remained unresponsive to public controversy and condemnation.

Meanwhile, the market for psychiatric drugs will eventually become saturated among middle and upper class Americans. As suggested by Zito's JAMA study, poor children in this country are beginning to provide another growing market for psychiatric drugs. At the same time, drug companies and drug advocates are successfully seeking to open new markets on other continents. Reports from my colleagues abroad indicate that the use of stimulants for the control of children is also rising in Australia, Great Britain, and the European continent. It will take a concerted international effort to stop the psychiatric diagnosing and drugging of children throughout the world.

Chapter 2

RITALIN IS NOT CANDY FOR THE BRAIN

Adverse Effects of Stimulant Drugs

[There are] thousands of American children who have been affected by the rush to Ritalin. The drug's use to treat ADD has become so rampant that at the slightest sign of trouble—a child keeps running back and forth to the water fountain, has an unruly week pushing other kids on the playground, plays drums on his desk with pencils—parents are circled by the school's teachers, psychologists, and even principal, all pushing Ritalin....

—Jeanie Russell, *Good Housekeeping* (1997)

Every day millions of parents must decide whether or not to start or to continue their children on stimulant drugs such as Ritalin, Dexedrine, and Adderall. These parents have usually been told that the drugs are safe and effective for treating children diagnosed with Attention Deficit-Hyperactivity Disorder (ADHD). The most important question for these parents is "How safe are stimulant drugs?"

The Stimulants

Stimulants are the drugs most frequently prescribed for ADHD in the hope of controlling behaviors described as hyperactivity, impulsivity, and inattention. With their chemical names in parentheses, the drugs include:

- Ritalin (methylphenidate)
- Concerta and Metadate (longer-acting preparations of methylphenidate)
- Dexedrine and DextroStat (dextroamphetamine, also called d-amphetamine)
- Adderall (a mixture of d-amphetamine and amphetamine)
- Desoxyn (methamphetamine)
- Gradumet (a longer-acting preparation of methamphetamine)
- Cylert (pemoline)

As already noted, except for Cylert all of these drugs have nearly identical effects and side effects, and are included in Schedule II of the DEA for the most highly addictive drugs. Ritalin and the amphetamines can for most purposes be considered one type of drug.

Amphetamine was synthesized in the late 19th century. In 1927 a form of amphetamine called Benzedrine was sold as an inhaler for asthma. In 1937 it became the first stimulant described in the professional literature as a psychiatric treatment for children.[1]

Ritalin has also been around for a long time. It was first synthesized in the mid-1940s and was approved by the Food and Drug Administration (FDA) in December 1955. Along with the amphetamines, it first came into widespread use for the behavioral control of children in the 1960s.

Cylert was approved by the FDA for "minimal brain dysfunction" in 1975. Until the recent increased concern about a number of cases of death from liver failure, Cylert had a small fraction of the market.[2] Prescriptions for Cylert will probably further decline as a result of recent warnings about liver failure.

Adderall has recently been marketed as an improved form of stimulant medication, but it is nothing more than a mixture of four old-fashioned kinds of amphetamine.[3] Parents who do not want to give their children Ritalin are sometimes encouraged by their doctors to accept Adderall as an alternative. However, Adderall is in no way safer than Ritalin. If anything, Adderall as an amphetamine is even more harmful to the brain than Ritalin (see chapter 3).

Concerta and Metadate, the longer-acting forms of Ritalin, may be more convenient for adults to give, because there may be no need for a lunchtime dose at school. However, longer-acting drugs tend to be more dangerous. When they cause an adverse reaction, a longer time elapses before they are cleared from the body. The child must therefore endure a lengthier exposure to the toxic agent.

Important Warnings Go Unheeded

The official FDA-approved label for Ritalin contains a prominent "WARNING" section. The reader can find a complete version of this label in any Physicians' Desk Reference, an annual publication sent to all physicians and owned by most libraries. The first two warnings in the section are of extreme importance to anyone concerned with the prescription or consumption of Ritalin.

The first warning states that "Ritalin should not be used in children under six years, since safety and efficacy for this age group have not been established." This warning, like the others in the label, remains in force today. But as we observed in chapter 1, it is increasingly ignored.

The second warning declares that "Sufficient data on safety and efficacy of long-term use of Ritalin in children are not yet available." The "PRE-

CAUTION" section of the label restates the warning: "Long-term effects of Ritalin in children have not been well established." This remains true. Recent efforts by NIMH to prove safety and efficacy over 14 months were flawed to the point of uselessness (discussed in chapter 8).

The consensus among researchers is the same as that proclaimed on the label. A recent review by two life-long researchers in the field laments "the difficulty of documenting long-term advantage" from using stimulants. Despite more than thirty years of effort and thousands of studies, advocates admit that they are unable to demonstrate the safety or the efficacy of stimulants beyond a few weeks. Our nation faces a potentially tragic situation with millions of children being exposed long-term to a drug whose long-term hazards have not been determined. There are also serious questions about Ritalin's short-term efficacy and safety.

If Your Child Is Already Stressed...

Acute stress can make a child overstimulated, anxious, upset, jumpy, and wary. The precaution section of Ritalin's label specifically warns that even if the child has ADHD-like symptoms, treatment with Ritalin is "not usually indicated" in acute stress reactions. This raises many issues in regard to the common practice of giving Ritalin to children when they are having difficulty adjusting to various stresses at school and at home.

In discussing "specific diagnostic considerations," the Ritalin label also declares, "Stimulants are not intended for use in the child who exhibits symptoms secondary to environmental factors." In other words, the drugs should not be given if the child's problem is created by the child's situation or circumstances in school or at home. This is very similar to the warning not to give Ritalin for acute stress. Prescribing Ritalin is based on the theory that the problem lies within the child rather than within a stressful, boring, difficult, or conflicted environment.

What if it turns out that most or all of the symptoms associated with ADHD are caused by environmental conflicts, stresses, or related difficulties? If so, the label for Ritalin states that it should not be prescribed.

As Safe As Candy?

Doctors frequently tell parents that Ritalin and other stimulants can be compared to aspirin or even eyeglasses in terms of both their safety and their usefulness. Side effects—called *adverse effects* in the scientific literature—are usually brushed off.

Ritalin is not "candy" for the brain. Nor does it "harmonize" brain chemicals. Ritalin and other stimulants produce gross impairments of brain function. There is a serious risk of permanent brain malfunction.

As I described in chapter 1, I was asked to be the scientific presenter on adverse drug effects in children at the NIH Consensus Conference on the

Diagnosis and Treatment of Attention Deficit Hyperactivity Disorder. In preparation for that conference, I updated my research on stimulant drugs and eventually published a series of articles reviewing the scientific literature.[5] The next several sections are based on those published papers. The papers contain even greater detail and the complete citations.

An Overview of the Adverse Effects of Stimulant Drugs

Table 1, Overview of the Harmful Reactions to Stimulant Drugs can be found on the following page. It presents an overview of the risks that a child or adult faces when taking these medications in routine doses.

In order to lend both scope and objectivity to the table, I combined information presented in several well-known professional sources, including tables from three textbooks, and information from the Drug Enforcement Administration (DEA) and the Food and Drug Administration (FDA).[6]

The stimulants are almost indistinguishable from each other in their basic adverse effects. Most of the items in the table have been reported with all of the stimulants, including Ritalin and the amphetamines such as Adderall and Dexedrine.

Negative effects on the brain and mind are by far the most common. Many children become sad, tearful, depressed, apathetic, and simply tired while taking stimulants. Many go through cycles of feeling energized and exhausted. Commonly they have difficulty sleeping.

Too often the doctor fails to recognize these adverse drug effects and mistakenly believes the child has now become depressed, leading to the prescription of an antidepressant that further worsens the child's mental condition.

Often children are lethargic when taking the drug during the day, but develop a "hyper" rebound at night that worsens their behavior and makes it hard for them to sleep. Once again, the physician may mistake this for the child's emotional problems. Instead of reducing or stopping the stimulant, the doctor may prescribe a sleeping medication, such as Klonopin, Dalmane or other sedative tranquilizers. Or, in keeping with the latest fad, the doctor may prescribe the adult anti-hypertensive agent, clonidine (Catapres), which has very sedative effects. I have seen children in my practice barely able to stay awake after their afternoon dose of clonidine.

Stimulants commonly interfere with the learning process. They focus the child in a narrow and obsessive way that may look good superficially, while real learning is impeded.

The stimulants can make children psychotic. They become suspicious and distrustful, imagine things that are unreal, and even hallucinate small insects or objects. They can become artificially energized into a state of mania, a condition characterized by grandiose plans, bizarre notions of invulnerability, poor judgement, and sometimes paranoia and violence. As I documented

Table 1: Overview of Harmful Reactions to Stimulant Drugs: Ritalin, Dexedrine, Adderall, Concerta, and Metadate

Brain and Mind Function
Obsessive-compulsive behavior
Zombie-like (robotic) behavior with loss of emotional spontaneity
Drowsiness 'dopey,' reduced alertness
Abnormal movements, tics, Tourette's
Nervous habits (picking at skin, pulling hair)
Convulsions
Headache
Stroke
Mania, psychosis, hallucinations
Agitation, anxiety, nervousness
Insomnia
Irritability, Hostility
Aggression
Depression, emotional, sensitivity, easy crying, social withdrawal
Confusion, mental, impairments (decreased cognition and learning)
Stimulant addiction and abuse

Gastrointestinal Function
Anorexia
Nausea, vomiting, bad taste
Stomache ache
Cramps
Dry mouth
Constipation, diarrhea
Liver dysfunction

Withdrawal and Rebound Reactions
Insomnia
Excessive sleep
Evening crash
Depression
Rebound worsening of ADHD -like symptoms
Overactivity and irritability

Endocrine and Metabolic Function
Pituitary dysfunction, including growth hormone and prolactin disruption
Weight loss
Growth suppression
Disturbed sexual function

Cardiovascular Function
Hypertension
Abnormal heart beat
Heart disease
Cardiac arrest

Other Functions
Blurred vision
Hair loss
Dizziness
Hypersensitivity reaction with rash

Modified from Breggin (1999a & c) by permission of Springer Publishing Company. Sources include Arnold and Jensen (1995, Table 38-5, p. 2306; Table 38-7; and p. 2307), Drug Enforcement Administration (1995b, p. 1217), Maxmen and Ward (1995, pp. 365-366), Dulcan (1994, Table 35-6, p. 23), and Food and Drug Administration (1997c, March).

in *Reclaiming Our Children* (2000) several of the school shooters were taking Ritalin, including T. G. Solomon from Heritage High School in Conyers, Georgia.

Too often the doctor fails to react properly to the development of psychosis or other serious mental disturbances in a child taking stimulant drugs. Instead of stopping the medication, the physician adds a dangerous antipsychotic drug.

Antipsychotics such as Haldol (haloperidol), Risperdal (risperidone), and Zyprexa (olanzapine) can cause permanent neurological disorders with potentially disabling twitches and spasms of the face, neck, torso, arms or legs, as well any other muscle group. While this book focuses on stimulants, the reader can find a review of the major adverse effects of all psychiatric drugs, including antipsychotics, in *Your Drug May Be Your Problem: How and Why to Stop Taking Psychiatric Drugs* (1999), which I wrote with co-author David Cohen.

It is common but tragic in my practice to see a child who was started on Ritalin or Adderall, and then prescribed additional drugs in an ever-increasing attempt to control the growing adverse drug effects. In this way, a stimulant like Ritalin or Adderall can become a gateway drug to multiple psychiatric medications and eventually to a lifetime on psychiatric drugs.

Stimulants frequently suppress growth. Since they do so not only by suppressing appetite but also by disrupting growth hormones, the growth suppression involves the entire body and all its organs. For this reason alone, giving stimulants to children is a bad idea.

Stimulants cause a variety of other problems listed in Table 1. They can cause irreversible tics and worsen existing ones. Skin rashes can become very serious and even life-threatening allergic reactions have occurred.

Stimulants can cause seizures.

They can disrupt the rhythm of the heart, leading to cardiac arrest and death. They can cause high blood pressure, a risk of special concern among African-Americans who suffer from a high rate of hypertension as young adults.

Stimulants frequently cause hair loss. Sometimes children on stimulants will pull out their hair, including their eyebrows. They also pick at their skin.

The Frequency of Adverse Drug Reactions to Stimulants

In preparation for my presentation at the Consensus Development Conference, I reviewed eight controlled clinical trials of stimulant drugs in order to obtain a general idea about the frequency of side effects. Although these studies were conducted by advocates of the stimulants who tended to minimize harmful effects, I was able to document a surprisingly high rate of adverse reactions. I have summarized these results in Table 2 on the following page.

Table 2: Harmful Reactions to Ritalin and Dexedrine (Amphetamine) in Children Diagnosed with "ADHD"

Summarized from Eight Controlled Clinical Trials

Authors	Group Size	Drugs	Duration	Salient Adverse Drug Reactions
1. Firestone et al.	41, age 4–6	Ritalin	7–10 days	Marked deterioration from placebo to 0.5 mg in Sad/unhappy (69% (1998) of children), Drowsiness (62%), Uninterested in others (62%), Loss of appetite 75%. Severe symptoms increased 12% for "Uninterested in others" and 28% for "Talks less with others." Nightmares increased 35%; tics or nervous movements increased 9%.
2. Mayes et al. (1994)	69, age 2–13	Ritalin	mean 8 days	6 discontinued because of adverse affects. 13 "significantly worse" on drug. 26% "irritability." 5.8% increase or emergence of "stereotypical behaviors, including hand-wringing, arm-waving, teeth-grinding and foot-tapping." 7% severe reactions with one manic-like. 18.8% experience lethargy: "Children with lethargy were variously described by raters as tired, withdrawn, listless, depressed, dopey, dazed, subdued, and inactive."
3. Barkley et al. (1990)	83, age 5–13	Ritalin	14–20 days	Decreased appetite, insomnia, stomachaches, and headaches. Proneness to crying increased at least 10% during low dose. Tics and nervous movements increased 10% at the high dose. Decreased appetite and insomnia "serious" in 13% and 18% at both doses. 3.6% dropped out due to "serious" drug reactions. One case of "excessive speech and disjointed thinking."

Continues...

Table 2 Continued...

Study	N, age	Drug	Duration	Findings
4. Schachar et al. (1997)	46, age 6–12	Ritalin	4 months	More than 10% drop out due to drug reactions. 3 due to "sadness and behavioral deterioration, irritability, withdrawal, lethargy, violent behavior, or rash;" 1 due to "withdrawal and mild mania;" 1 due to "withdrawal and dysphoria." 45% experienced at least 1 drug reaction ($p < 0.005$). Increased severity of emotional drug reactions (mostly withdrawal, sadness, crying) ($p < 0.01$). Increased severity of physiological drug reactions (mostly anorexia and stomachaches) ($p < 0.005$).
5. Gillberg et al. (1997)	62, age 6–11	Dexedrine	4–15 months	3 cases of hallucination, 1 with severe tics. 32% abdominal pain occasionally or often. 56% poor appetite.
6. Borcherding et al. (1990)	46, age 6–12	Ritalin & Dexedrine	3 weeks	Studied compulsive and tic drug reactions. 58% develop abnormal movements. 51% develop obsessive-compulsive or perseverative drug reactions. 1 persistent tic. Many severe OCD drug reactions. See Table 3.
7. Solanto and Wender (1989)	19, age 6–10	Ritalin	3 separate days	Studied cognitive functions. 42% "over-aroused" with "cognitive perseveration" (over-focused obsessive-compulsive reaction).
8. Castellanos et al. (1997)	20, age 6–13 all with Tourette's	Ritalin & Dexedrine	3 weeks	25% developed obsessive drug reactions on Ritalin. 3 stopped medications at completion due to increased tics. One third experienced worsened tics.

Each of the trials was double-blind, placebo controlled, except Mayes (1994) where only the preschoolers were double-blind. Most of the doses were in the low to average clinical range, and are summarized in Breggin (1999a & c). Ritalin is methylphenidate and Dexedrine is dextroamphetamine. This table was modified from Breggin (1999a & c) and is reproduced by permission of Springer Publishing Company.

Notice the frequency of symptoms along the spectrum of apathy, sadness, and depression.

In the study by Firestone (Table 2) involving the youngest children, a relatively small dose of Ritalin produced a worsening or deterioration in regard to sadness or unhappiness in 69% of the youngsters. While noting that the problem has not been sufficiently studied, the Drug Enforcement Administration (DEA) (1995b) noted reports that over 20% of children become depressed on stimulants. In their handbook on psychiatric drugs, Maxmen and Ward estimated that 39% of children on amphetamines become depressed while 8.7% on Ritalin become depressed. While estimates vary widely, they confirm the danger that stimulant drugs will commonly cause children to be depressed.

Can Ritalin Turn Kids into Zombies?

Stimulants constrict, flatten, or suppress a child's mental activity and behavior, often making the child more obedient or compliant. This constellation of symptoms is related to the depression produced in these children. It is a part of what Davy and Rodgers (1989) referred to as the child becoming "hypoactive," "too quiet," and "depressed," so that he "loses his sparkle."

L. Eugene Arnold is professor emeritus of psychiatry at Ohio State University and holds the post of "special expert" on children and adolescents at NIMH. We have already met Peter Jensen in chapter 1 as an avid advocate of stimulant drugs. As co-authors of the chapter on ADHD in the 1995 *Comprehensive Textbook of Psychiatry*,[7] Arnold and Jensen made a remarkable admission:

> The amphetamine look, a pinched, somber expression, is harmless in itself but worrisome to parents, who can be reassured.

What sort of medical mind-set can dismiss a child's "pinched, somber expression" as "harmless in itself"? Of course the effect is worrisome to parents—but should the doctors try to reassure them?

Arnold and Jensen further observe:

> The behavioral equivalent, the "zombie" constriction of affect and spontaneity, may respond to a reduction of dosage, but sometimes necessitates a change of drug.

In admitting that Ritalin can produce a zombie-like inhibition of feeling and spontaneity, many questions are left unanswered by these NIMH experts. How can they dismiss this drastic suppression of a child's feelings and vitality? Is the zombie effect an unusual adverse reaction or is it the main effect? Does Ritalin have its "therapeutic" effect by producing relative degrees of robotic conformity? The next several chapters will answer these questions with a further look at the zombie effect.

Causing Obsessions and Compulsions

Stimulant drugs impair the function of a portion of the brain called the basal ganglia. Dysfunction in the basal ganglia results in a variety of mental and physical symptoms, including impaired higher mental functions, obsessions and compulsions (OCD), and abnormal movements.

A study by Borcherding and his colleagues at NIMH specifically looked for the production of OCD symptoms and abnormal movements caused by both Ritalin and amphetamine. (It was a crossover study so that each of the children was exposed to each drug at different times.) The researchers found that 23 of 45 (51%) of children developed symptoms of OCD. Some of the OCD symptoms were extremely severe. One child became so obsessed with doing a good job raking the leaves, he would wait for each one to fall from the tree. Another played Legos for a 36-hour period without breaking to eat or sleep. Table 3 contains a summary of these drug-induced obsessive-compulsive reactions.

The NIH study was double-blind and placebo controlled, and specifically looked for obsessive-compulsive reactions. Most clinical studies don't focus on these drug-induced symptoms and instead completely overlook them.

Borcherding also found a high rate of drug-induced abnormal movements. Thirty-four of the 45 (76%) children suffered from either tics or obsessive-compulsive reactions caused by the drugs and many had a combination of both (see below).

Borcherding's results are confirmed by Castellanos, who found that 25% of children developed OCD while taking Ritalin. Solanto and Wender (Table 2) discovered that a single dose of stimulant drugs produced an obsessive over-focusing in 42% of children. The children were sometimes unable to stop performing the tasks that were assigned to them.

The production of OCD in children taking stimulants is typically mistaken for an "improvement." If the child sits stoically in his or her classroom seat while bearing down hard on the pencil obsessively copying every detail from the book, the teacher considers it an improvement. If a child endlessly plays the same game on his computer, his parents may feel relieved by the child's absence. In fact, as Borcherding notes, parents and especially teachers almost never report drug-induced OCD as an adverse effect. Instead, they think it's an improvement. But drug-induced OCD is a form of *severe brain dysfunction*. It is an involuntary obsession that the child often cannot stop on his or her own. It enforces social isolation and will not lead to genuine learning. Chapter 4 looks in more detail at how adverse drug reactions are confused with improvement in children treated with stimulant drugs.

Table 3: Obsessive-Compulsive Harmful Drug Reactions to Ritalin and Dexedrine (Amphetamine)

23 of 45 children (51%) in a Controlled Clinical Trial

	Age	Drug	Adverse Drug Reaction
1.	6	Dexedrine	Perseverative [obsessive-compulsive] drawing and writing at home; counting puzzle pieces
2.	6	Dexedrine	Perseverative play with Legos and puzzles (36-hours with Legos with no break to eat or sleep)
3.	6	Ritalin	Perseverative playing of piano
4.	6	Dexedrine	Perseverative speech
5.	7	Dexedrine	Rewriting work; over-erasing; repetitive checking of work; overly neat and organized at home
6.	7	Ritalin Dexedrine	Rewriting work Compulsively lining up crayons
7.	8	Ritalin	Overly detail oriented
8.	8	Ritalin Dexedrine	Coloring over and over the same area Repetitive checking of work; frantically goal-oriented; solitary activities
9.	8	Ritalin Dexedrine	Perseverative playing of video games Cleaning room compulsively, buttoning and then folding dirty laundry
10.	8	Dexedrine	Repetitive checking of work; perseverative with work in school
11.	8	Ritalin Dexedrine	Over-erasing; redrawing; excessive pressure on pencil Over-erasing
12.	8	Ritalin	Markedly detail oriented in drawings

13. 9	Dexedrine	Over-erasing; making lists (TV shows, model cars)
14. 9	Dexedrine	Cleaning room compulsively; overly orderly at home
15. 9	Dexedrine	Perseverative at school
16. 9	Ritalin	Over-erasing; rewriting; excessive pressure on pencils and crayons; perseverative speech
	Dexedrine	Overly meticulous; inability to terminate school & play activities; perseverative speech
17. 9	Ritalin	Inability to stop school and play activities; repetitive erasing and redoing projects; overly detail oriented
18. 10	Dexedrine	Cleaning room compulsively; folding dirty laundry
19. 10	Dexedrine	Repetitive checking behavior; lining things up; excessive pressure on pencil; repetitive erasing and rewriting
20. 11	Dexedrine	Overly meticulous work; overly neat and organized; cleaning room compulsively; raking leaves for 7 hours and then as they fell individually
21. 11	Dexedrine	Lining up crayons; repetitive erasing and redrawing
22. 11	Ritalin	Repetitive erasing; "perfectionistic;" excessive pressure on pencil and crayons
23. 12	Dexedrine	Overly detail oriented; excessive pressure on pencil & crayons

Data taken from Borcherding et al. (1990). Both drugs increased the likelihood of "repetitious, perfectionistic, overfocused behaviors" ($p<.01$). Ritalin caused a combination of abnormal movements and obsessive-compulsive reactions ($p=.009$).

Causing Tics

The production of tics can also become a serious problem. These stimulant-induced abnormal movements commonly disfigure the face. These abnormalities can make a child look strange and harm his self-esteem and social acceptance. On occasion, the tics can become permanent.

Borcherding found a rate of 58% for tics and abnormal movements in his study of 45 children on stimulants. As already mentioned, many also had obsessive-compulsive symptoms. Castellanos reported a worsening of pre-existing tics.

A group led by Paul Lipkin (1994) from the Long Island Jewish Medical Center and Albert Einstein College of Medicine did a retrospective evaluation of 122 children with ADHD currently or recently treated with stimulants. They found that 9% of the children developed tics or dyskinesias. Other tics and dyskinesias found in the study included mouth movements (5 children), eye blinking, rolling, or deviation (4), throat clearing or vocalizations (2), eye "bugging" (1), neck turning (1), and face rubbing (1). Five of the children had more than one type of dyskinesia or tic. One child did not recover. He developed an irreversible syndrome with "facial twitching, head turning, lip smacking, forehead wiping, and vocalizations."

The development of at least one permanent severe neurological disorder among 122 children treated with stimulants at ordinary doses should give pause to many parents before starting their own child on the drug.

Stimulants should not be started if a person already has a history of tics and should be stopped if tics develop during treatment. The official label for Ritalin states that Ritalin is contraindicated "in patients with motor tics or with a family history or diagnosis of Tourette's syndrome." Remember, a contraindication is an absolute prohibition against using the drug under the specified conditions.

A study by Mark Schmidt (1994) from NIMH, and a string of other researchers, found changes in calcium and magnesium concentrations in the blood during treatment with Ritalin and Dexedrine. They suggested that this might be the cause of abnormal movements produced by the stimulants. These findings once again emphasize that the harmful impact of these drugs is widespread in the body and little understood.

Curing or Causing ADHD?

Ritalin and amphetamine are stimulants. As such they can produce the very symptoms they are supposed to control: hyperactivity, impulsivity, and inattention. When a child becomes stimulated while taking the drug, a parent or doctor can mistakenly believe that the child's "ADHD" is getting worse. In a destructive cycle, this can lead to further increases in the stimulating medication.

Nurses, for example, are warned in regard to Ritalin toxicity that "Behavioral clues include anxiety, agitation, restlessness, insomnia, inability to concentrate, and personality changes.... The person will become easily distracted, unable to concentrate. Often he'll complain of feeling jittery or on edge."[8] This, of course, is exactly what ADHD is supposed to look like. How is the nurse, or anyone else, to determine if the child is getting worse due to "ADHD" or due to the drug? Often, the worsening condition of the child is mistakenly blamed on "ADHD" rather than on the drug.

ADHD-like symptoms are also produced by long-term exposure to Ritalin in people who become dependent on it. The American Psychiatric Association (1987) *Diagnostic and Statistical Manual of Mental Disorders-III-Revised* describes Ritalin dependence as causing "irritability," "attentional disturbances," and "memory problems," as well as a variety of more severe psychological disorders, including depression and social withdrawal.[9]

To avoid dependency and long-term toxicity, some experts recommend stopping Ritalin when a child reaches puberty.[10] Unfortunately, the growing tendency is to keep children and adults on the medication for years at a time.

Stimulant drugs frequently cause agitation—a state of tension and anxiety often accompanied by hyperactivity, such as pacing, handwringing, or foot jiggling. The agitated individual looks nervous and perturbed, and sometimes develops an aggressive "edge." Drug-induced agitation looks very much like "ADHD."

The official label for Ritalin warns about the danger of the drug worsening agitation. In the "**CONTRAINDICATION**" section, the label states: "Marked anxiety, tension, and agitation are contraindications to Ritalin, since the drug may aggravate these symptoms." The theme is repeated in the precaution section of the label which states, "Patients with an element of agitation may react adversely." Agitated states are also seen as contraindications in the labels of the amphetamines, Dexedrine and Adderall.

When a drug is contraindicated, it means it should *never* be used under the specified conditions. Yet doctors too often mistakenly prescribe stimulants to children who are suffering from conditions that the drugs can worsen, including anxiety, tension, and agitation. As already noted, they can then fail to realize that the worsening of the child's ADHD-like symptoms is caused by the drug itself.

People are often surprised that a "stimulant" drug is given to children to "calm" them. They wonder why the drug doesn't make the children more over-active and over-excited. To some extent, it depends on dosage. With larger doses, the agitation tends to become more frequent and more obvious. However, different children can react to the same drug dose very differently. At relatively low doses many develop a more subdued reaction but some will become agitated.

A similar variability is seen in adult responses to the relatively mild stimulant, caffeine. Some adults can drink a pot of coffee without any noticeable stimulation. They may even feel more calmed or relaxed, and more able to focus their attention on work. Hence coffee machines are available in many workplaces. Other people cannot drink a partial cup without becoming jittery, jumpy, and even touchy and aggressive. Children taking Ritalin respond with similar variability. One child may seem quieted by a dose that will cause severe stimulation in another child.

Drug-induced agitation is a dangerous state that can lead to aggressive and violent behavior. Some of the most horrendous crimes I have evaluated as a medical expert have resulted at least in part from agitated patients being treated with drugs that worsen their agitation. I have described these dangers in *Talking Back to Prozac* (1994), *Brain-Disabling Treatments in Psychiatry* (1997), and *Your Drug May Be Your Problem* (with David Cohen, 1999).

Can Ritalin Cause Cancer?

Cancer concerns have recently flared up in regard to Ritalin. There has been no reported increase in cancer rates in humans treated with stimulants. There is, however, a report of cancer tumors in the liver of mice receiving very large doses of Ritalin in a two year study from the National Toxicology Program, a branch of the National Institutes of Health (NIH).[11] The tumors, called hepatoblastomas, are rare in humans, usually striking children under age four. This should add to cautions against prescribing Ritalin to younger children. The FDA forced the drug company, CibaGeneva (now a division of Novartis) to add the finding to its label for Ritalin. In a more extreme step, the agency also required the company to send a "Dear Doctor" letter to 100,000 physicians throughout the country.[12] Overall, however, the FDA played down the risk in its 1996 "Talk Paper" where it labeled the cancer report a "weak" signal.

The FDA's conclusion was disputed among the researchers themselves. One of the three principal investigators in the cancer study disagreed with the characterization of "some" evidence of carcinogenic activity and wanted the report to conclude that there was "clear evidence."[13] An amendment to change the conclusion to "clear evidence" was proposed to the entire panel. It was defeated by a narrow 4-3 vote with two abstentions. The manufacturer, CibaGeneva, was happy with the result.[14] Especially given the two abstentions, as well as political factors that will be examined in this book, it may be reasonable to ask if something other than "pure science" affected the vote.

Can Stimulants Cause Addiction?

There is agreement among knowledgeable pharmacologists and physicians that there is a basic similarity between the effects of Ritalin and the amphetamines (Dexedrine, Adderall, Desoxyn, Gradumet). For example, the International Narcotics Control Board (1996b) has declared:

Methylphenidate's pharmacological effects are essentially the same as those of amphetamine and methamphetamine. The abuse of methylphenidate can lead to tolerance and severe psychological dependence. Psychotic episodes, violent and bizarre behavior have been reported.

The DEA and the International Narcotics control Board agree that Ritalin and the amphetamines are highly addictive and frequently abused. We shall examine this issue further in a chapter of its own. Right now it is important to remember that new research described in chapter 1 has confirmed the inevitable—that children who are prescribed Ritalin or other stimulants will have a higher risk of cocaine addiction in young adulthood.

What Professionals Are Reporting to the FDA and Ciba

Through the Freedom of Information Act (FOIA), I obtained a summary of computerized reports of "adverse drug experiences" compiled by the FDA's Spontaneous Reporting System (SRS) from 1985 through March 3, 1997.[15] The FDA now calls this program MedWatch. The reports were originally sent to the FDA or to Novartis, the drug company that makes Ritalin. Most of these adverse reaction reports come from busy pharmacists and physicians who were concerned enough about a drug reaction to take the time to write a letter to the drug company or to fill out a special form provided by the FDA. In recent years, about one-third of the reports come from consumers.[16] More than 2,700 reports were made but these reflect only a tiny fraction of the total number of adverse reactions that occur throughout the country.[17]

The reports demonstrate the expected problems such as headache, nervousness and agitation, various mental disturbances, insomnia, increased heart rate and blood pressure, and growth suppression.

There are some drug reactions that don't frequently get mentioned in textbooks and reviews:

(1) **Hair Loss** (250 reports of alopecia or hair loss). Since most of the patients were probably children, this is an especially remarkable finding. Hair loss is not a widely known side effect but it could cause considerable embarrassment to patients of any age. I am also aware of cases of children pulling out their hair, including their eyebrows, as an adverse reaction to Ritalin.

(2) **Drug Dependency, Addiction, and Withdrawal** (87 reports of drug addiction and dependence, plus 30 reports of drug withdrawal symptoms).

(3) **Skin Disorders** (over 100 reports of skin problems under a variety of categories including acne, rash, and urticaria or hives). There were many additional reports of a variety of potentially serious skin conditions.

(4) **Blood Disorders.** There were many reports of various blood disorders. These included several kinds of anemia and bleeding disorders that produce ecchymosis (bruis-

ing). There were more than 50 reports of leukopenia (low white cell count).

(5) **Liver Disorders**. There were many reports of abnormal liver function tests and several liver disorders. This is not a widely recognized adverse effect. It is consistent with recent NIH animal studies which show that large doses of Ritalin produce not only higher rates of liver cancer but other liver pathology, including hypertrophy (abnormally increased weight).

(6) **Abnormal Movements** (almost 150 reports of twitches). There were nine reports of oculogyric crisis, a potentially agonizing and terrifying experience involving spasms of the eye muscles.

(7) **Convulsions** (69 reports, including 18 grand mal seizure reports). It is known that all stimulants can cause convulsions.

Reports of Harmful Effects to the Brain and Mind

The reports sent to the FDA included many abnormal mental reactions to Ritalin. Confirming my analysis of the literature and my clinical experience, there were 48 reports of depression and 11 reports of psychotic depression for a total of 59 depression reports in response to Ritalin. Closely related to depression, there were more than 50 reports in the combined categories of overdose, overdose intentional, and suicide attempt.

There were also a striking number of personality disorders (89) reported. A sampling of some of the other frequently reported mental reactions includes agitation (55), hostility (50), abnormal thinking (44), hallucinations (43), psychosis (38), and emotional lability [instability] (33). There were also reports of amnesia, anxiety, confusion, nervousness, neurosis, stupor, and paranoid reactions. There were a few reports of manic reactions.

Can the Drug Make a Child Crazy?

Although "toxic psychosis" is mentioned as an adverse effect on the official Ritalin label, it receives too little attention. Yet these drug reactions have been recognized in regards to stimulants for more than two decades.[18] These psychoses have also been reported during withdrawal from long-term stimulant therapy.[19] Hallucinations, if they occur during stimulant treatment, are commonly visual and may involve seeing and feeling small creatures, like bugs. The experience is usually terrifying.

The onset of drug-induced psychosis is often abrupt and often associated with starting, increasing, or stopping the medication. Recovery can be relatively rapid after the drug is stopped, although symptoms may persist in some cases. The patient usually has no idea that the drug is causing the problem.

Even if full recovery seems to occur, the individual may be left with a variety of fears and anxieties. I have evaluated patients who were considered fully recovered by previous physicians but who continue to display residual effects, including recurrent strange ideas or sensations, insecurity, and fearfulness.

Until recently, the frequency of stimulant-induced psychotic reactions has usually been estimated at less than 1%. However, these relatively low estimates were based on relatively unreliable clinical impressions rather than research studies. A new study by Cherland and Fitzpatrick in the October 1999 issue of the *Canadian Journal of Psychiatry* retrospectively reviewed the charts of 98 stimulant-treated children over a five-year period. *A striking 9% of children who took stimulants (mostly Ritalin) developed "psychotic symptoms" during treatment.* Because of under-reporting, the authors consider this to be an underestimate of the actual rate. No cases of psychosis were reported in a comparison group of children diagnosed with ADHD who were not treated with stimulants. Cherland and Fitzpatrick concluded that "despite careful screening, psychotic side effects may occur and occur at rates higher than previously reported."

Alexander Lucas and Morris Weiss (1971) described the reaction of a six-year-old girl whose dose of Ritalin was raised to 15 mg per day over nine days. She developed "grossly bizarre behavior" with glassy-eyed withdrawal, babbling, grimacing, and body distortions. She recovered a few days after termination of the medication. In another case, a 10-year-old boy received four doses of Ritalin 10 mg spaced over five days. He was described as talkative, wild-looking, arching his arms and legs, and physically abusive. He reported headache, ringing in his ears, abdominal pain, hallucinations, and feelings of great power. He then became depressed. After stopping the drug, he was almost fully recovered in two days.

Because Ritalin and other stimulants are promoted as relatively free of adverse effects, the development of a severe mental disturbance can be mistaken for the surfacing of further "mental illness." Drug-induced psychoses often involve seeing and feeling small creatures, especially bugs. Yet even these classic cases are sometimes improperly diagnosed as due to the child's psychiatric condition.

In the first of two cases reported by J. Gerald Young (1981), the physicians initially missed the cause of the child's psychosis and restarted him on the Ritalin:

At that time he complained about mosquitoes, spiders, and other bugs, which he thought were getting into his ears, eyes, and nose. He said he could hear the bugs. His methylphenidate dose during this period ranged from 20 to 30 mg/day. He reported that "At camp I saw them—gnats, flies, and mosquitoes—they were really true! At the beginning of school, they were really there."

When his Ritalin was stopped, the "bug problem" ceased. His doctors tried him on Ritalin again, and once again the toxic psychosis returned until his medication was once again terminated.

In the second case, the initial signs of the drug intoxication were also missed:

When the dose reached 7.5 mg/day, the child began to complain that he saw horseflies and became very passive. His parents thought that his complaint was related to a tingling or itching that also preoccupied him. As the dosage was further increased to 20 mg/day, he became fearful, his agitation increased, and he clung to his mother. He no longer wanted to go outside the house and continued to talk about horseflies.

When the medication was stopped, his hallucinations and fearful behavior disappeared.

A similar case was reported in 1997 by McGinnis in the *Wall Street Journal*:

One day in April 1994, after he'd been taking 60 milligrams of Ritalin per day for about seven months, Tim ran to his mother as she talked on the phone, jumped on her and screamed. "The bugs are going to get me!" Hundreds of bugs were falling on him from the ceiling, he told her.

Tim's mother had to find a new pediatrician who would reduce her son's dosage, putting an end to a series of drug-induced episodes of psychosis.

Young (1981) reminded us that clinicians in general were slow to realize that amphetamines can cause toxic psychoses. Two decades later, they are still too slow.

In the official label for Ritalin, the manufacturer, Novartis, states that Ritalin is a "mild" stimulant. The myth that Ritalin is a relatively "mild" stimulant is contradicted by the fact that it may have a greater tendency than other stimulants, including cocaine and amphetamine, to exacerbate or cause schizophrenic-like symptoms.[20] Wouter Koek and Francis Colpaert (1993) observe that Ritalin "induces a psychopathology that seems to mimic schizophrenic psychosis more closely than that induced by amphetamines and cocaine."

In adults, doses commonly used in children can produce severe mental aberrations. According to a team headed by C. Thomas Gualtieri (1981), at doses of 0.6 mg/kg, "toxicity, such as hallucinations and severe insomnia, occurred quite frequently." They did not get the same disastrous results with children in this dose range, but children would be less able to recognize or describe mental symptoms.

A Schizophrenogenic Drug?

All of the stimulants, including Cylert, can cause psychoses that mimic schizophrenia with paranoia, hallucinations, and delusions. Stimulant-induced psychosis has frequently been investigated as a model for schizophrenic and manic psychoses.[21] These drug-induced psychoses at times look so much like schizophrenia that a strong argument has been made that stimulant abuse sometimes causes "chronic schizophrenia."[22] These schizophrenic-like and manic-like reactions to stimulants can lead to violence as well as to depression and suicide.

Extreme psychotic reactions to stimulants have been known for decades through the experience of drug abusers who use large doses of stimulants. A recent study of amphetamine addicts,[23] for example, found that at the start of their drug abuse they experienced depression (79%), anxiety (76%), paranoia (52%), hallucinations (46%), and violent behavior (44%). Mania was also common.

Adverse reactions during drug abuse are, of course, likely to be more frequent and severe than adverse reactions during treatment with smaller doses in clinical practice. However, these more extreme reactions can tell us what to look for, usually with reduced frequency and severity, in patients for whom the drug is prescribed. Many stimulant-treated children end up with a mistaken diagnosis of psychosis or schizophrenia when they are really suffering from an adverse drug reaction.

"Why Does My Child Get Worse Later in the Day?"
Rebound and Withdrawal from Ritalin

If a stimulant drug is abruptly stopped, withdrawal symptoms frequently set in, potentially causing a severe worsening of behavior. Withdrawal is called rebound if the reaction is worse than the child's original or "baseline" behavior. Some children can become psychotic on withdrawal from Ritalin and other stimulants. Other children will "crash," becoming depressed and even suicidal. There is a wide variety of withdrawal reactions across the spectrum from excitement to exhaustion and hypersomnia (excessive sleeping). On the other hand, many children seem to withdraw relatively easily from stimulants, sometimes with little more than a few days of increased irritability or tiredness. Some parents commonly take their children off the drugs on weekends. No one can explain this marked variation in the severity of withdrawal reactions, but parents and doctors should be especially cautious when removing children from long-term exposure to large doses.

A parent, teacher, or doctor is likely to mistake symptoms of drug withdrawal for a worsening of the child's "ADHD." Increased doses of Ritalin,

Adderall, or Concerta are prescribed by unwitting physicians when the child really needs to be more gradually withdrawn from it. A vicious circle is generated, with withdrawal-induced inattention, hyperactivity or impulsivity causing the doctor to prescribe more medication, all the while blaming the problem on a defect within the child.

Withdrawal results from the brain's resistance to the effects of a medication. Alcohol is a familiar example. People who drink 2–4 oz. of alcohol to suppress the brain to induce sleep at midnight are likely to awaken at 4 AM as the alcohol effect wears off. The brain, struggling to remain awake and alert despite the alcohol, now becomes hyper-awake in the absence of the alcohol. Many sleeping medications, such as Halcion, also produce this kind of rebound. The drug suppresses the brain, the brain reacts, and the insomnia worsens.

With relatively short-acting stimulants, such as Ritalin, Dexedrine, and Adderall, rebound can occur a few hours after taking the drug, making the child more inattentive or hyperactive than before taking the medication. Citing the literature, Lawrence Scahill and Kimberly Lynch (1994) from the Yale Child Study Center provide a summary of stimulant rebound effects:

> Some children being treated with stimulant medications demonstrate a behavioral rebound 5–10 hours after the last stimulant dose. This rebound may be characterized by excitability, insomnia, hyperactivity, and garrulousness. Evidence from double-blind studies suggests that this rebound effect is not simply a return to baseline behavior. Indeed, some children may exhibit higher levels of activity and impulsivity compared with baseline.

Notice that the rebound occurred as long as 10 hours after the last dose of Ritalin. Because Ritalin typically has a half-life and an estimated duration of action of no more than a few hours, doctors will tell parents that the drug cannot adversely affect the child many hours or days later. In fact, rebound symptoms can persist for *days* after a drug has left the body. When the drug use has been prolonged, rebound symptoms may persist for months as the brain continues to recover in the absence of the drug. Alcohol and cigarettes are well-known examples. Although they have short half-lives, the brain can continue to rebound for weeks or months, causing abstinence symptoms, such as agitation and craving.

Rebound frequently occurs in normal children and can be severe after only one dose of stimulant! It often occurs within a few hours after taking the drug. A controlled, double-blind study from NIMH gave normal children age 6 to 12 one typical therapeutic dose of amphetamine.[24] The degree of rebound from one dose was startling:

A marked behavioral rebound was observed by parents and teachers starting approximately 5 hours after medication had been given; this consisted of excitability, talkativeness, and, for three children, apparent euphoria. This behavioral overactivity was reported (by diary) for ten of the 14 subjects following amphetamine administration and for none of the group following placebo.

This is an extraordinary finding: Most of the children had severe rebound, reaching proportions that could be diagnosed as bordering on mania (hypomania). *Science*, the journal in which this report was published, is one of the world's most widely read and respected journals. A single warning would have reverberated around the globe. Judith Rapoport, a career advocate of drugs for children, was the senior author. She issued no warning. As far as I know, neither did any of her four co-authors from NIMH and NIH. Nor did any of the numerous professionals in the ADHD/Ritalin community who must have read this study.

There are several reasons why withdrawal from Ritalin and other stimulants has been minimized.[25] Stimulants do not produce the dramatic physical withdrawal reactions that are seen with morphine, alcohol, or minor tranquilizers such as Xanax or Valium. Instead, they produce psychological symptoms, such as excitement and hyperactivity or despair and depression. While these reactions are based on physical changes in the brain due to drug withdrawal, they are more easily overlooked than obviously physical symptoms, such as vomiting, sweating, or seizures.

Cognitive Toxicity: Can Ritalin Worsen My Child's Thinking and Learning?

The literature on stimulants and learning was extensive by the mid-1970s and was already largely negative in regard to real-life classroom learning. Rie and his team (1976a) made clear that Ritalin *interferes* with learning: "The reactions of the children strongly suggest a reduction in the commitment of the sort that would seem to be critical for learning." While suppressing "disapproved behaviors" that can interfere with learning, the researchers conclude, the drug also suppresses "desirable behaviors that facilitate it."

In their double-blind study, the authors documented the suppression of behavior. Even when the children's behavior was rated as improved, they found no improvement in scholastic achievement. In fact, they found that teachers confused behavioral changes with academic ones, and mistakenly imagined improvements in learning. Rie and his colleagues recommend against giving the medication to children with learning problems.

Among ADHD/Ritalin advocates, James Swanson is a leader. Yet, after reviewing the literature, Swanson and his colleagues (1992) warned that "cognitive toxicity may occur at commonly prescribed clinical doses of stimulant medication." They warn about "zombie-like" behavior. In a paragraph laced with citations to the literature, they make the following points about Ritalin's adverse effects on mental and social functioning:

> In some disruptive children, drug-induced compliant behavior may be accompanied by isolated, withdrawn, and overfocused behavior. Some medicated children may seem "zombie-like" and high doses which make ADHD children more "somber," "quiet," and "still" may produce social isolation by increasing "time spent alone" and decreasing "time spent in positive interaction" on the playground.

They attribute many of these problems to "overfocusing of attention which may impair rather than improve learning if taken to an extreme." They seem to be saying that a little "overfocusing" is good but that a lot is bad. A more realistic appraisal suggests that this is a continuum of toxicity. The initial stage of brain malfunction makes a child focus persistently on boring tasks while more obvious brain malfunction makes the child's obsessive, robotic behavior more embarrassingly apparent to adult observers.

Swanson indicates that the problem of "cognitive toxicity" from Ritalin is not rare. It is common! Bolstered with additional research citations, the review concludes that using parent and teacher reports as a basis for determining the stimulant dose can "produce cognitive toxicity in as many as 40% or more of the typically treated cases."

Swanson is not alone in finding that stimulants can impair learning. While less concerned than Swanson, Whalen and Henker (1997) observe, "Especially worrisome has been the suggestion that the unsalutary effects occur in the realm of complex, higher-order cognitive functions such as flexible problem-solving and divergent thinking."

Our children are subjected to a tragic reality. There is no evidence that Ritalin or any other stimulant enhances real-life learning and academic performance, while there is convincing evidence that it can impede them. Yet escalating numbers of children are being prescribed the drug to improve their performance in school.

Can Ritalin Make My Child More Withdrawn?

Chapter 4 will take a more detailed look at how Ritalin and amphetamines compromises and blunts mental capacity, including curiosity, "novelty-seeking," and socializing in both animals and humans. It will be shown that these drugs often cause social withdrawal.

Jacobovitz and her colleagues (1990) reviewed the effects of Ritalin on social relationships with other children: "Studies of the immediate effects of stimulant medication [on peer relations] show few significant positive effects and a high incidence of negative effects." They pointed to a study indicating no improvement in behavior with peers as measured by direct observation and peer evaluations. Citing additional research,[26] they suggest, "This could be because methylphenidate leads to decreased social interactions and adversely affects mood, with medicated children rated as less happy and pleased with themselves and more dysphoric."

This is a searing indictment of Ritalin's effect on children and adolescents. There are no improvements in peer relations and there are negative effects associated with feeling less happy and self-satisfied, a worsened mood, and painful emotional feelings. Jacobovitz warns, "At present, no studies have examined the effects of drug treatment during the school years on children's formation of friendships during adolescence. There is a critical need for additional research here." Once again, the most basic questions about the drug's effects remain unanswered—even unexplored.

If My Child Is Developmentally Disabled or Delayed...

Researchers have found a greater rate of adverse effects from stimulant medication, especially social withdrawal, in developmentally disabled or delayed children with relatively low IQ.[27] Benjamin Handen and a group from Pittsburgh report on adverse Ritalin effects in a population of 27 children diagnosed with ADHD and developmental disability. Despite the greater difficulty these children would have in communicating about drug-induced impairments, the authors found an increased rate of adverse effects. Medication had to be discontinued because of motor tics in three children and "severe social withdrawal" in two.

Effects on Growth Hormone and Growth

There is now a mountain of evidence that stimulants disrupt growth hormone production on a daily basis and that they also can reduce the child's overall growth, including height and weight. Nonetheless, many ADHD/Ritalin advocates continue to make light of this danger, usually by emphasizing the hope that growth may rebound if and when the drug is stopped.

Many parents and health professionals assume that stimulant-induced growth suppression is the result of the obvious suppression of appetite that takes place in many children and adults who take stimulants; but there is yet another more insidious and potentially dangerous cause. Dozens of studies have demonstrated that Ritalin disrupts the normal cycle of growth hormone production in the body. This indicates that all of the organs of the body, including the brain, are affected by the growth inhibition.

By the mid 1970s, the effect of Ritalin and other stimulants in disrupting growth hormone levels in most subjects was already "unequivocal."[28] The adverse effect on growth hormone is so regular and predictable that it can be used as a measure of whether or not the Ritalin is active in the child's body.[29]

It is much easier to assay blood samples for changes in hormone concentrations than to evaluate long-range changes in height and weight in children who are growing at varying rates. As early as 1977, a Norwegian team led by D. Aarskog demonstrated abnormal growth hormone responses to clinical doses of Dexedrine and Ritalin. They attributed it to stimulant-induced disruption of dopaminergic neurotransmission to the pituitary, and gave a largely unheeded warning:

> The findings indicate an acute and probable long-term effect of dextroamphetamine and methylphenidate on the homeostasis of growth hormone. The possible long-term adverse effects of these drugs on the growth of children indicates the need for caution in the widespread use of these agents.

Citing scientific references, Deborah Jacobovitz and her colleagues (1990) did show some concern:

> Research reveals that methylphenidate stimulates daytime release of growth hormone, disrupting the usual nocturnal release. This is troublesome since disturbances in the normal release of growth hormone may not only influence height velocity but may also impact on other critical aspects of physical development such as sexual maturation.

Jacobovitz and her team warn that the effects on sexual growth might be an important consideration when giving the medication to adolescents. For some reason, Jacobovitz does not mention that brain development will also be affected by the disruption of the growth hormone cycle.

Although stimulant growth suppression is a well-known phenomenon, extreme drug advocates have tried to reassure professionals that it's not really a problem. A team lead by Spencer and Biederman (1996) tried to prove that ADHD, rather than Ritalin, causes growth suppression. However, the study only measured each child's height and weight one time during the entire study. It then used flawed statistical analyses to try to make something out of this relatively useless data. By contrast, studies showing growth suppression have used multiple measures of height and weight over time. They have also studied compensatory rebound when the child is removed from the drugs.

In their 1991 textbook, psychiatrists Stuart Yudofsky and Robert Hales, and co-author Tom Ferguson, suggest that the growth lag induced by Ritalin is temporary "in most cases." But they acknowledge that some doctors are much more worried about the hazard. They observe, "However, the effects on growth that the long-term use of stimulants has on children lead some physicians to believe that this drug should never be prescribed for children."

What Happens to the Growing Brain?

Animal research has confirmed the obvious danger—that Ritalin-induced suppression of growth can be measured in a variety of organs in the body, including the brain. One research team showed that "neonatal rats treated with MPH [Ritalin] show a reduction in femur length and a reduction in thyroid, pituitary, testes, adrenal gland, and brain weights immediately following drug cessation." [30]

When a child's overall growth is impaired, we need to be concerned about the growth of the brain and mind as well. Since the growth suppression results from a generalized impairment in growth hormone production, all organs of the body are likely to be affected. Not only height and weight, but head size—and brain size—are being reduced. This is an obvious point I have *never* seen mentioned in my review of hundreds of articles and books by Ritalin advocates.

Will My Child Recover from Growth Inhibition?

Growth rebound after stopping stimulants is taken as a positive sign by ADHD/Ritalin advocates.[31] However, rebound does not necessarily mean that the child has fully recovered from the suppression and delay of growth. Rebound, if anything, is a powerful sign that the body has been harmed and is trying to recuperate. In one study,[32] Ritalin reduced the expected monthly weight gain by 25%. When Ritalin was stopped, the rebound produced weight gain that was 68% more per month than expected. This indicates drastic abnormalities in growth rate during and after the drug exposure. Height rebound was also significant but less dramatic. It is very misleading to suggest to parents that it is somehow harmless, or even normal, to go through a drastic growth reduction followed by a drastic growth escalation; both processes are abnormal.

Recapturing lost growth will depend on how long the children remain on the drug and then how long they are off the drug. It will also depend on age. Increasing numbers of children are being continued on the medication into young adulthood and even later. Under such circumstances, there will be no significant rebound.

Parents and doctors sometimes defend the use of Ritalin by saying, "He's still bigger than his siblings." The child's size relative to other children is not a good measure of what the drug has done to his growth. The drug may have made him considerably smaller than he was genetically programmed to be. Larger children may suffer a proportionally greater loss of height and weight.[33] Their initially larger size can mislead doctors and parents into underestimating the amount of drug-induced growth suppression.

In summary, growth studies indicate that stimulant drugs profoundly interfere with normal growth processes, producing suppression on the one hand and then abnormal rebound on the other. Many organs of the body, including the brain, are probably affected.

Disruption of Prolactin Secretion

It is known that Ritalin and amphetamines not only disrupt growth hormone, they also suppress the production of prolactin in children and in adults of both sexes.[34] As in growth hormone, the dysfunction is produced by over-stimulation of the dopamine nerves to the pituitary gland. The effect of Ritalin on prolactin, like the effect on growth hormone, is regular and predictable.[35] Almost no effort has been made by drug advocates to study the impact of disrupting prolactin on the sexual development of children of either sex.

Prolactin is best known as the hormone that initiates lactation but it also affects a variety of other functions, including menstruation and pregnancy.[36] Prolactin receptors have been identified in many tissues of the body including, of course, the breast, as well as the hypothalamus, liver, testes, ovaries, and prostate. The functions of prolactin in these various organs are poorly understood. More seems to be known about excessive prolactin production than about reduced production such as occurs during stimulant treatment. Almost no concern has been shown by ADHD/Ritalin advocates about causing suppression of this hormonal system in children and adolescents and little research has been conducted.

Graver Consequences with Younger Children

With the increasing tendency to give Ritalin to younger children, including preschoolers, it is important to remember that they are even more vulnerable to harmful drug effects. This is one reason not to allow children to use alcohol and other "recreational" drugs. Furthermore, while younger children are more adversely affected, they are less able to understand or to communicate what is happening to them.

A controlled study of twenty-eight three-to-four year olds at the Montreal Children's Hospital led by Michael Schleifer (1975) described the potentially devastating emotional effects of Ritalin on small children. Observations were made in nursery school and at home by professionals, including teachers and psychiatrists, who were blind concerning drug and placebo conditions:

> Clinical observations indicated that methylphenidate very often had a negative effect on the child's mood and also on his relationships with peers, causing less social behavior and interaction. These almost always appeared and were reported as unwanted side effects of the drug, including sadness, irritability, excessive hugging and clinging, and increased solitary play, as well as the more usual side effects of poor appetite and difficulty getting to sleep....

These adverse reactions to Ritalin were so severe that the psychiatrists and the parents discontinued treatment in all but three of the twenty-eight children. The results are consistent with the findings of the more recent 1998 study by Firestone described earlier in the chapter.

Dulcan and Popper (1991) confirm that "In preschool children, stimulant efficacy is more variable, and the rate of side effects is higher, especially sadness, irritability, clinging, insomnia, and anorexia."

Despite findings like these, many doctors continue to prescribe stimulants for increasingly younger children. These physicians seem oblivious to the threat to the child's physical brain, as well as to the child's psychological and social development, during these formative years.

As described in chapter 1, NIMH is planning to subject very young children to clinical trials with stimulant drugs, and this will surely increase the willingness of doctors in clinical practice to do the same.

Other Issues of Concern

Although the Ritalin label is used as a main source of many of the following observations, keep in mind that they also apply to amphetamines such as Dexedrin and Adderall.

More about Contraindications and Cautions

We have already seen that Ritalin is contraindicated—not to be given under any circumstances—to children suffering from "marked anxiety, tension, and agitation," because it may worsen these symptoms. It is also contraindicated in children who have tics or Tourette's, or who develop them during treatment. It is also contraindicated in children with a family history of these disorders.

According to the official label, Ritalin is also contraindicated in individuals with glaucoma.

Ritalin is contraindicated with certain other drugs, including stimulants and MAOI antidepressants (see below).

Problems with Hypertension

As the drug label confirms, caution should be used when prescribing Ritalin to hypertensive patients. Special concern should be shown in regard to giving Ritalin to African-American children who may eventually be at higher risk for hypertensive disorders, including life-threatening kidney failure. Ronald Brown and Sandra Sexson (1988) conducted a placebo-controlled study of 11 black male adolescent boys taking 6 weeks of Ritalin at doses of 0.15 mg, 0.30 mg, and 0.5 mg/kg. They showed a significant rise from a placebo mean of 69 diastolic blood pressure to a drug mean of 83 at the higher doses. The authors expressed concern about the long-term effects and recommended closer monitoring of adolescent boys.

The dangers of even a slight, chronic increase in blood pressure have recently been underscored by a National Institute of Aging press report. It indicated that elderly patients with hypertension suffer increased rates of brain atrophy with loss of cognitive function, such as memory.[37] Stimulants pose special problems for anyone with cardiovascular disease. They are also especially dangerous to patients suffering from hyperthyroidism, narrow-angle glaucoma, and kidney disease (nephritis and renal failure).

While this book is about children, it is worth noting that the older persons are also at higher risk from Ritalin adverse reactions.

If My Child Starts to Have Trouble Seeing

As the label for Ritalin recognizes, the drug can cause "visual disturbances" with difficulties focusing and blurred vision. The label states that it is "rare."

Can Stimulants Cause Seizures?

The label for Ritalin warns that epileptic seizures can be caused by the drug, usually but not always in patients who have a history of prior seizures or abnormal brain waves. The drug should be stopped if seizures occur.

Why Not Give Stimulants for Fatigue?

The official Ritalin label warns that it should not be used for "the prevention or treatment of normal fatigue states." Much like huge doses of caffeine, Ritalin and other stimulants can mask fatigue. This can cover up underlying problems in children that are causing tiredness, including physical illness, emotional stress, and insomnia. It can also lead to impaired functioning when the fatigue is masked. This can make a child accident prone and turn an adolescent into a menace when driving an automobile.

Nonetheless, many adults do find that an occasional stimulant, from coffee to amphetamine, can help them temporarily overcome fatigue. Since their inception, stimulants have been used by armed forces to overcome fatigue. They were even used by aircraft pilots on an "occasional" basis during Desert Storm in Iraq.[38] The single doses of 5 mg were relatively small, especially for adults. The occasional use of small doses of amphetamine to overcome fatigue during brief combat missions does not seem like a good recommendation for its routine, daily use—often in much larger doses—for children in classrooms and homes.

What If My Child Is Diabetic?

Stimulants can alter the response to insulin and should be avoided in diabetic patients. If they are prescribed, careful monitoring of blood and urine sugar levels is required.

What about Taking Stimulants with Other Drugs?

There are sufficient problems combining stimulants with other medications, even over-the-counter preparations, to require concern whenever a drug is added to the regimen of a child taking stimulants. Ritalin can inhibit the breakdown in the body of several classes of medications, including anticonvulsants (e.g., phenobarbital, diphenylhydantoin, primidone), anticoagulants or blood thinners (e.g., Coumadin), the anti-inflammatory agent phenylbutazone, and drugs used to treat depression, including the tricyclics (e.g., imipramine, clomipramine, desipramine). The effect of these drugs can be increased to dangerous levels by combining them with Ritalin. For example, in a child who is taking phenytoin (Dilantin) for seizures, Ritalin increases the blood level of the anticonvulsant, potentially causing toxicity. Similarly, the combination of Ritalin and imipramine (Tofranil) can raise the blood levels of the latter several-fold, resulting in increased rates of side effects.[39] There have been reports of severe mental deterioration when Ritalin is combined with imipramine.[40]

Combination with the antihypertensive agent, guanethidine, should be avoided, since Ritalin can decrease the antihypertensive effect.[41]

Ritalin may increase adverse reactions when combined with other drugs that have stimulant effects, such as those used to treat asthma and colds. These include theophylline, ephedrine, and various nasal drying agents. Ritalin and caffeine together can also increase their mutual stimulating effects, and should be avoided.

Ritalin should not be combined with the monoamine oxidase inhibitors (MAOI's) used to treat depression, such as isocarboxazid (Marplan), tranylcypromine (Parnate), and phenelzine (Nardil). The combination can result in life-threatening hypertensive crises.

Once again, all of the stimulants pose similar dangers when combined with other drugs.

I have seen cases in which the combination of stimulants with selective serotonin reuptake inhibitors (SSRI's), such as Prozac, Zoloft, and Paxil, has worsened agitation.

The official labels for the amphetamines, such as Dexedrine and Adderall, offer even more elaborate descriptions of potential adverse drug reactions. The labels can be found in the *Physicians' Drug Reference* which is updated annually.

Are Stimulants Safe During Pregnancy?

Exposure to amphetamines can harm the fetus of a mother who abuses the drugs.[42] Children of mothers who abused Ritalin during pregnancy have a variety of developmental disabilities when tested through ages 14–15. These disabilities include diminished overall academic achievement as well as specific delays in language and mathematics. The difficulties develop regardless of whether or not the children are raised by their biological mother. The prenatal effects of cocaine and methamphetamine can cause lasting effects on the brain and behavior.[43] Ironically, exposure to stimulants in utero can result in developmental problems similar to "ADHD."[44]

If the fetus can be harmed by exposure to large doses of stimulants, then it's logical that the growing child may also be at risk. Pregnant women should not take Ritalin. Women who are breast feeding should not take Ritalin.

Stimulants and Alcohol

Stimulants and alcohol are frequently abused together. Sometimes they are used as an upper-downer combination by taking alcohol or other sedatives in the evening to sleep and stimulants in the morning to wake up. But the two drugs in combination can also produce an enhanced global intoxication that some drug abusers seek.[45] It is not uncommon to find adolescents abusing both drugs in combination or at different times. It has been known for some time that in large doses the combination can cause extreme, dangerous agitation.[46]

Children Like to Chew

There have been a few reports in the literature of children being made toxic by chewing Ritalin.[47] Chewing tablets exposes the child to a rapidly absorbed dose through the mucosa of the mouth. Chewing a Ritalin-SR (slow release) tablet exposes the child to a larger dose at once than anticipated and could cause severe adverse reactions.[48] This may become an increasing problem with the development of other long-acting forms of methylphenidate, such as Metadate ER and Concerta. I have not seen any reports of chewing Ritalin as a form of abuse. However, considering all the other ways by which Ritalin is abused, including nasally and intravenously, some teenagers may be tempted to experiment with chewing it. Stimulant abuse will be further discussed in chapter 5.

Cylert (Pemoline): Less Effective and Potentially Life-Threatening

Cylert (pemoline) is thought to produce most of the stimulant effects typical of Ritalin or Dexedrine but less frequently. Cylert is considered a weaker stimulant and a less effective drug. In studies performed for FDA approval, it consistently had less effect on behavior than amphetamine or Ritalin.[49] Advocates for the drug emphasize that it has less addictive potential than Ritalin or amphetamine. As a schedule IV drug, it also has fewer regulations governing its prescription. It requires only one daily dose.

Cylert frequently produces abnormal liver function tests with more than a dozen reported deaths from liver failure since the drug was marketed in 1975. The actual number is probably higher than reported. Adverse reactions in general are rarely reported and there may be a misleading time-delay between the drug administration and later liver toxicity.

The risk of death from liver failure led the FDA to force Abbott Laboratories (1996) to put a boxed warning in the drug's label and to send a "Dear Doctor" letter to all physicians with the following warning: "Because of its association with life threatening hepatic [liver] failure, CYLERT should not ordinarily be considered as a first line drug therapy for ADHD." I was a medical expert in a Cylert liver death case that was settled. It was, of course, a devastating tragedy for the family of the young child.

Information from FDA's Spontaneous Reporting System indicates that 1,284 adverse reaction reports for Cylert have been submitted as of March 10, 1997. In addition to liver problems, the summary of the Cylert adverse reaction report discloses a very high number of abnormal movements and adverse mental effects.

The abnormal movement reports included twitches (55 separate reports), dyskinesia [abnormal movements] (50), dystonia [muscle spasms, sometimes very painful and disabling] (18), choreoathetosis [various abnormal motions that can be disabling] (14), ataxia (12), movement disorder (10), oculogyric crises [a very severe and disabling spasm of the eye muscles] (8), and a variety of others. Hyperkinesis [excessive motor activity] was reported 51 times. Except for one report of tardive dyskinesia, a persistent or irreversible drug-induced dyskinesia, there's no indication if any of these movement disorders proved permanent after the drug was stopped.

Reports of mental malfunction in association with Cylert included the following: insomnia (80), agitation (39), hallucinations (37), nervousness (34), hostility (29), aggravated reaction (25), personality disorder (24), psychosis (22), emotional lability [unstable emotions] (15), confusion (13), abnormal thinking (12), central nervous system stimulation (11), paranoid reaction (11), depression (11), anxiety (8), and many other categories.

There was also a relatively large number of reported grand mal convulsions [epileptic seizures with unconsciousness] (20). Hair loss [alopecia] was reported 19 times.

Cylert is often said not to produce withdrawal problems but a withdrawal syndrome was reported 11 times.

What Do Doctors Tell Their Patients?

What is the profession's perception of the dangers of these drugs? Recently I picked up a brochure from a learning disabilities center in the Washington, DC area. After defining ADHD as a "neurologically-based learning problem," it recommended drugs. "Medications," the brochure announces to parents, "are a safe way to help many children overcome their learning problems." As this book will document, ADHD is not neurologically-based; Ritalin is not "safe;" and stimulants do not help children learn better.

Why Do So Many Adverse Effects
Show Up After the Drug Is Marketed?

Pharmaceutical companies must present evidence that a new drug is safe and effective before the FDA approves the product, but safety and efficacy are relative. To its credit, the FDA has increasingly emphasized that its stamp of approval does not mean that a drug is completely or ultimately safe. [50] At a meeting sponsored by the FDA that I attended in 1995, the agency handed out black and white posters with the following warning emblazoned on it:

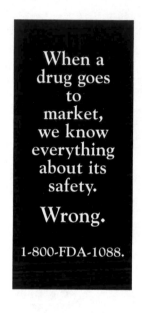

When a
drug goes
to
market,
we know
everything
about its
safety.

Wrong.

1-800-FDA-1088.

The FDA confirms that controlled studies used for FDA approval are too short in duration, too small in patient numbers, and too limited in the range of patients and clinical conditions to rule out all potentially serious adverse reactions before a drug is put on the market.[51]

Major new side effects show up months or years after a drug's initial approval, occasionally leading the FDA to withdraw the product from the market. A Government Accounting Office report (1990) disclosed that 50% of drugs approved between 1976 and 1985 were later found to have "serious" undetected adverse effects. Of fifteen psychiatric drugs approved during that period, nine turned out to have serious, previously undetected toxic effects. One of the drugs, nomifensine, was withdrawn after more than eight years of worldwide use. In addition, drugs approved for other purposes but used in psychiatric practice, including valproic acid and bromocriptine, were also found to have previously undetected serious adverse effects.

Recently the public was made aware that Seldane, a widely used antihistamine, was being withdrawn after 12 years of use due to fatal cardiac arrhythmias.[52] Another even more widely used drug, the Novartis laxative called Ex-Lax, was recently withdrawn from the market. The FDA concluded that its principal ingredient, phenolphthalein, is a potential cancer risk.[53] Phenolphthalein had been in use in varying preparations for almost *one hundred years*!

In September 1997 fenfluramine (Pondimin) and its newer relative dexfenfluramine (Redux) were withdrawn from the market because of drug-induced abnormalities of heart valves. Fenfluramine was widely used in combination with phentermine as "fen-phen" in weight reduction programs and centers throughout the country. These drugs are cousins of Ritalin and amphetamine.

The reader may be wondering, "How can one class of drugs, the stimulants, cause so many different adverse effects and pose so many threats to the health of the child?" The answer lies in the impact that stimulants have upon the structure and function of the brain. The next chapter examines the effect of Ritalin, Dexedrine, Adderall and other stimulants on brain anatomy, blood flow, energy utilization, and biochemistry. We shall find that, far from correcting biochemical imbalances, the stimulants cause them.

Chapter 3

Gross Brain Malfunctions and Cell Death Caused by Stimulants

Animal studies indicate that amphetamines can cause constriction of brain vessels, increase the likelihood of convulsive seizures, and influence carbohydrate metabolism in an unknown way. They also alter the output of growth hormone, and affect the sensitive biochemical balance in the brain and central nervous system. It may well be that stimulant drugs produce greater harm in the long run than the hyperactive symptoms they are meant to control....

—Sidney Walker, III, Psychology Today (1974)

In monkeys the toxic effects of chronic amphetamine use include damage to cerebral blood vessels, neuronal loss, and microhemorrhages.

—Jerome Jaffe, Comprehensive Textbook of Psychiatry (1995)

As chapter 2 documented, stimulant drugs can cause a broad array of adverse drug reactions from growth inhibition to psychosis. They can worsen ADHD-like symptoms or produce robot-like inhibition of children. But there is a yet more ominous threat to taking stimulants—their impact on the fabric of the brain itself, including brain structure, biochemistry, blood flow, and energy utilization. There is strong evidence that stimulants deform and destroy brain cells.

While it is disturbing enough to know that children can *sometimes* be made zombie-like and even psychotic by Ritalin and other stimulants, it is even more disturbing to realize that children *always* suffer from persistant brain malfunction when taking these drugs.

Much of the material in the following sections has been added to this edition of the book. The research was initially reviewed for a series of peer-reviewed professional articles that I wrote as a result of my scientific presentation to the National Institutes of Health Consensus Development Conference on the Diagnosis and Treatment of Attention Deficit Hyperactivity Disorder.[1]

This chapter first describes the biochemical effects of the stimulants, and then proceeds to examine the accumulating evidence for acute and persistent brain damage and dysfunction caused by these drugs. Parents, teachers, health professionals, and other caregivers will be provided a scientific basis for refusing to subject children to Ritalin, Concerta, Adderall, or any other stimulant drugs.

Biochemical Abnormalities Caused by Stimulants

Stimulant drugs cause major changes in brain neurotransmitter systems. Neurotransmitters are the chemical messengers between brain cells or neurons. They are released by one brain cell (neuron) usually in order to cause an adjacent neuron to fire. In this way, impulses travel along the neurological "wiring" of the brain. Neurotransmitters are often described as the "messengers" between cells. Most excite brain cells but some inhibit them.

Neurons communicate across a tiny space called the synapse or synaptic cleft. Within each synaptic cleft is a soup of multiple neurotransmitters and other chemical agents that control nerve function.

The neurotransmitter released from one neuron attaches to receptors on a nearby neuron, stimulating that adjacent cell to fire. In other words, neuron "A" releases a chemical into the space between itself and neuron "B." If the neurotransmitter attaches to its receptor on neuron "B," in most cases it contributes to that nerve cell's tendency to fire.

Individual brain cells typically have 10,000 or more connections to other cells. There are several hundred billion cells, adding up to trillions of synapses. Nerve transmission and the relationship among nerve cells involve very complex processes that are, at this time, very poorly understood.

Brain cells can be named or categorized according to the neurotransmitter chemicals they synthesize and release into the synapse. The most studied neurons in regard to stimulant drugs are the following: dopaminergic (producing the neurotransmitter dopamine), noradrenergic (producing norepinephrine), and serotonergic (producing serotonin). The common stimulants—Ritalin, Dexedrine, and cocaine—cause an increased presence of these three neurotransmitters in the synapse, activating the adjacent nerves that can receive them. The nerves that the stimulants activate reach into every part of the human brain. They are likely to impinge on a vast array of neurological processes that affect thinking, feeling, and acting.

Studies show that Ritalin (and other stimulants) "bind" or attach to receptors throughout most of the forebrain.[2] The forebrain is the most highly developed and specifically human part of the central nervous system. It includes the cortex or surface of the frontal lobes where functions related to intelligence take place.

Ritalin and other stimulants also profoundly disrupt the reticular activating system in the core of the brain, causing impairments in energy level, alertness, and responsiveness to external stimulation. The person becomes more apathetic and less aware of the world around them.

Diagram 1, "Areas of the Brain Affected by Stimulants," sketches regions of the brain that are affected by stimulants. Table 4, "Functions of the Brain Impaired by Stimulants," lists some of the activities of the brain that can be adversely affected by these drugs. The diagram and table document how stimulant drugs can potentially impair widespread functions throughout the entire brain.

How Stimulants Impair Neurotransmitter Systems

Keep in mind that there are hundreds of neurotransmitters and other substances actively participating in brain function, many of which have not yet been identified. Also keep in mind that our understanding of even the most carefully studied neurotransmitters—including the three known to be energized by stimulant drugs—is relatively rudimentary. For all we know, the main impact of these drugs on the brain has not yet been discovered. Nonetheless, we know enough to make some informed observations.

The stimulants increase the activity of nerves in two known ways. First, they increase the amount of neurotransmitter released into the synapse and,

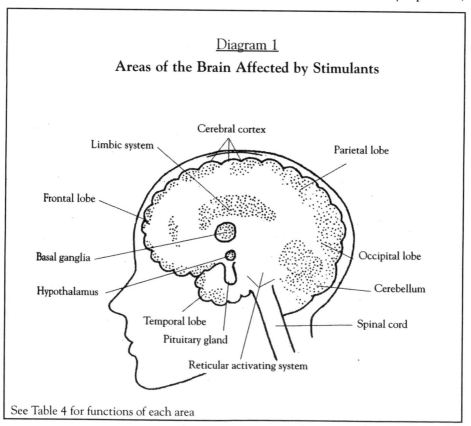

Diagram 1
Areas of the Brain Affected by Stimulants

Cerebral cortex
Limbic system
Parietal lobe
Frontal lobe
Basal ganglia
Occipital lobe
Hypothalamus
Cerebellum
Temporal lobe
Spinal cord
Pituitary gland
Reticular activating system

See Table 4 for functions of each area

Table 4

Functions of the Brain Impaired by Stimulants

Area	Where Located	Effects of Dysfunction
Cerebral Cortex	Outer surface of the brain	Dysfunction within the cerebral cortex impairs higher mental activities, including intelligence and sensory perception.
Frontal Lobes	Front of the brain	Dysfunction within the frontal lobes impairs initiative and autonomy, reason, empathy and social awareness, insight and judgment—in short, the most human functions. It can cause emotional blunting and zombie-like or robotic behavior.
Limbic System	Widespread, beneath the frontal lobes	Dysfunction within the limbic system affects regulation of emotions, and usually produces indifference and apathy or euphoria. It can cause zombie-like or robotic behavior.
Basal Ganglia	Middle of the brain	Dysfunction within the basal ganglia causes abnormal movements, and can cause emotional blunting, and zombie-like or robotic behavior.
Temporal Lobes, including Hippocampus	Lower side and undersurface of the brain	Dysfunction within the temporal lobe impairs memory and learning.
Parietal Lobe	Toward the back surface of the brain	Dysfunction within the parietal lobe impairs integration and understanding of sensory perceptions, language, and sense of self.
Cerebellum	Lower posterior of the brain	Dysfunction within the cerebellum affects regulation of muscular tone, posture, gait, and skilled coordination.
Hypothalamus	Small area of undersurface of brain above the pituitary gland	Dysfunction within the hypothalamus impairs temperature control, appetite, and hormonal function, including the pituitary gland.
Pituitary Gland	Base of the brain	Dysfunction of the pituitary gland can impair growth, thyroid, adrenal, and sexual functions, and the overall reaction to stress.
Reticular Activating System	Core of the brain	Dysfunction within the reticular activating system blunts energy, alertness, self-awareness, and responsiveness.
Spinal Cord	Begins at base of brain and extends downward through	Dysfunction within the spinal cord affects nerves that spread throughout the body; especially

Each of these functional areas of the brain is labeled in Diagram 1. This chart gives only a partial review of the various regions of the brain impaired by stimulant drugs.

second, they reduce the rate of its removal from the synapse. This is a kind of one-two punch, first increasing the amount of neurotransmitter dropped into the synapse and second making it remain longer in the space. The synapse becomes flooded with unusually large amounts of the chemicals. There are variations between the amphetamines and Ritalin in how they generate increased amounts of neurotransmitters, but the differences are of no consequence to this discussion.[3]

Dopamine Pathways in the Brain

The ability of stimulants to cause hyperactivity of dopamine neurotransmission is thought to cause some of the most serious adverse effects of stimulants on the brain and mind. Hyperactivity of dopamine neurotransmission seems to play a major role in causing drug abuse and addiction. It probably plays a primary role in the "therapeutic" effects as well—the suppression of spontaneous behavior in favor of rote performance. Dopamine nerves originate in two areas deep within the brain, the substantia nigra and the ventral tegmentum. Dopamine nerves in the substantia nigra reach into the basal ganglia which control motor activity. These clusters of cells, called ganglia, also influence mental processes. They are richly connected to the energizing core of the brain, the reticular activating system, and to the emotion-regulating centers of the brain, the limbic system. Impairments in these systems can cause robotic or zombie-like behavior. Dopamine fibers from the ventral tegmentum go directly to the highest centers of the brain that control thinking and feeling, including the frontal lobes and limbic system (nucleus accumbens and amygdala).[4] This neurotransmitter system affects portions of the brain involved with the processes most essential to being human.

Dopamine nerves also reach the hypothalamus and pituitary gland, where they control many hormonal processes, including those involved in growth and reproductive functioning. Studies have demonstrated that stimulants cause major impairments in the functioning of dopamine, and that amphetamines and methamphetamine cause permanent damage.

Norepinephrine Pathways in the Brain

Ritalin and amphetamine also energize the noradrenergic system of the brain—neurons that release norepinephrine into the synapse. This drug-induced stimulation is thought to be most closely related to over-activity of the cardiovascular system, and to some symptoms of drug withdrawal as well.

Most noradrenergic (norepinephrine-generating) nerves originate in an area of the brain called the locus coeruleus. Nerves in the locus coeruleus send their fibers into the higher brain, including the cerebral cortex, as well as into the reticular activating system.[5] These nerves have widespread pathways throughout the brain. The reader may wish to review the brain function table. Most functions are affected by this neurotransmitter. Once again, it becomes apparent that the hyperactivity produced in the nervous system by stimulants will have widespread but poorly understood effects.

Serotonin Pathways in the Brain

Ritalin and amphetamine also induce hyperactivity of the serotonin neurotransmitter system. Some researchers believe that this may contribute to the production of more extreme mental aberrations, including psychosis with hallucinations and delusions.[6] In *Talking Back to Prozac*, I have described the effects of the serotonergic neurotransmitter system on all higher human activities, as well as its effects on a variety of basic physiological functions. These widespread connections affect every part of the brain and every brain function described in Diagram 1 and Table 4.

The serotonin system seems especially vulnerable to drug-induced damage. Stimulants and other drugs that affect this neurotransmitter often cause permanent harm, including cell loss.

It is important to re-emphasize that there are hundreds of substances that control brain function. Dopamine, norepinephrine, and serotonin are among the most extensively studied, but we know only the most rudimentary facts about how they work and almost nothing about their relationship to overall mental function. At present the effects of stimulant drugs on the brain and mind are literally beyond comprehension. We do, however, know enough to understand that widespread disruption of normal mental processes is the mechanism by which stimulants induce a condition interpreted as a "therapeutic effect."

Cylert (Pemoline)

Pemoline, hopefully, will be used less since it has been associated with fatal liver damage.[7] Its chemistry is different from that of Ritalin and the amphetamines. It also has a much longer half-life of twelve hours compared to Ritalin's half life, estimated at 1–3 or 2–4 hours. Pemoline can take up to three or four weeks to have its maximum effect. Ritalin and the amphetamines, on an empty stomach, can start affecting a child in less than an hour.

Little is known about pemoline's mechanisms of action in the brain, but it probably gains some of its impact by stimulating dopaminergic nerves. This is probably why it has most of the same hazards as other stimulants, although it is much less subject to abuse and addiction.

Can Stimulants Cause a Permanent Loss of Brain Tissue?

A team led by Henry A. Nasrallah (1986) from Ohio State found shrinkage of the brain in more than 50% of twenty-four young adults with hyperactivity since childhood. Shrinkage—or the more technical term, atrophy—indicates that brain tissue has become withered and reduced in volume. All of the subjects had been treated with stimulants in childhood. The authors propose that "cortical atrophy may be a long-term adverse effect of this treat-ment."[8] The cortex of the brain, as already noted, is critical to higher men-tal functions, including intelligence. This study should have raised serious concerns within the profession about stimulant drugs causing permanent brain shrinkage. Instead, medication advocates have flooded the profession-al arena with unfounded claims that ADHD is somehow the cause of any observed brain damage.

The public continues to be bombarded with media misinformation about brain scans supposedly showing abnormalities in the brains of children diag-nosed with ADHD. Indeed, several brain scan studies have claimed to demonstrate brain abnormalities associated with ADHD.[9] Most of the stud-ies have found relatively small brain abnormalities in frontal lobes and basal ganglia in children diagnosed with ADHD. (These areas are among those known to be damaged by stimulant drugs.) The differences were based on comparisons between groups of normal children and groups of children labeled ADHD. The findings were not detectable on a case-by-case basis and cannot be used for diagnostic purposes. There are no physical defects associ-ated with the ADHD diagnosis.

The differences found between normal brains and those of children diag-nosed with ADHD are almost certainly due to medication effects. For exam-ple, a typical study is entitled "Evaluation of Cerebellar Size in Attention-Deficit Hyperactivity Disorder."[10] According to its summary, it finds that children with ADHD have abnormalities in the cerebellum, a lobe at the back of the brain.

However, in the text of the report the following information is provided about the twelve children with ADHD: "Seven of the patients with ADHD had... received methylphenidate in the past. One of these seven individuals had also received dextroamphetamine and pemoline. Another had received clonidine."[11]This is actually a study of drug-treated children diagnosed with ADHD, and the failure to indicate this in the title or the abstract indicates a Brain Scan Scam. Even in their discussion, the authors fail to mention that drug exposure is a likely confounding factor and the most probable cause of any damage to the cerebellum. Yet they do mention that stimulants increase the metabolic activity in the cerebellum, so they are aware of potential drug effects.

At the recent NIH Consensus Development Conference on Attention Deficit Hyperactivity Disorder, Swanson presented a paper co-authored by Castellanos (1998). The study reviewed the whole range of brain scan reports that supposedly show a "Biological Basis of ADHD." A number of the stud-ies involved Swanson's co-author, Castellanos.[12] Some studies failed to men-tion prior drug treatment while drawing on populations, such as the NIH clinics, where the children are likely to have extensive prior drug exposure.[13]

Other studies alluded to previous drug treatment without attempting to correlate it with the brain changes.[14]

As mentioned in chapter 1, in the public discussion following Swanson's presentation, Swanson was asked if *any* of the studies in his review involved children without a prior history of drug treatment. Swanson could not name a single study based on untreated patients. He had to admit that *all* of the studies involved children who had been exposed to stimulants and other psychiatric drugs. He tried to wriggle off the hook by explaining that untreated children are difficult to obtain in the United States. His response, of course, was nonsense. So many children are diagnosed with ADHD, it would be easy to give hundreds of them brain scans before they received any psychiatric medication. Besides, as I've already emphasized, Swanson behaved unscientifically and unethically when he failed to mention that the children in the brain scan studies had been previously exposed to drugs that are toxic to the brain.

After hearing all the scientific presentations and discussions, the consensus conference panel concluded "there are no data to indicate that ADHD is due to a brain malfunction."[15] The conclusion was so threatening to the establishment that the National Institute of Mental Health edited it out of the final version after the consensus panel had already disbanded and gone home. However, the failure of brain scans to show any distinct abnormality attributable to ADHD is reconfirmed by the American Academy of Pediatrics (2000) in its official report.

As this chapter will document, stimulants have toxic effects on both gross and biochemical functions of the brain, including the frontal lobes and basal ganglia. They are known to cause lasting brain changes, including cell death. In addition, stimulants are known to disrupt growth hormone which could affect brain development.

By contrast, any association between ADHD and brain pathology remains speculative at best. No valid ADHD syndrome has been demonstrated and no neurological or other physical defects have been found in association with the "ADHD" label.

Brain structural abnormalities found in children diagnosed with ADHD and treated with stimulants—to the extent that they are valid findings—are almost certainly due to the stimulants and other psychiatric medications to which they have been exposed. These studies add to the accumulating evidence that psychostimulants cause irreversible brain damage.

Do the Researchers Know It's a Brain Scan Scam?

When I give workshops or participate in radio talk shows, parents frequently tell me that they have been informed that ADHD is a brain disease that shows up on brain scans. Often they cite CHADD as their source.

CHADD is the parent group that has many biological psychiatrists on its board and that takes money from drug companies (see chapter 14 for details).

At CHADD's annual conference in 1995, NIMH's Judith Rapoport presented pre-publication information about a new study that claimed to find brain structure differences in children diagnosed with ADHD. CHADD put out a press release that gave no hint that the brain abnormalities might be due to the drugs the children had been taking.

Castellanos, Giedd and a team of NIMH scientists published the misleading study in 1996. They found a reduced cerebral volume in children with ADHD. This is entirely consistent with the Nasrallah study showing shrinkage or atrophy caused by prior exposure to stimulants.

The scientists realized that their study was flawed. They knew it could not prove that the brain abnormalities were caused by ADHD rather than by exposure to psychiatric drugs, including stimulants. Tucked into their "Comment" sections, the NIMH scientists offered the following observation, "Because almost all (93%) subjects with ADHD had been exposed to stimulants, we cannot be certain that our results are not drug related." This, of course, is a huge admission. The authors followed it with a promise that "A replication study with stimulant-naïve boys with ADHD is under way." That, of course, piqued my interest.

I wrote to Freedom of Information at the NIH and asked them to send me all available information on the research to which Castellanos referred. In response on August 3, 2000 I received a package "about an ongoing research project conducted by F. Xavier Castellanos at the National Institute of Mental Health and involving magnetic resonance imaging and/or other physiological measures of the brains of stimulant naïve boys with ADHD." The information described a study entitled "Neurobiological Correlates of Stimulant Drug Treatment in Hyperactive Children."

Unfortunately, there is nothing in the materials sent to me to indicate that Castellanos and his colleagues are in fact planning to compare the brains of stimulant-naïve and stimulant-treated children. They are not likely to do so. They do not want to conduct a study that is likely to show that the drugs are causing the brain abnormalities in children diagnosed with ADHD. Nonetheless, I continue to use Freedom of Information to pursue the elusive study.

The following sections examine some of the animal literature that confirms lasting brain dysfunction and damage following exposure to stimulant medication.

Animal Studies of Brain Damage Caused by Amphetamines (Adderall, Dexedrine)

Adderall is one of the most highly promoted stimulants on the market and is replacing Ritalin as the most commonly prescribed. Some parents who are concerned about giving Ritalin to their children are misled into accepting Adderall as a "newer" or "safer" drug. Some doctors may even believe that Adderall is "newer" or "safer," but only because they believe everything they are told by drug company sales representatives.

In reality, Adderall is a mixture of four old-fashioned variants of amphetamine. Amphetamines are, if anything, more toxic to the brain than Ritalin. For example, there is more evidence showing that amphetamines cause cell death. Dexedrine is another FDA-approved amphetamine for treating behavioral problems in children. It has been around for four decades. Adderall, as a mixture of amphetamines, is no newer or safer than Dexedrine. It's merely the beneficiary of a very expensive and successful marketing campaign.

Evidence that amphetamines are toxic to brain cells has been documented for more than thirty years and the mechanism continues to be refined.[16] Several animal studies, including some involving rhesus monkeys, have shown that relatively small doses of amphetamine over several days or weeks will produce a lasting loss of receptors for the neurotransmitter dopamine. When a neurotransmitter system is over-stimulated by amphetamine, there is a compensatory die back of the receptors for the neurotransmitter.[17] Studies have shown a persistent reduced output of dopamine after the initial stimulation by amphetamine.[18] This, too, is a compensatory mechanism to stop the over-stimulation of the dopamine system. Persistent changes have also been found in the norepinephrine neurotransmitter system after relatively small, short-term doses of amphetamine. The authors of the study concluded that amphetamine produces biochemical adaptations that far outlast the acute drug effects and may account for both transient and more persistent discontinuation effects in humans.[19]

Permanent structural changes have been found in the brains of animals treated with amphetamine twice a day for 5 days a week for a total of only 5 weeks. Thirty-eight days after stopping the amphetamines, the investigators found lasting structural deformities in brain cells, including those in the frontal lobes where the highest human functions take place.[20]

A team led by Melega (1997b) used Positron Emission Tomography (PET) in monkeys to determine if persistent brain-cell dysfunction follows the administration of two relatively small acute doses of amphetamine (2 mg/kg, four hours apart). These two doses produced persistent, marked decreases in dopamine synthesis and concentration up to three months later. One animal showed continued dysfunction when last measured, eight months later. The authors concluded that these limited amphetamine doses produced long-lasting "neurotoxicity."

In another study using larger, more chronic doses (4–18 mg/kg over 10 days), another team led by Melega (1997a) found a gradual, long-delayed recovery from neurotoxicity in the brain over a two year period after termination of treatment.

Amphetamines have been demonstrated to cause irreversible brain damage. They maim and destroy brain cells. On this basis alone, amphetamine stimulants such as Adderall and Dexedrine should not be prescribed for children.

Animal Studies of Brain Damage Caused by Methamphetamine (Gradumet, Desoxyn)

Especially if a child has not responded to other stimulants, methamphetamine is sometimes prescribed. A slight variation on the amphetamine molecule produces methamphetamine which is also FDA-approved for the treatment of ADHD. It is sold by Abbott Laboratories under the names Desoxyn and Gradumet (long-release dose form).

On the street, methamphetamine is called "speed" in pill or powder form and "ice" when smoked. Federal agencies have become increasingly concerned about the widespread abuse of this drug.[21] It is known for its addictive qualities, and its capacity to produce bizarre and dangerous behavior, including paranoia and violence.

Methamphetamine is FDA-approved for the treatment of behavioral disorders in children despite the fact that its capacity to cause neurotoxicity—including the destruction of brain cells—has long been demonstrated in animals. Animal research shows that chronic exposure to methamphetamine can produce irreversible loss of receptors for dopamine and/or the death of dopaminergic and other neurons in the brain.[22] Melega and his colleagues (1997b), for example, found persistent "neurotoxic" changes in dopamine function (dopamine depletions of 55–85%) in monkeys lasting at least three months after doses that were relatively small and brief.[23]

Larger chronic doses of methamphetamine and the related diet drug, fenfluramine, caused the death of serotonergic nerves in animals. The changes are described as "long-lasting neurotoxic effects with respect to both the functional and structural integrity of serotonergic neurons in the brain."[24] Additional studies have shown that the drug also causes permanent impairment in norepinephrine neurotransmission.[25] Thus methamphetamine causes destructive changes in all three of the neurotransmitter systems that are made hyperactive by the drug.

Autopsy studies of stimulant addicts provide evidence of damage from methamphetamine. A 1996 study from Toronto's Clarke Institute confirms that methamphetamine depletes dopamine in the brains of people who abuse the drug.[26] The researchers did not demonstrate permanent degeneration, but they believe that the deterioration they found could produce emotional disturbances. In an interview with the *Toronto Star*,[27] one of the Clarke Institute researchers, Steven Kish, made a remarkable admission. Kish said that the effects of long-term Ritalin use in ADHD children "would logically be similar" to the long-term effects of methamphetamine, since the two drugs are so similar.

On the basis of animal research and human addiction studies, methamphetamine should never be prescribed to children for any purpose. Yet it is FDA-approved as Desoxyn and Gradumet without any warnings about its toxic and even lethal effects on brain cells.

Animal Studies of Brain Damage and Dysfunction Caused by Ritalin

Many different kinds of studies indicate that Ritalin has very similar effects on the brain as amphetamine, methamphetamine, and cocaine.[28] Therefore, the studies we have reviewed showing persistent brain dysfunction from amphetamines and methamphetamine should prepare us to anticipate similar findings in regard to Ritalin. However, the Ritalin literature is much more sparse, and the trend indicates substantial acute changes and less persistent ones.

One study found that the dopamine neurotransmitter system becomes less sensitive (down-regulation) after Ritalin administration to animals.[29] Unfortunately, it did not test the animals after stopping the Ritalin to determine if any receptor recovery took place. There is evidence for dramatic and possibly irreversible changes in the adrenergic (norepinephrine) neurotransmitter system after Ritalin treatment. The density of the norepinephrine receptors is reduced after treatment with Ritalin.[30] This means the receptors have disappeared or died off. The danger of irreversibility looms large. Another study found that after seven days of Ritalin treatment in rats, the locus coeruleus, the site of origin for adrenergic nerves, becomes less responsive to further stimulation.[31] The percentage of neurons decreased and it became harder to stimulate the remaining ones. The changes persisted at the last testing, 18 hours after the drugs were stopped. The authors note that these changes could ultimately impact on cells in the cerebral cortex, the area of the brain most associated with intelligence. They were able to record "altered responses" in these neurons during Ritalin administration.

Mice and rats given very large doses of Ritalin seem to develop a tolerance to some of its effects. For example, the animals eat less for a week or more but then return to normal consumption levels. This may reflect the development of down-regulation.[32]

Other Ritalin studies have demonstrated the short-term disruptive impact on the animal brain, but have not tested for a more lasting effect.[33] The few studies that have tested for longer-term changes have failed to document it.[34] However, this does not rule out irreversible neurotoxicity. Given the findings of short-term abnormalities, the lessons from amphetamine and methamphetamine must raise concern that irreversible changes are also caused by Ritalin. This is consistent with mounting evidence from human brain scans cited earlier in this chapter indicating that Ritalin causes shrinkage in the brains of children treated with the drug.

Recognition of Brain Damage from Ritalin and Amphetamines

Everett H. Ellinwood, M.D., is Professor of Psychiatry and Pharmacology at the Duke University Medical Center. Addressing the use of stimulants for the treatment of children, Ellinwood (1996) and his co-author concluded: "Drug levels in children on a mg/kg basis are sometimes as high as those reported to produce chronic CNS changes in animal studies"[35].

Jerome Jaffe, M.D., is Adjunct Clinical Professor of Psychiatry at the University of Maryland School of Medicine and a research scientists in the field of drug abuse. Writing in *The Comprehensive Textbook of Psychiatry*, Jaffe (1995)[36] summarized the irreversible brain changes caused by stimulants:

> In animals chronically administered high doses of amphetamines [the drugs] produce long-lasting depletion of brain norepinephrine, and more selective but even longer-lasting depletion of dopamine, alterations in dopamine uptake sites, and reduction in serotonergic activity. Methamphetamine in particular seems capable of inducing damage to serotonergic fibers.... In monkeys the toxic effects of chronic amphetamine use include damage to cerebral blood vessels, neuronal loss [brain cell death], and microhemorrhages.

Remember, Jaffe is talking about a class of drugs, the amphetamines, routinely given to children. He singles out methamphetamine—a drug that is FDA-approved for ADHD—but clearly indicates concern about the amphetamines in general. Remember, too, that Ritalin is closely related to amphetamines.

Jaffe's warnings are not heeded in textbooks that advocate stimulant drugs. For example, Arnold and Jensen have a chapter on treating ADHD in the same 1995 textbook in which Jaffe voiced his concerns; but Arnold and Jensen make no mention of any danger of permanent brain dysfunction and damage from these drugs. I reviewed numerous psychiatric textbooks and could not find a single chapter on stimulant medications that referred to the studies reviewed in this chapter concerning brain damage and dysfunction.

The reader of this chapter has already learned much more about the dangers of stimulant drugs to the brain than most practicing psychiatrists, pediatricians, or family doctors are likely to know. Unfortunately there's more to come.

Constricting Blood Flow to the Brain

From early studies it is known that Ritalin can decrease blood flow to selected parts of the brain, in particular the area of the cortex (brain surface) that controls conscious movement.[37] To study the effects of Ritalin on overall cerebral blood flow, investigators from the Brookhaven National Laboratory in Upton, New York used the PET scan.[38] They measured the effect of clinical doses of Ritalin on blood flow in normal volunteers. Ritalin, like cocaine, decreased the overall flow of blood into the brain. The loss was large: 23–30% in all areas of the brain, including the higher brain centers in the frontal lobes, as well as the basal ganglia deeper in the brain. The changes were sufficiently dramatic to be grossly apparent in the before and after photos reproduced in a medical journal. They attributed the reductions in blood flow to constriction of the blood vessels, probably related to the drug's impact on dopamine.

The Ritalin reduction in blood flow to the brain lasted for *at least* thirty minutes after the injection, the point at which the study ended. It is probable that the effects of *oral* doses of Ritalin would be similar but less intense and more prolonged.

The researchers warned that these Ritalin effects "should be considered when prescribing this drug chronically and/or when giving it to subjects with cerebrovascular compromise." Of course, the drug is routinely given "chronically" to children diagnosed with ADHD.

Compromising the Brain's Energy Utilization

The brain can utilize only one food, glucose (a sugar), to meet its energy needs. By radioactively labeling glucose, the rate of metabolism (energy consumption) can be measured. This can be used as a gross indicator of activity in various parts of the brain. NIMH's Laboratory of Cerebral Metabolism studied the effects of Ritalin in the brains of conscious rats.[39] They found "significant dose-dependent alterations in metabolic activity" occurring "throughout many portions of the brain," and especially those affected by dopaminergic nerves. The energy consumption increases in these areas are consistent with known effects of Ritalin in causing hyperactivity in dopaminergic nerves in the brain. This includes impairment of emotional responsiveness and mental functions.

The NIMH researchers also point out that "the response of both normals and hyperactives [sic] to stimulants is similar." The study demonstrates the effect that stimulant drugs will have on the brain of any animal or child, regardless of the presence or absence of an ADHD diagnosis.

The Brain Says "No!" to Drugs

How does the brain respond when a drug over-stimulates its neurotransmitter system? It acts as if it must defend against an invasion by a harmful foreign substance. Despite the claim by drug advocates that stimulants correct an imbalance in the brain, in reality they cause drastic imbalances. Instead of welcoming these intrusions as "enhancing" brain function or "correcting biochemical imbalances," the brain tries to compensate for them. These compensations can lead to permanent biochemical imbalances.

The stimulant drugs, as already described, give out a single message, "Go!" The brain, however, tends to react against the message and to reply, "Stop!"

The brain's attempt to compensate for drug effects produces an inherently unstable condition. It is often difficult to determine if the patient's mental state is the result of a direct drug effect or the result of the brain's attempt to compensate for the drug effect.[40] A person who takes a few drinks of alcohol each day, for example, may at varying times and in varying combinations experience the direct toxic effect (sedation) or undergo the brain's attempt to overcome the effect (stimulation).

The brain compensates in at least two ways against a stimulant drug's attempt to flood the synapses with excess neurotransmitters.[41] First, neuron "A," the one that releases the extra neurotransmitter, receives feedback signals that cause it to shut down. This compensatory effect then reduces the amount of neurotransmitter that the brain cell releases into the synaptic space. Second, neuron "B," the nerve that receives the neurotransmitter, tries to blunt the overstimulation by destroying its own receptors for the neurotransmitter.

The process in which nerve "B" reduces its capacity to receive stimulation is called down-regulation. The result is called subsensitivity. The nerve turns itself down in order to become less sensitive to the abnormal rate of stimulation produced by the stimulants. The disappearance or dying off of the neuron's receptors can actually be measured in animals in laboratory experiments and provided the basis for some of the studies cited in this chapter.

Sometimes the compensatory changes in the brain can become permanent, leading to irreversible malfunction. This chapter has documented irreversable changes in animals exposed to relatively small doses of amphetamine (brand names Adderall and Dexedrine) and methamphetamine (Desoxyn and Gradumet), and raised concerns about the same dangers in regard to methylphenidate (Ritalin and Concerta).

Escaping from Their Own Findings

Recent research has disclosed some of the adverse effects of cocaine on the brains of addicts.[42] In a theme we shall hear repeated in this book, the researchers describe their technology as "achieving a sort of Holy Grail of psychiatry"—the discovery of an actual biological basis for a psychiatric disorder, cocaine addiction. The investigators claim that "brain imaging has for the first time given researchers a peek at precisely what is going wrong biologically inside the head during an attack of a mental disorder, in this case, drug addiction."

In reality, the brain scan showed nothing about the origin of mental illness. Instead, it displayed the harmful impact of a stimulant drug on the brain—a stimulant with very similar effects on the brain as Ritalin and amphetamine. Some of the brain stimulation outlasted the presence of the cocaine, suggesting long-lasting drug-induced impairments of function.

Lessons from the FDA's Withdrawal of Redux and Pondimin

The diet drugs fenfluramine (Pondimin) and its newer relative dexfenfluramine (Redux) were recently withdrawn from the market when it was found that they cause abnormalities of the heart valves. Fenfluramine was a component of "fen-phen" which was widely used in weight reduction programs. Pondimin and Redux had been given to millions of patients over twenty years.

Fenfluramine and dexfenfluramine are closely related chemically and clinically to Ritalin and amphetamine which also cause weight loss. Furthermore, in a somewhat similar fashion to both stimulants and to Prozac-like drugs, they increase availability of serotonin in the synapses of the brain. It is thought that increased serotonin in the heart might be the cause of the heart valve abnormalities.[43]

More relevant to the impact on the mind—and to the dangers of Ritalin and other stimulants—NIH research found that Redux and Pondimin "have been demonstrated to damage brain serotonin neurons [brain cells] in animal studies."[44] The axons or main fibers of the nerves were irreparably damaged. The doses that caused brain toxicity in animals are the same as those used in human beings for weight reduction.

It is interesting and important that the FDA made no official response to these disastrous findings of brain cell maiming and destruction from Pondimin and Redux. Why not? The answer in part lies in the politics of the FDA which will be examined in chapter 15. As already noted, similar permanent damage to brain cells has been demonstrated in regard to amphetamine and methamphetamine, drugs approved for the treatment of ADHD, and signs of the same possibly irreversible reactions were also described in regard to Ritalin. The FDA and the drug companies have ignored these findings as well.

When drugs affect mental function, even serious drug-induced disorders are likely to be blamed on "mental illness" and hence forever overlooked or denied. The fenfluramines, Redux and Pondimin, were allowed to remain on the market despite mounting evidence that they destroy brain cells but were taken off relatively quickly when they were shown to be harming the heart.

Once again, we have a warning against experimenting on children with the widespread use of drugs that affect the brain and mind.

Developmental Toxicity—Bathing the Child's Brain in Chemicals

When psychiatric drugs are administered to a child, the intensity of exposure to their toxic effects is far greater than the intensity of exposure to many other agents in the environment that we worry about, such as lead, pesticide residues, and air pollutants. We know that drugs can disrupt the child's psychological, social, cognitive, and educational development. In a standard textbook on the treatment of children, Mina Dulcan (1994)[45] warns:

> The term developmental toxicology refers to unique or especially severe side effects caused by interaction between a drug and the process of growth and development. Children and adolescents are growing and developing not only physically but also cognitively and emotionally. It is important that medications not interfere with learning in school or with the development of social relationships within the family or with peers.

Dulcan points out that developmental toxicity can affect the child *before* more obvious side effects become apparent:

> Behavioral toxicity, the worsening of preexisting behaviors or affective [emotional] states or the provoking of new ones that are undesirable, often develops before physical side effects are observed, especially in young children.

Once a child begins to take a medication that changes his or her brain, it becomes nearly impossible to differentiate drug effects from other causes of the child's evolving or worsening difficulties.

Making a Malformed Brain?

In 1995 the National Institute of Mental Health (NIMH) and the Food and Drug Administration (FDA) held a conference on the future testing and use of psychiatric drugs for children. The government funded the conference to cooperate with the pharmaceutical industry in its effort to increase psychiatric drug marketing to children. This is consistent with the government's more recent efforts, described in chapter 1, to conduct clinical trials of stimulant drugs on toddlers age 2–4 years old.

Some token concern about drugging children was shown at the conference. Benedetto Vitiello, head of NIMH's pediatric psychopharmacology program, pointed out that "By issuing psychotropics to children, we do, in fact, create an interaction between the chemical, the drug, and the developing organism, and in particular the developing brain, which is the target organ of a psychotropic." Even without the interference of medications, he observed, there are dramatic changes going on in the organization of the major neurotransmitters. He specifically mentions the adrenergic, dopaminergic, and serotonergic systems—the three most affected by stimulant drugs. This "interaction of the drug with a developing brain" can lead to unusual and sometimes more severe adverse drug reactions in children.

Vitiello made a dramatic and important disclosure:

Now, we know from work in animals that if we interfere with these neurotransmitter systems at some crucial times, like the prenatal or the perinatal or the neonatal phase of their lives, we can change in the animals
the destiny of the neurotransmitters forever. We can cause permanent
changes.

These studies focus on the period of time around the birth of the animal
when permanent changes are most likely to be detected but he makes clear
that this raises broader concerns for the entire period of childhood and adolescence.

According to Vitiello, "If one looks at the literature, one can find that
really there are very few studies that have been specifically designed with the
purpose of long-term safety of psychotropics." How different from the public's
image of the safety of the drugs that patients take for months and years at a
time, including children on Ritalin.

Those few long-term studies that have been conducted have yielded
frightening results. Vitiello described an NIH study of 200 children taking
phenobarbital, a sedative, for the control of seizures due to fever. The study
came up with two startling results. First, phenobarbital proved to be no better than the sugar pill in controlling febrile seizures. Second, after two years
of treatment, "the group on phenobarbital had an IQ which was about eight
points lower than the placebo group." Phenobarbital, assumed safe and effective for decades, when actually studied in a controlled trial, turned out to be
useless and to be associated with a drop in the children's IQ.

Vitiello concluded that "we have a number of animal data that show that
if we manipulate their neurotransmitter systems at some developmental
stages, we can cause permanent changes, but we don't know exactly how to
extrapolate these data to humans."

Thomas Laughren, an FDA official involved with overseeing the approval
of psychiatric drugs, summarized Vitiello's remarks in order to emphasize
them. He, too, called for more attention to the effects of drugs on the child's
developing brain, "since I think everyone agrees that children and adolescents, given that they are going through so many physiological changes, are
probably more vulnerable." He ended on that note.

As a parent, I would be very careful about putting my child on any drug
that affects the brain and mind. It's a gamble and we can never be sure of the
results.

The Vulnerability of the Child's Brain

The size of the child's brain increases three times from birth until age five,
reaching nearly its adult weight.[46] There is an enormous elaboration in the

branching and the connections between the brain cells, much of it in response to the child's environment.

Between the ages of five to fifteen—the period of time when most Ritalin is prescribed—the brain undergoes new and striking changes in its function and even composition. Frequently used nerve pathways are firmed up while others are allowed to disappear from lack of use. There is a pruning back of up to 40% of the brain connections (synapses) in the frontal lobes of the brain—the part that most fully expresses human nature and human ability. Moreover, as described in chapter 1, new research discloses that the adolescent and young adult brain goes through yet another burst of growth and development.

Environmental influences profoundly impact on the development of the brain. Enriched environmental experiences, for example, increase the number and complexity of connections among brain cells. The term "plasticity" has been used to emphasize the brain's responsiveness to environmental input. If environmental influences, such as the frequency and quality of cuddling and communication, can influence brain development—what does bathing the child's brain in drugs do to it? It is incredible that so many doctors are willing to soak the child's brain in drugs during these periods of astonishing growth and change.

Child development researchers have eloquently described how neurotransmitter systems are permanently changed by the child's environment and how emotional trauma can build negative responses into the brain.[47] Can a child or adolescent brain drenched in these drugs develop in a normal fashion? It seems—at the very least—improbable.

Even after the Drug is Gone

Doctors who prescribe Ritalin often ease the fears of parents by telling them that Ritalin washes out of the body in three hours. First of all, only *half* the drug washes out in the first three or four hours. It takes yet another three-to-four hours for half of the remaining amount to wash out, and then another three hours for half of that to wash out. It's a gradual process.

More important, drugs can have long-lasting, even irreversible effects, after they have left the body, in some cases producing a permanent loss of receptors and even brain cells.

Do Stimulants Always Cause Brain Malfunction?

ADHD/Ritalin advocates frequently claim that Ritalin enhances or improves nerve transmission in the brain by correcting biochemical imbalances. These are unfounded speculations aimed at justifying the use of medication. Instead of improving brain function, Ritalin and other stimulants create severe biochemical imbalances. They do not "normalize" the brain; they render it abnormal. This cannot be over-emphasized: Stimulants produce pathological malfunctions in the child's brain. Whenever these drugs have any direct effect on the child's mind or behavior, they do so by disrupting brain function. In short, effective doses of Ritalin, Adderall, and similar drugs always cause malfunctions in the brain.

Stimulants such as Ritalin and amphetamine also have grossly harmful impacts on the brain—reducing overall blood flow, disturbing glucose metabolism, and possibly causing permanent shrinkage or atrophy of the brain. They produce a loss of receptors for various neurotransmitters and, in some cases, this is known to become permanent. Stimulants have been shown to deform and to destroy brain cells.

It is worth re-emphasizing that the scientific studies and data covered in this chapter are largely unknown to the overwhelming majority of professionals who claim to be experts on stimulant drugs in the treatment of children. Even the "authorities" who write medical textbooks and who conduct research on children don't know—and seemingly don't want to know—about the damaging effects of these drugs. You won't find anything like this review in any other book.

While the "experts" and "authorities" know little about the damaging effects of the drugs they advocate, the average psychiatrist, neurologist, pediatrician, and family doctor knows even less. Doctors who routinely prescribe stimulants to children are almost wholly ignorant about what these agents do to the brain. However, parents, teachers, and ethical health professionals should find in this chapter sufficient scientific basis for refusing to subject any children to stimulant drugs.

Chapter 4

How Stimulants Really Work

If a parent forced a child to take alcohol, a depressant, in the mistaken belief that he was curing a "chemical imbalance" in the child's brain, we would not hesitate to have the child removed from home. Yet millions of children are forced to take mind-altering drugs in the equally mistaken belief that depression and other mental illnesses are biologically caused, for which there is not a shred of scientific evidence.

—Keith Hoeller, editor-in-chief,
Review of Existential Psychology and Psychiatry (1997)

Students who take their medication do become more tractable, completing more repetitive "work," such as worksheets with fill-in answers and drills on math problems. In most studies conducted thus far, however, drugs per se do not make them score better on tests of academic achievement or of higher-level thinking and problem-solving. Some studies have even shown that the level of dosage needed to make teachers approve a child's behavior is so high that it actually dulls reasoning ability. These findings raise questions, not only about the type of "work" dominating many classrooms, but also about the real source of the problem.

—Jane M. Healy, author, *Endangered Minds* (1991)

ADHD/Ritalin advocates often claim that no one knows how Ritalin and other stimulants produce their supposedly beneficial effects on behavior. In fact, there is solid evidence from both animal and human research showing how stimulants work. Unfortunately, it's not good news for children or for adults who care about them.

Dispelling the Myth of Paradoxical Effects

It is sometimes said that stimulants have a paradoxical effect on children compared to adults, by calming instead of exciting them. At other times it is claimed that stimulants only work if the child suffers from "ADHD." In reality, the effects on all children and adults, and even on animals, are basically the same. This has been agreed upon by clinicians and researchers for many years.[1] James M. Swanson and his colleagues from the ADD Center at the University of California, Irvine, refer to the "outdated notion that the response to stimulants is different (or 'paradoxical') in children compared to adults." Stimulant drug effects are also the same whether or not the individual child or adult has ADHD-like symptoms.[2]

The confusion has been due in part to the size of the doses given children. With larger doses, Ritalin and amphetamines become more obviously stimulating for children and adults alike. Also, young children tend to dislike the mental effects of the drug while adults, especially when abusing them, more often tend to interpret them as positive.[3] Furthermore, as described in chapter 2, many children do become over-stimulated by the drugs, even in the usually prescribed doses. Most important, as we shall see, stimulation is not the sought-after therapeutic effect.

Subduing Hospitalized Children

In the very first paper published on the use of amphetamines for the control of children, Bradley (1937) noted a marked change in behavior in half the youngsters.[4]

Fifteen of the 30 children responded to Benzedrine by becoming distinctly subdued in their emotional responses. Clinically in all cases this was an improvement from the social viewpoint.

More than once, Bradley uses the word "subdued" to describe the children. Bradley was also among the first to speak mistakenly of the effect as paradoxical: "It appears paradoxical that a drug known to be a stimulant should produce subdued behavior in half of the children." Given that these children were confined in a mental hospital, the Emma Pendleton Bradley Home in Rhode Island, it is understandable that Bradley equates subdued behavior with improved behavior.

Snuffing Out Enthusiasm

Again turning to the early literature for more truthful accounts of stimulant effects, a team led by Herbert Rie from the Ohio State Department of Pediatrics[5] carried out a double-blind study of 28 children given placebo or Ritalin for twelve-week periods each. Despite ratings of improvement by parents and teachers, Rie found no objective evidence for improvement from Ritalin on any of the tests of learning or performance. Instead, the children endured "the typical suppressive behavioral effects" of the drug. There was a reduction in spontaneous behavior (responsivity) and a flattening of emotions. The children became:

distinctly more bland or "flat" emotionally, lacking both the age-typical variety and frequency of emotional expression. They responded less, exhibited little or no initiative and spontaneity, offered little indication of either interest or aversion, showed virtually no curiosity, surprise, or pleasure, and seemed devoid of humor. Jocular comments and humorous situations passed unnoticed. In short, while on active drug treatment, the children were relatively but unmistakably affectless, humorless, and apathetic.

Snuffing Out Curiosity and Initiative

Nancy Fiedler and Douglas Ullman (1983) reviewed literature showing that Ritalin inhibits the exploratory drive which they characterize as consisting of "curiosity, initiative, spontaneity, emotional responsiveness." They cite Rie's work showing that Ritalin can make children "more manageable in the environment, but less interested in it." They state that "Educators, as well, have hypothesized that stimulants suppress curiosity in the classroom, while parents have commented that the medication makes the child too somber and apathetic."

By reducing the most highly developed aspects of human nature—the impulses for freedom, spontaneity, curiosity, initiative, emotional expression, and sociability—Ritalin makes children more manageable in boring, unstimulating, and otherwise frustrating environments.

More about the Zombie Effect

Arnold and Jensen's observations on what they call the "zombie" effect of suppressing emotions and spontaneity were quoted in chapter 2. As already noted, the zombie or robot theme also appears in a discussion by James Swanson (1992) and his colleagues of "cognitive toxicity" caused by Ritalin. It is worth repeating their summary of the more extreme effects on children:

> In some disruptive children, drug-induced compliant behavior may be accompanied by isolated, withdrawn, and overfocused behavior. Some medicated children may seem "zombie-like" and high doses which make ADHD children more "somber," "quiet," and "still" may produce social isolation by increasing "time spent alone" and decreasing "time spent in positive interaction" on the playground.

Studies confirming stimulant-induced social isolation can be found in the literature from the 1970s to today. Charles E. Cunningham and Russell Barkley (1978) examined the effects of Ritalin on "hyperactive identical twins." Although the authors consider it a positive outcome, they find that

"Both children showed a marked drug-related increase in solitary play and a corresponding reduction in their initiation of social interactions." This drug-induced inhibited mental state made it easier for the mother to handle the twins.

Even when ADHD children are rated improved in their peer or social relationships, they suffer from drug-induced increased "social inhibition—passive and submissive behaviors."[6] The child who becomes more socially inhibited by drugs becomes a more compliant member of large, structured classrooms. Stimulants "work better in a structured environment such as a classroom than in a free play situation."[7]

According to Peter Schrag and Diane Divoky (1975), Ritalin researcher Herbert Rie told them that "the youngsters on drugs are far less responsive and enthusiastic, and far more apathetic, humorless and zombie-like. It's there and you can see it and measure it, and we don't know why it hasn't been picked up before."

Compliance and the Zombie Effect

Compliance is a euphemism for blind obedience to all authority. Only an occasional stimulant-treated child will become obviously robotic or zombie-like; but most children on Ritalin become more docile and obedient. Over the years, Barkley has been especially forward about describing "ADHD children" as noncompliant—that is, rebellious or autonomous in nature. He wrote that "Methylphenidate produced a marked increase in compliance and sustained attention to the activities assigned during the structured task sessions."[8]

Barkley also observed mother-child interactions in a controlled study of twenty hyperactive boys: "It has been reported that stimulant drugs reduce the child's interest in social interactions. Several observations in this study would support this notion."[9] The medication made the boys socialize less and play alone more. They were less interactive and less responsive to other children during free play. They were also less responsive to their mothers, so that the parents had to supervise them less. "Thus, reduced sociability appears to be a response of these boys to methylphenidate."

These studies describe drug-induced *abnormal behavior*. As with any toxic effect, it tends to be dose dependent. As Barkley also wrote, "Only the high dose (0.7 mg/kg given twice daily) was effective in improving the compliance of ADD-H [hyperactive] children to their mother's commands or the duration of that compliance."[10]

Author Louise Armstrong (1993) remarks:

The alleged "improvement" was that some children placed on the drug [Ritalin] became markedly more subdued, less obstreperous. If I am not mistaken, in the not so long ago, mothers figured out the same thing about moderate amounts of brandy. However, when the doctors prescribe a drug, it is evidently science. What mothers did, we now consider an outrage.

Making Good Caged Rats

In the short term at least, stimulants make children more compliant—more willing and able to obey adult commands, especially in regard to carrying out boring, repetitive classroom tasks or homework. There are striking parallels in animal research.

The effects of Ritalin and other stimulants on animals have been demonstrated by countless studies over several decades.[11] The drugs inhibit exploration, spontaneity, novelty-seeking, and overall interest in the environment. At the same time, they induce repetitive, meaningless behaviors, such as rearing up for no apparent reason, pacing, posturing, or chewing.[12]

By 1970, Randrup and Munkvad were already comparing stimulant-induced repetitive behavior in animals to obsessive and compulsive behaviors seen in humans taking the same drugs. Later investigators compared these effects on animals to the same effects on school children.

Ritalin and amphetamines inhibit spontaneous, exploratory, and social behavior. The animal's activities become compulsive, repetitive, inflexible, narrowly focused, meaningless, and ultimately useless. Stimulants also obliterate spontaneous social interactions in animals at relatively small doses, making them more socially isolated.

When I was selected by the National Institutes of Health (NIH) to be the scientific presenter concerning the mechanism of action and adverse effects of stimulants for the November 1998 NIH Consensus Development Conference on ADHD and its treatment, I took the opportunity to review the animal literature in further depth. I published the results in *Ethical Human Sciences and Services* (1999b) an in the *International Journal of Risk and Safety in Medicine* (1999c). Citing two dozen scientific reports,[13] I was able to succinctly summarize the two basic effects of stimulants on animals (and children):

First, stimulants suppress normal spontaneous or self-generated activity, including curiosity, socializing, and play.

Exploration, novelty seeking, curiosity, purposeful locomotion, and escape behaviors are diminished. Inhibitions in socialization are demonstrated by reductions in approach behavior, interactions, mutual grooming, and vocalizations. There may be avoidance of contact with the cage mate, obliviousness to other animals, and increased fearfulness. Play is inhibited.

Second, stimulants promote stereotyped, obsessive-compulsive, overly-focused behaviors that are often repetitive and meaningless.

These effects may be demonstrated by limited or constricted pacing, reduced or localized self-grooming, staring out the cage, staring at small objects, repetitive head movements, and other compulsive behaviors, such as picking, scratching, gnawing, or licking limited areas of the body or objects.

In the animal literature, stimulant-induced repetitive, compulsive activity is called *stereotypical* behavior or *perseveration*—an involuntary, pathological repetition of activities. It is important to realize that this drug-induced behavior is *involuntary* and *abnormal*. This is the same stimulant-induced behavior that is considered an "improvement" in children.

Psychostimulant Behavioral Effects On Humans

For the NIH Consensus Conference, I also reviewed twenty clinical trials to develop a list of stimulant adverse effects, such as depression or apathy, that are easily mistaken for improvements in the behavior of children diagnosed with ADHD. That is, I looked for harmful drug effects on brain function that are often misinterpreted as "beneficial" by parents, teachers, and doctors.

Many of the adverse effects that I found parallel the effects reported in animal studies. Overall, spontaneous and social behaviors, along with humor and play, were suppressed, while obsessive, perseverative behaviors were caused or increased.

The abnormal movements seen in the animals are also seen in stimulant-treated children, including rhythmic head movements, picking or rubbing the body, and lip movements (see chapter 2).

The twenty clinical trials are cited in my two papers (1999b&c). They provide the basis for Table 5: Harmful Stimulant Drug Reactions Commonly Misidentified as 'Therapeutic' or 'Beneficial' for Children Diagnosed with ADHD.

Making Children Obsessed with Meaningless Robotic Activities

In a study of Ritalin's impact on cognition, Mary Solanto and Esther Wender (1989) were surprised to find some children persisting at their assigned tasks in a compulsive and self-defeating manner. As already discussed, perseveration—compulsive, inflexible, narrowly focused, meaningless behavior—is a sign of drug-induced brain malfunction. It is an aspect of stereotypical behavior seen in animals and people treated with stimulants. Solanto and Wender observed this "cognitive perseveration" in eight of nineteen of the children. They say the children appear "compulsive" with "difficulty stopping after a reasonable period of time:"

As the children continued, the quality of the response appeared to decline, with an increase in the number of responses that did not make

Table 5: Harmful Stimulant Drug Reactions Commonly Misidentified as 'Therapuetic' or 'Beneficial'

Selected from Twenty Controlled Clinical Trials Involving Children Diagnosed with ADHD

Obsessive Compulsive Effects	Social Withdrawal Effects	Behaviorally Suppressive Effects
Compulsive persistence at meaningless activities (called stereotypical or perseverative behavior)	Social withdrawal and isolation	Compliant in structured environments; socially inhibited, passive and submissive
Increased obsessive compulsive behavior (e.g., repeating chores endlessly and ineffectively)	General dampened social behavior	Somber, subdued, apathetic, lethargic, dopey, dazed, and tired
Mental rigidity (called cognitive perseveration)	Reduced communication and socialization	Bland, emotionally flat, humorless, not smiling, depressed, and sad with frequent crying
Inflexible thinking	Decreased responsiveness to parents and other children	Lacking in initiative, spontaneity, curiosity, surprise or pleasure
Overly narrow or excessive focusing	Increased solitary play and diminished overall play	

Modified From Breggin (1999b & c), reprinted by permission of Springer Publishing Co. References to twenty clinical trials provided in Breggin (1999b & c).

sense, were vague, tangential, or repetitive. The phenomenon was observed to occur at all dosages.

Solanto and Wender present a most extraordinary description of stereotypical behavior: The drug-impaired child compulsively repeats tasks to the point of diminishing returns and can hardly be stopped. It once again confirms how the drug works—by obliterating spontaneous and social behavior in favor of compulsive, narrow, meaningless and ultimately self-destructive behaviors. This is an aspect of drug-induced robotic or zombie-like behavior.

The authors should not have been surprised by their findings. Several years earlier, a team led by Dyme (1982) from the New England Medical Center found a similar result. They studied "perseveration induced by methylphenidate" in a group of hyperactive children who were thought to be doing well on treatment. Using a single dose of 1 mg/kg, they found that four out of five children "worsened in a measure of flexibility of thinking." The increased focus of attention seen in these children was "accompanied by increased perseveration (difficulty in changing mental set from one idea to another)." Teachers and parents continued to rate their behavior improved, even when the children displayed this "excessive focusing of attention." This is a sad commentary on the expectations of many teachers and parents for their children.

Defenders of Ritalin claim that perseveration with inflexible thinking and obsessively focused attention occur only at higher doses and are therefore not relevant to clinical practice. But 1 mg/kg is within the range of clinical practice; and the study used only one dose. More importantly, the effect takes place across a continuum from imperceptible to grossly apparent. The child who seems to have improved attention in class is suffering from the same basic brain malfunction as the child who can't stop focusing even when asked to stop.

Solando and Wender conclude, "Clinicians should be aware that psychomotor stimulant drugs may produce over-focusing of attention or perseveration in hyperactive children." In reality, this over-focusing or perseveration is the basis of the "therapeutic effect" itself. Perseveration of a more subtle kind, with its relative inflexibility of the mind, is precisely what makes the children more willing and able to focus on boring, repetitive, uninspiring classroom materials. It also makes them more able to sit for hours over their homework at home when they'd much rather be doing something else.

Stimulant Addiction and Robotic Behavior

Stimulants produce "over-focusing" in drug addicts and drug abusers in much the same way that they produce it in a less obvious fashion in drug-treated children. More than thirty years ago, John Scher (1966) observed of amphetamine addicts:

An individual who is "hung-up" will literally get stuck in a repetitious thought or act for hours. He may sit in a tub and bathe all day, clean up the house or a particular item... The danger of getting "hung up" in this way seems to be peculiar to the amphetamines, although it may occur to a lesser extent in the course of a psychedelic "trip."

Except for the *degree* of drug-induced impairment produced in addicts and drug abusers, there is no essential difference between the addict who gets "hung up" for hours by himself in his isolated apartment and the child who sits dutifully performing boring tasks in class.

John Kramer (1970) compares the stereotypical behavior of animals to similar reactions in human beings:

Perhaps the most curious effect of amphetamines is their capacity to induce behavior which is persisted in or repeated for prolonged periods. If the activity is not too disorganized, the activity may, on the surface at least, be useful.

Notice the author's remark that the behavior may "on the surface at least, be useful." Kramer describes how "dwellings may be cleaned, automobiles polished, or items arranged to an inhuman degree of perfection." It is no wonder that some parents and teachers find their children more willing to persist at boring, compulsive activities when taking these same drugs. Kramer specifically compares these abnormal drug reactions to stereotypical behavior in stimulant-treated animals.

Schiørring (1981) also describes the stereotypical behavior seen in stimulant abusers:

Reactions to close stimuli can be increased in the speed user, while more distant stimuli in the same room (even crying or aggression) do not affect him, possibly indicating a kind of autism or withdrawal. Stereotyped movements or actions, including mental activities, lacking variation and without relevant goal-direction, are well known features of "speed" use. Simple repetitions or perseverations are found...

Addiction expert Everett Ellinwood[14] points out that stereotypy may be the sought-after effect in treating children with stimulants:

[T]hey are no longer hyper-responsive to their environment and, for the first time, they focus on the object or task before them. For the first time in their lives they can accomplish a task like reading, which requires concentration, without responding to someone who's talking in the room. Some adults also take amphetamines before going to a party, because it cuts down on the peripheral distraction and the noisy background din.... Cats who are in this stereotypy mode cannot be distracted by stimuli in their periphery; you can wave your arms, etc., to no avail.

The Biochemical Mechanism for Producing Robotic Behavior

Stimulants disrupt dopamine functions in the basal ganglia, areas of the brain that are involved in the exertion of will and the initiation of spontaneous movement. Therefore, it is sometimes hypothesized that this is the mechanism for producing stereotypy or perseveration—an aspect of robotic or zombie-like behavior.[15] The basal ganglia have intimate connections to both the emotion-regulating limbic system and to the frontal lobes.[16] Drug-induced dysfunction in these regions would dampen overall energy as well as will power, initiative, and spontaneity. The basal ganglia also have indirect connections to the reticular activating system of the brain. Ritalin is known to suppress the reticular activating system of the brain which modulates the overall activity of higher brain cells.[17] This inhibitory action could further subdue both emotional life and motor activity.

Ritalin can cause reduced energy usage as measured by glucose metabolism in some parts of the brain, especially the motor cortex which controls conscious movement.[18] The study also found that Ritalin caused stereotypical behavior in the animals at the same doses. The authors hypothesize that reduction in energy consumption in the motor area may "explain the underlying mechanism of action of methylphenidate in attention deficit disorder." The study fails to underscore that this drug-induced reduction in energy usage is a severe *malfunction*. In fact, stereotypical behavior can also be produced by brain lesions and sometimes by severe psychotic disorders.[19]

Many Drugs Can Suppress a Child

While this book focuses on stimulants, it is important to realize that there are many ways to suppress a child's brain, to reduce the child's spontaneity, and to make the child more docile or compliant. Almost any form of induced brain dysfunction will, to some degree, accomplish the goal. Even multiple psychosurgical brain mutilations have been used to control "hyperactivity" in children.[20]

Arnold and Jensen (1995) list 29 drugs in a table entitled "Some Drugs Studied and Sometimes Used for ADHD." It's easier to list the drugs that they don't recommend: "Most minor tranquilizers, including benzodiazepines," and barbiturates. Barbiturates, such as phenobarbital and amytal, are contraindicated because they "can even cause it [ADHD]."

In a book for parents, physician Patricia Quinn (1997) lists the following additional drugs as possible treatments for ADHD: buproprion (Wellbutrin), an atypical antidepressant; imipramine (Tofranil) and desipramine

(Norpramin), older tricyclic antidepressants; clonidine (Catapres), an anti-hypertensive agent that also can be applied as a transdermal patch; and guan-facine (Tenex), another antihypertensive agent.

In the past, antipsychotic drugs—especially those with more sedative effects such as Mellaril, Navane, and Thorazine—were often used to subdue children labeled ADHD. Mellaril is still sometimes mistakenly prescribed for behavior control, even though it often causes severe and irreversible neuro-logical disorders, including tardive dyskinesia and neuroleptic malignant syn-drome.[21] It is unfortunate that the new neuroleptics, such as Zyprexa, Risperdal, and Seroguel, are now too often used in a medically negligent fash-ion to control behaviors in children. MAOI (monoamine oxidase inhibitor) antidepressants, such as Parnate, Nardil, and Marplan, have also been rec-ommended but they have many adverse effects and require dietary restric-tions. Anticonvulsants, such as Dilantin and Tegretol, are a mainstay in insti-tutions, although they suppress cognitive processes. The sleeping medication, chloral hydrate, has been tried, but the benzodiazepines and other sedatives often tend to aggravate the behavior of children. The atypical antianxiety agent, buspirone (BuSpar), has also been recommended. And of course, many physicians are enamored with the latest group of fad drugs, the sero-tonergic antidepressants such as Prozac, Zoloft, Paxil, and Effexor.

Although the stimulants are the only ones with official FDA approval for the treatment of children with ADHD, almost any drug that disrupts brain function—including every psychiatric drug—automatically becomes a candi-date for the behavioral control of children.[22]

A British Voice for the Ethical Treatment of Children

While many American advocates for Ritalin act as if there is no scientif-ic controversy surrounding its use, British physicians and scientists are much more skeptical about controlling children through the use of stimulant drugs. In the *Oxford Textbook of Clinical Psychopharmacology and Drug Therapy*, Grahame-Smith and Aronson (1992) indicate that stimulants probably affect children in the same way they impact on rats—by "inducing stereo-typed behavior in animals, i.e. in reducing the number of behavioural responses…"[23] The British textbook authors observe with a hint of disdain for the practice, "It is beyond our scope to discuss whether or not such behav-ioural control is desirable."

The Importance of Spontaneous Activity in All Living Creatures

What is called "spontaneous" behavior, including exploration and novel-ty-seeking, is at the heart of normal functioning for animals and humans. Any animal—including monkeys, rats, mice, or pigeons—has a natural curiosity or tendency to explore its environment. These animals also have a natural tendency to congregate and to relate to each other. Their investigative or exploratory drives, as well as their social drives, are basic life forces—central features of thriving animals and people.

ADHD/Ritalin advocates view children through a narrow behavioral eye-glass that leaves no room for the child's natural desires for play, for exploration, and for variety. As a healthy antidote to such a narrow behavioral vision, it is worth recalling that I. P. Pavlov (1957), the Russian behaviorist, recognized that animals, as well as humans, display drives to investigate, to explore, and to be free. He spoke of the "freedom reflex" as well as the "investigatory reflex" and "inquisitiveness." With humor, Pavlov also declared, "I sometimes call it the 'What-is-it?' reflex."[24]

Pavlov considered these spontaneous drives to be among the most important in life. Without freedom-affirming impulses, "life, one might say, would always hang by a thread." Human beings do not thrive by virtue of their compulsive, rote behaviors but through their exploratory, experimental, and more daring activities.

It is basic to a child's survival and growth to want to socialize with other children and with adults, to explore, to play, and to learn all there is to learn about the surrounding environment. Ritalin and other stimulant drugs suppress this whole range of behavior—the spontaneous, exploratory, investigative, playful, and social activities of animals… as well as children.

It is bad enough that Ritalin and amphetamine cause so much harm to the brain and mind, but there are more hazards to be concerned about. The next chapter documents that Ritalin and amphetamine are highly addictive and subject to abuse.

Chapter 5

VITAMIN R

The Road to Addiction and Abuse

"Out of 10 people I know, maybe one has seen or tried cocaine but nine of them have done Ritalin."

—High school student, Bethesda, Maryland[1]

Producing cocaine-like stimulant effects, snorted or injected Ritalin is just the latest trend in a resurgence in abuse of stimulant drugs that recalls the "Speed Freak" era of the late 1960's... Even when taken according to the prescription directions, there is a risk of developing dependence and tolerance to the drug.

—William J. Bailey, Indiana Prevention and
Resource Center at Indiana University (1995)

The documentation in this report directly contrasts to the assertions that methylphenidate is a benign, mild stimulant that is not associated with abuse or serious side effects.

—Drug Enforcement Administration (DEA) of the
U.S. Department of Justice (1995c)

The most widely prescribed stimulant, methylphenidate, has significant abuse potential... Clinical studies have reported abuse in young patients for whom stimulants have been prescribed, although the notion is unpopular.

—Charles A. Dackis and Mark S. Gold,
Advances in Alcohol and Substance Abuse (1990)

Soon after Ritalin was first marketed in the mid-1950s it became recognized as highly addictive and subject to widespread abuse. Several waves of Ritalin addiction and abuse swept parts of the world, including the United States and Japan, during the 1960s and 1970s. More than four decades have confirmed that addiction and abuse are a serious problem with the amphetamine and amphetamine-like stimulants used in the treatment of ADHD, including Ritalin (methylphenidate), Metadate ER and Concerta (long-acting forms of methylphenidate), Dexedrine and DextroStat (d-amphetamine), Adderall (d-amphetamine and amphetamine mixture), and Desoxyn and Gradumet (methamphetamine). The increasing availability of these drugs to so many people has resulted in a new wave of stimulant addiction and abuse among American children and young adults who obtain the drug illegally. It is shocking that many ADHD/Ritalin advocates continue to deny the addictiveness of stimulants and to show very little concern about making these drugs of abuse readily available to so many children as well as to the friends, and families of the children.

Are Parents Misinformed by Doctors?

Parents are often misinformed by doctors who tell them that Ritalin is not addictive and not abused. Gene Haislip, the recently retired head of diversion control at the Drug Enforcement Administration (DEA), has warned, "A lot of people don't know Ritalin is like cocaine."[2] Haislip "found parents abusing their kids' prescriptions, kids selling to kids, illegal drug rings, illicit trafficking. Mexican smuggling rings, even." In a formal analysis of the dangers of Ritalin, a DEA publication (1995c) declared:

> The majority of the literature prepared for public consumption and available to parents does not address methylphenidate's abuse liability or actual abuse.

> How do Ritalin advocates respond to the mass of evidence concerning Ritalin addiction and abuse? Few, if any, ADHD/Ritalin books for parents give proper emphasis to the drug's addictive capacities.[3]

Russell Barkley, one of the world's most quoted ADHD experts, recently declared, "No, Ritalin is not addictive—when taken orally. For this drug to be potentially addictive, it has to be crushed and inhaled nasally, or injected, and that has to be done repeatedly."[4] Similarly, in his 1997 book Barkley stated there is "no risk of addiction" when the drug is "taken orally as prescribed."

Barkley takes a most extraordinary and unprecedented position when he declares that Ritalin—or any highly addictive drug—can be addictive by one route of administration but not by another. In regard to all of the stimulants, this is patently false. All of them are known to be addictive when taken orally.[5]

Barkley is also wrong in suggesting that there is "no risk of addiction" when Ritalin, or any addictive drug, is taken as prescribed. The risk of addiction *begins* with taking the drug as prescribed, and then *escalates* when and if the individual develops a tolerance or craving for it. Exactly as the first step to narcotics addiction commonly begins with taking prescription analgesics for pain, the first step to stimulant addiction can begin with taking Ritalin, amphetamine, or methamphetamine as prescribed for "ADHD."

Barkley (1991) gives especially dangerous and misleading information when he states "Ritalin and Cylert are nonamphetamines."[6] Medication experts and narcotics control agencies link Ritalin with the amphetamines— and not with Cylert—in terms of clinical effects, including the potential for addiction and abuse. Ritalin is placed along with amphetamines in Schedule II by both the DEA and the International Narcotics Control Board. Schedule II indicates the highest possible abuse potential for a prescription drug. The American Psychiatric Association's *Diagnostic and Statistical Manual of Mental Disorders, IV* classifies Ritalin with the amphetamines as a drug that has "amphetamine-like action." It categorizes it together with amphetamine and methamphetamine ("speed"), as well as cocaine, for purposes of examining patterns of addiction, abuse, and toxicity.[7] Similarly, the American Psychiatric Association (1989), *Treatments of Psychiatric Disorders*, observes that cocaine, amphetamines, and methylphenidate are "neuropharmacologically alike."[8] As evidence, the textbook points out that abuse patterns are the same for the three drugs; that people cannot tell their clinical effects apart in laboratory tests; and that they can substitute for each other and cause similar behavior in addicted animals.

An editorial comment in the *Archives of General Psychiatry* (1995) states, "Cocaine, one of the most reinforcing and addictive of abuse drugs, has pharmacological actions very similar to those of MPH [methylphenidate], one of the most commonly prescribed psychotropic medications for children in the United States." The remarks were inspired by a report in the same issue of the journal by a team led by N. D. Volkow (1995) from the Brookhaven National Laboratory. Using the PET scan, the researchers found that the distribution of cocaine and methylphenidate in the brain are identical, but that Ritalin remains for a longer period of time. More recently Volkow and his colleagues (1997) observed:

> MP [methylphenidate], like cocaine, increases synaptic dopamine by inhibiting dopamine reuptake, it has equivalent reinforcing effects to those of cocaine, and its intravenous administration produces a "high" similar to that of cocaine.

Given the facts that Ritalin is pharmacologically related to the amphetamines, and that it is clinically equivalent to amphetamine, it is unconscionable for Barkley or any other expert to say that Ritalin is a "nonamphetamine" like Cylert. Statements like these have lulled parents and teachers, as well as misinformed health professionals, into a false sense of security about Ritalin.

Do Prescribed Stimulants Predispose to Stimulant Drug Abuse?

Are Ritalin, Adderall, Dexedrine, Concerta, and Metadate ER gateway drugs to later stimulant abuse, including cocaine? As this chapter will document, there is stong evidence that prescribed stimulants will promote future abuse of stimulants, including Ritalin itself, amphetamines, methamphetamine, and cocaine. All of these stimulants affect the same three neurotransmitters in the brain, all can cause long-lasting changes in brain function and even structure, all cause addiction and abuse, and all are used interchangeably by addicted animals and humans.

The Drug Enforcement Administration (1995b) has shown considerable concern about "the possibility of drug abuse as a consequence of methylphenidate treatment." It finds that "a number of recent studies, drug abuse cases, and trends among adolescents from various sources, indicate that methylphenidate use may be a risk factor for substance abuse." The DEA (1995c) cites research that the stimulants sensitize the brain to each other. Individuals obtain greater effects from cocaine, amphetamine, or Ritalin if they have been previously exposed to any of them.[9]

Recently, additional scientific confirmation has been found for these concerns. Nadine Lambert, Ph.D. is Professor of Cognition and Development and Director of the School Psychology Program at the Graduate School of Education of the University of California, Berkeley. She has for many years been conducting a unique long-term study comparing future drug abuse in two groups of children labeled ADHD. The study compares one group who had been prescribed stimulants as children with another group that had not been given medication.

Lambert presented her results at the 1998 Consensus Conference and in a research study published in 1998 with co-author Carolyn Hartsough. Lambert found a significant correlation between *stimulant treatment in childhood* and later drug abuse. Lambert told the conference that the prescriptions of stimulants to children for a year or more was correlated with increased "lifetime use of cocaine and stimulants." Stimulant treatment in childhood resulted in increased rates of "cocaine dependence, lifetime use of stimulants, and a combined measure of lifetime use of both cocaine and stimulants."

Lambert also found that prescription use of stimulants encouraged increased rates of smoking in adulthood. Presumably, exposure to stimulants in childhood cause a sensitization of the brain that predisposed the individual to seek later use of these drugs. She concluded in her NIH paper that childhood use of stimulants "is significantly and pervasively implicated in the uptake of regular smoking, in daily smoking in adulthood, in cocaine dependence, and in lifetime use of cocaine and stimulants."

A Death in Roanoke from Snorting Ritalin

Given the lack of information made available to parents about the dangers of Ritalin, imagine the shock in Roanoke, Virginia, when parents awoke to the following news story. One early morning on April 14, 1995 a group of teens were partying when they began to crush and to snort Ritalin. The teenagers thought Ritalin had to be safe or it wouldn't be given out so freely to the younger children. After drinking a couple of beers, 19-year-old Lucas Lawson snorted some Ritalin and collapsed. By the time his friends got him to the emergency room, he was in cardiac arrest. He was resuscitated and put on life support but died eighteen hours later.

Reporter Diane Struzzi (1995) of the *Roanoke Times* interviewed the students:

> His friends say Lawson had no idea that the abuse of Ritalin could be fatal. Why would he, they asked? The use of it has become so common that teens have seen their peers snort up during class or in the bathroom. Some refer to it as Vitamin R—the wonder drug that can keep you up, make you study longer and party harder. Others have been known to take it in the belief it will increase their SAT scores.

Teens told the reporter that it was easy to swipe the drug from their younger siblings or to buy it at $3 to $5 a pill. One high school student explained, "You've got kids who are sick and tired of taking it and they're handing it out to their friends." As quoted at the head of the chapter, another elaborated, "Out of 10 people I know, maybe one has seen or tried cocaine but nine of them have done Ritalin." The students had been warned about dangerous drugs by their parents and by a drug education class in school, but not about Ritalin.

A series of articles over the next year and a half continued to make disclosures concerning Ritalin abuse in the Roanoke schools.[10]

Not Only in Roanoke

One of the most heart-rending legal cases in which I was an expert witness involved a young boy who was started on Ritalin as a child and then turned to other stimulants when taken off Ritalin as a teenager. Eventually he deteriorated into a severe abuser of multiple substances and committed murder for hire in order to support his habit. He was sentenced to death in part because of "expert" testimony by a psychologist (not a medical doctor) that Ritalin was not addictive and could not have contributed to his problems. In a death penalty appeal, I testified to a number of mitigating factors, including the impact of Ritalin on his life. Unfortunately, the judge dismissed the appeal on technical grounds. I am now a medical expert in another case involving a boy who turned to cocaine when his Ritalin was stopped, and who then murdered another child.

I know a number of teenagers who are recovering addicts in the Washington, DC area who tell me that Ritalin is often abused along with other drugs. For some of them, prescribed Ritalin was their first drug. The similarity of our metropolitan area to Roanoke in regard to Ritalin abuse is made clear in an article in the *Washington Post* by Laura Sessions Stepp (1996). Stepp observed, "Because it's a legal drug, many young people see no harm in either snorting it or gulping down larger-than-therapeutic doses." The young people in our area also call it "Vitamin R" as well as "R-ball" and "the smart drug." In some private schools, students have been discovered selling their prescribed Ritalin to classmates:[11]

> Students report that at two prestigious Virginia boarding schools, boys with prescriptions for Ritalin—a drug for attention deficit disorder—have been selling their pills to classmates looking to get high. At one school, a student said, "Ritalin rivals acid and marijuana."

School nurses are warned to be careful of students diverting Ritalin for abuse purposes: "The potential to abuse MPH [Ritalin] is always present."[12]

In the last few years there has also been a marked increase in Ritalin abuse among teenagers and young adults. I recently talked to reporters who were able to obtain Ritalin pills for a dollar or two a pill from college students within minutes of setting foot on campus. Ritalin is commonly used to facilitate all-night cramming for exams and also as a recreational stimulant at parties.

Continued Warnings from the DEA

At the November 1998 Consensus Development Conference, DEA-representative Gretchen Feussner warned:

> However, recent reports of MPH [Ritalin] misuse/abuse among adolescents and young adults are particularly disturbing, since this group has the freest access to this drug. Reports from numerous states and local municipalities indicate that adolescents are giving and selling their MPH medication to friends and classmates, who frequently crush the tablets and snort the powder like cocaine. Anecdotal reports from students and faculty on college campuses indicate that MPH is being used as a study aid in the same manner that amphetamine was used in campuses in the 1960s.

Feussner concluded, "Physicians, parents, and school officials need to be alerted to take the necessary steps to safeguard against the diversion and abuse of this drug."

Ritalin's Long History
as a Drug of Addiction and Abuse

By the early 1960s there were widespread reports of abuse and psychosis associated with Ritalin. Soon many addicts were considering Ritalin the most highly addictive of all stimulants.[13] Some used it intravenously, exposing themselves to the additional risks of internal damage from tiny fragments of the binders and other inert contents of the pills.

In 1968 Sweden withdrew Ritalin from the marketplace due to its escalating abuse. According to Einar Perman (1970), Swedish doctors and medical students felt "considerable resentment" toward American medical journals that continued to advertise the drug: "Swedish doctors see no reason why similar abuse of central stimulants could not appear in other countries if their serious abuse potential is not carefully weighed against their rather limited therapeutic application."

In 1970, the FDA belatedly began to call for curtailment of the production and use of amphetamine drugs, including Ritalin. George Cahill, Jr. (1970) warned that stimulant "drug abuse is an epidemic that to date has found the focus of public health helpless and unprepared." Also in 1970 the Food and Drug Administration reviewed Ritalin, which had been grandfathered into use on the basis of its approval during the 1950s. The FDA placed greater limitations on its approved uses and emphasized more of its adverse effects.[14]

The World Health Organization (WHO) concluded that Ritalin, amphetamine (Dexedrine), and methamphetamine were pharmacologically similar among themselves and to cocaine in their abuse patterns. In 1971 it placed Ritalin along with the other stimulant drugs in Schedule II—the most addictive drugs in medical usage: "Methylphenidate, due to its high abuse potential, was one of the first substances to be placed under international control in Schedule II of the 1971 Convention on Psychotropic Substances."[15]

In 1971, the U.S. Department of Justice also placed Ritalin in Schedule II of the Controlled Substances Act due to its very high potential for abuse. Ritalin joined morphine, opium, and barbiturates in Schedule II. The DEA explained (1995c): "It was found that methylphenidate's pharmacological effects are essentially the same as those of amphetamine and methamphetamine and that it shares the same abuse potential as these Schedule II stimulants."[16] Treaty obligations require the United States to provide the United Nations with data on the production, distribution, and consumption of Ritalin, including its exportation and importation.

By 1971 the FDA was already considering reports of death and blindness from the injection of crushed Ritalin tablets by addicts and drug abusers.[17] It was accepted that "The abuse of amphetamine, methamphetamine, methylphenidate ... is well recognized."[18]

In 1979, the first case of Ritalin addiction and abuse resulting from routine therapy for hyperactivity was reported. The thirteen-year-old boy who had been treated for two years, reaching a maximum dose of 60 mg per day, would get "high," "numb," and develop a "buzz" on larger doses that he stole from his mother.

The FDA's Neurologic Drug Advisory Committee (1977) met more than two decades ago to consider the question of withdrawing amphetamine from the market because of its addictiveness. At that time, clinical toxicologist and drug abuse expert David Smith testified about the stimulants that "all of them, including Ritalin, have high abuse potential."[19] Before other stimulants, including cocaine, became more popular, methylphenidate was one of the most commonly abused street drugs.[20] Stricter federal guidelines then produced a sharp reduction in prescriptions during the latter part of the 1970s,[21] but Ritalin abuse continued to be a significant problem in the addict population.[22] Since then there have been waves of abuse of cocaine, amphetamine, and Ritalin. Addicted adults have used their children's Ritalin prescriptions to foster their own habit.[23]

Ritalin Makes the "Most Wanted List" of Drug Culprits

The International Narcotics Control Board (INCB) (1995, 1996) is an agency of the United Nations that monitors drug addiction and abuse throughout the world. In recent years, it has become gravely concerned about the over-prescription of Ritalin in the United States, as well as the diversion of Ritalin for illegal use as a drug of abuse and addiction.

In its 1995 report, the board warned about increasing abuse of the drug:[24]

The abuse of methylphenidate in the United States has increased and cases have been reported of serious damage to health as a result of such abuse. Methylphenidate is mainly abused by adolescents who illegally obtain the substance in tablet form from children undergoing treatment for ADD.

In its 1996 report, the board continued its warnings:

With respect to abuse, according to estimates of the Drug Abuse Warning Network (DAWN) of the United States, the number of methylphenidate-related emergency room mentions for persons aged 10–14 has since 1990 increased more than 10 times and in 1995 reached the level of cocaine-related mentions for that age group.

The board (1996a) underscored a global escalation in the production of Ritalin from less than 3 tons in 1990 to more than 10 tons in 1995. It anticipated a rise to 13 tons in 1997.[25] The INCB showed particular concern about the United States which it found responsible for 90% of world-wide consumption. Canada was in second place. According to the Board (1996a), Ritalin "is among the top 10 controlled drugs involved in drug thefts and is diverted and abused by health professionals as well as drug addicts." The rising prescription rate for Ritalin has made it readily available for abuse among teenagers. In 1994, 10% of high school seniors reported using amphetamines without a doctor's prescription. Of those, 16.6% were using Ritalin. More recent INCB reports continue to warn about the danger of Ritalin over-prescription and abuse in the United States.

Ritalin—Among the Worst Addictions

The DEA recently reviewed the question of Ritalin's potential for abuse.[26] After a lengthy review of animal research and clinical data, the DEA concludes:

> Like amphetamine and cocaine, abuse of methylphenidate can lead to marked tolerance and psychic dependence. The pattern of abuse is characterized by escalation of dose, frequent episodes of binge use followed by severe depression, and an overpowering desire to continue the use of this drug despite medical and social consequences. The abuser may alter the mode of administration from oral use to snorting or intravenous injection to intensify the effects of the drug. Typical of other CNS stimulants, high doses of methylphenidate often produce agitation, tremors, euphoria, tachycardia, palpitations and hypertension. Psychotic episodes, paranoid delusions, hallucinations and bizarre behavior characteristic of amphetamine-like psychomotor stimulant toxicity have all been associated with methylphenidate abuse. Severe medical consequences, including death, have been reported.... Clearly, the literature indicates that addiction produced by methylphenidate abuse is neither benign nor rare in occurrence, and is more accurately described as producing severe dependence.

Intoxication with stimulant drugs such as Ritalin, amphetamine, and cocaine can produce particularly vicious symptoms in the abuser, including psychosis with paranoia, hallucinations, and delusions. Psychosis is common as a result of abuse of stimulant medication in general and may last for months after termination of the abuse.[27] Chronic users suffer from anxiety, loss of impulse control, and impaired judgment. Feelings of euphoria may give way to severe, suicidal depression. Lives are frequently ruined.

Craving for stimulants usually occurs in two phases—a "crashing" phase immediately after stopping the drug and a more lasting or persistent phase for a lengthy period afterward.

Stimulants produce a particularly rapid addiction. Individuals who use them may become addicted in a much shorter period of time than abusers of alcohol and sedative drugs.[28] Animal studies and clinical observation confirm that addiction to stimulants is commonly much worse than addiction to opiates, sedatives; or alcohol.[29]

Special Dangers of Intravenous Ritalin Abuse

Ritalin abuse can cause many adverse reactions. Often Ritalin has been used intravenously as a drug of abuse. Some of the adverse reactions have been due to the fillers and binders in the ground up tablets that get injected along with the methylphenidate and cause damage to various organs including the lungs, brain, liver and eyes.[30] Cerebral hemorrhages can be produced by abuse of oral Ritalin as well as injected Ritalin.[31]

The Craving for More

Ritalin, amphetamine, methamphetamine and cocaine, as we have described, all stimulate dopamine nerves. Stimulation of the dopamine system is thought to cause or contribute to euphoria—an artificial high. Following stimulation, there is a relative loss of activity in the same dopaminergic system, and this is thought to produce craving, a sense of desperate need for more of the drug-induced stimulation.

Dackis and Gold (1990) theorize that stimulants excite and then deplete dopamine, causing a cycle of euphoria followed by craving. They call this stimulating and depleting the "pleasure circuitry in the brain."

Methamphetamine:
The Most Addictive Stimulant
Approved for ADHD

Methamphetamine is marketed as Desoxyn and Gradumet for the treatment of ADHD. Yet it is notorious for its capacity to cause addiction, abuse, and disturbed behavior. More recently, it has been proven to cause permanent brain damage and cell death (see chapter 3). Because of the similarity of their names, it is easy to confuse methylphenidate (Ritalin) with methamphetamine. Methamphetamine is closely related to both amphetamine and methylphenidate.

Methamphetamine pills are frequently called "speed," while the crystalline form, called "ice," is smoked like "crack" cocaine. Methamphetamine was associated with many episodes of psychoses and violence in the Haight-Ashbury district in California during the 1960s.[32]

Addiction to methamphetamine is on the increase again. According to the International Narcotics Control Board (1995):[33]

In the United States, clandestine manufacture of, illicit traffic in and abuse of methamphetamine are on the increase and constitute significant problems.

Methamphetamine, unlike Ritalin, can be easily manufactured, starting with a readily available drug, ephedrine.

The White House Office of National Drug Control Policy issued a warning that in some areas of the country methamphetamine is becoming the drug most commonly abused by people seeking treatment for addiction and abuse.[34] It vies with another stimulant, cocaine. The report estimates that about 2.5 million Americans use cocaine occasionally and about 400,000 are hardcore users who usually favor crack, an especially addictive form.

The effects of methamphetamine, like those of cocaine, are largely indistinguishable from Ritalin. Amphetamine and methylphenidate abuse is again growing world-wide, including Germany, Great Britain, and Australia.[35] The symptoms associated with abuse, including paranoia and depression, are often more severe for amphetamine than for cocaine.

When is Treatment a Form of Drug Abuse?

It is remarkable that the "Just Say No" campaign against stimulants has faded away into the "Just Say Yes" campaign for stimulants. It can be hard to tell the difference between dependence on prescribed Ritalin and dependence on illegally obtained Ritalin. The American Psychiatric Association's *Diagnostic and Statistical Manual Of Mental Disorders-III-R* description of Ritalin abuse sounds like the use of Ritalin to treat children:[36]

> Chronic daily, or almost daily, use may be at high or low doses. Use may be throughout the course of the day or be restricted to certain hours, e.g., only during the working hours or only during the evening. In this pattern there are usually no wide fluctuations in the amount of amphetamine used on successive occasions, but there is often a general increase in doses over time.

Similarly, writing in the *Journal of the American Medical Association* more than thirty-five years ago, P. H. Connell (1961) spoke about the dangers of amphetamines and amphetamine-like drugs. Connell describes "The individual who takes 2 or 3 tablets a day and cannot carry out the normal tasks of life without them, and who may or may not be distressed at the inability to do without the drugs." While two or three tablets a day is not the most serious level of abuse, Connell believes that the individual "would certainly be better off without them." Connell's description matches exactly the situation of millions of children in America who are being forced to take these drugs for the control of their behavior.

When Your Child Stops Ritalin: Withdrawal Symptoms

As with any addictive drug, when Ritalin use is abruptly stopped, the user can experience withdrawal symptoms. Since the drug's effects begin to wear off after two to four hours, withdrawal can begin to occur a few hours after the child's most recent dose.

Ritalin and amphetamine, as documented in chapter 2, can cause severe withdrawal symptoms, including "crashing" with depression, exhaustion, withdrawal, irritability, and suicidal feelings, or excitability, euphoria, and hyperactivity. Psychosis can be precipitated by withdrawal from stimulants. Typically parents will not recognize a withdrawal reaction when their child gets upset or disturbed after missing even a single dose. They will mistakenly believe that their child needs to be put back on the medication or needs more of it.

According to the Drug Enforcement Administration (1995c):[37]

> Abstinence from psychomotor stimulants, such as d-amphetamine and cocaine, after chronic use results in the appearance of withdrawal signs within one to three days, including depression, sleep disturbances, anxiety, fatigue, anger/hostility, dysphoria, psychomotor agitation, confusion and drug craving. Case studies document the same type of syndrome with methylphenidate abstinence after chronic use.

Stimulants produce less intense *physical* withdrawal reactions than some other agents, such as alcohol or opiates. This has led to the mistaken notion that they do not produce withdrawal at all. But it is now recognized within the addiction field that the intense craving or need for stimulants, and other painful emotional reactions to withdrawal, are not "merely psychological." They constitute a physically-based withdrawal syndrome.

Tolerance and Sensitization

Constant exposure to stimulant drugs can produce tolerance, or a reduction in drug effect, as the brain compensates for the effects. Thus, the drugs may lose their tendency to produce euphoria, requiring increased doses to achieve an equivalent effect. At the same time, some brain functions seem to become more sensitive to stimulation. This may be why stimulants can cause seizures, cardiac arrhythmias, and psychotic symptoms such as hallucinations and delusions. The result can be confusing as the child becomes seemingly less affected by the drug while some adverse effects actually worsen.

How to Withdraw a Child from Stimulants

When withdrawing a child from any psychiatric or psychoactive drug, it is always best to do so with experienced clinical supervision. The professional who supervises the process should know about drugs without being compulsively devoted to them. Often this is a difficult combination to find. A parent may wish to provide this book to the professional since it contains information that is not otherwise readily available.

Partly because it is so difficult to locate professionals who are willing to help parents withdraw their children from psychiatric drugs, many parents proceed on their own. In regard to stimulant drugs administered in doses approved by the FDA and by textbooks, it is often possible for children to come off these drugs without severe consequences.

Many, many parents simply stop giving their child the prescribed Ritalin or amphetamine, especially when it has been given for only a few weeks or months in routine doses. Sometimes this withdrawal is uneventful, but sometimes problems arise. Similarly, parents often stop their children's drugs "cold turkey" on weekends and in the summers without any serious adverse effects. But it is better to be cautious and to withdraw more slowly under clinical supervision.

The longer the child has been exposed and the higher the doses, the more caution the parent must use, and the more need there is for gradual withdrawal and for experienced clinical supervision. The more troubled a child has been, the more cautious a parent needs to be during withdrawal. It is common for behavior to worsen temporarily.

All stimulants tend to produce withdrawal symptoms. This is true of Ritalin, methamphetamine, and amphetamine, which are highly addictive, and also Cylert (pemoline) which is rarely addictive. The main danger in withdrawing children from these drugs is "crashing," with various mental disturbances, especially fatigue or inertia, depression, and suicidal tendencies. More rarely, a child may become paranoid and psychotic during withdrawal. The child may sleep and eat an enormous amount.

Withdrawal from stimulants is rarely physically life-threatening. However, withdrawal can be psychologically life-threatening if it results in depression and suicide or, more rarely, paranoid or psychotic reactions.

There is also the danger of the child turning to other drugs for relief of emotional tensions that worsen during withdrawal. Children may resort not only to illegal stimulants but to caffeine, alcohol, or sedatives. Many young drug abusers mix a variety of seemingly contradictory combinations of drugs.

There is no simple rule for withdrawing from stimulants. Parents and other adults should remain in close touch with the child, check regularly on how the child is feeling, and provide as much emotional support as needed. Nothing is more important than a trusting relationship with an adult during this time.

Each child will react differently to withdrawal from stimulant drugs. The best way to evaluate your child's reaction is to partially reduce the dose for one day while carefully staying in touch with his or her feelings and responses. While many children can be withdrawn in a few days of gradual dose reduction, I would suggest at least one month's duration of gradual withdrawal. Even if your child has come off the drugs abruptly without problems in the past, withdrawal problems may have become worse as the treatment period has lengthened or as the dose has been increased.

In no case, should withdrawal be continued if a child begins to feel emotionally disturbed, paranoid, highly fatigued, depressed, or suicidal. Obviously, clinical consultation and supervision become even more necessary at such times. However, the parent should be cautious about starting the child on an alternative drug to replace the Ritalin or to treat the withdrawal symptoms. This is likely to further compromise the child's brain function, further delaying the withdrawal process.

Remember that your child's behavioral problems are very likely to worsen during withdrawal. This can be due to rebound from the drug or due to the resurfacing of problems that were masked by the drug. Children need our attention—almost always more attention than we feel we have the time to give. During drug withdrawal, children especially need our attention. Give as much as you can. You may find that it sets a precedent that you and your child will continue to enjoy and to benefit from in your life together.

For parents and professionals who want to know more about how to withdraw children from stimulant medications, I have devoted a whole chapter to the subject in a recent book co-authored with David Cohen, *Your Drug May Be Your Problem: How and Why to Stop Taking Psychiatric Medications* (1999).

Controls over Ritalin Prescription

Due to its addiction and abuse potential, many countries have an *upper* age limit (as well as a lower) for the prescription of Ritalin.[38] In the United States, there is no upper limit, and there is an increasing trend to prescribe it for adults. Some nations also have limits on how many years the drug can be prescribed but again this is not so for the United States where the tendency is to prescribe stimulants for increasingly longer periods of time.

All countries place some restrictions on Ritalin prescriptions, including the United States, where a prescription must be renewed in writing each month. In some countries, it requires a special license to prescribe Ritalin but in the United States any doctor can do so. In many countries, including Austria, Finland, France, Ireland and Norway, more than one expert opinion is required before prescribing Ritalin. In Australia the policy varies from state to state.

Most countries report that additional therapies are required when Ritalin is prescribed. While this view is advocated by experts in the United States, "few children are treated with anything other than methylphenidate" in the U.S.[39] Now of course, the amphetamines, especially Adderall, are increasingly used instead of Ritalin.

Are We Institutionalizing Drug Abuse?

ADHD/Ritalin advocates pay almost no attention to the fact that Ritalin and amphetamine are highly addictive and frequently abused drugs. Ritalin and Dexedrine, when prescribed by doctors, can become gateway drugs to the abuse of stimulants and other substances. Earlier in the chapter, I described research indicating that children who take prescribed stimulants are more prone to stimulant and cigarette abuse in young adulthood.

Youngsters give away or sell their prescribed stimulants to friends who then abuse the drug. Sometimes parents steal their children's medications. U.S. and international drug control agencies are expressing deep concern about the over-prescription of these potentially addictive drugs. But there's a different kind of gateway that Ritalin opens up—the gateway to other psychiatric drugs. In the long run, this may prove its greatest danger—teaching children to think of themselves in psychiatric diagnostic terms and to handle their problems and conflicts with drugs.

Dackis and Gold (1990) explain, "the marketing of cocaine is greatly facilitated by its safe mythology, so that both dealers and addicts are quick to promote the idea that this stimulant is safe and non-addictive." They remind us, "The controversy over stimulant addictiveness has therefore varied with the mystique surrounding particular agents and the time period in question." Right now the mystique surrounding Ritalin and amphetamines for children tends to gloss over, or to deny, their serious addiction and abuse potential.

Michael Parry (1997), a concerned citizen, wrote to his local newspaper:

> While we challenge our youth to "Just Say No" to one form of drug abuse, have we institutionalized another? Is it any less a national tragedy?

The "Just Say No" campaign was aimed at discouraging children from taking dangerous and addictive drugs such as amphetamine and methylphenidate (Ritalin). We viewed with loathing those who "pushed" these stimulant drugs on children. Yet today there are more children taking Ritalin and amphetamine from doctors than ever received them from illegal pushers. Furthermore, the ready availability of prescribed stimulants has led to their increasing illegal use by children and youth. The medical profession has led the way in creating a tidal wave of stimulant abuse among our children and youth, first by prescribing the drugs directly to millions of them, second by propagandizing teachers, parents, and children in general to believe that the drugs are safe and useful, and third by flooding the black market with these substances through their over-prescription.

Chapter 6

"THEY NEVER LIKE THE MEDICATION"

How Children Feel about Taking Ritalin and How Adults React to Them

The child can conclude that he is not responsible for his behavior: "I can't help being bad today. I haven't had my pill." The child comes to believe not in the soundness of his own brain and body, not in his growing ability to learn and to control his behavior, but in "my magic pills that make me into a good boy and make everybody like me."

—L. Alan Sroufe and Mark A. Stewart,
New England Journal of Medicine (1973)

But guess what? A lot of kids don't want to take their medication. For four juniors I found hanging out near Bethesda-Chevy Chase High School in an affluent suburb of Washington, refusal is rebellion. "People should talk to their kids, not just give them pills," says David, 16, who says he was urged to take antidepressants because he was staying in his room all the time after his alcoholic mother left the family. "They thought I was depressed or gothic or something," he says. "I think I was just unhappy."

—Arthur Allen, journalist (1997)

The look in the eyes of a child on Ritalin is like the look in Peter Pan's eyes when Tinkerbell is mortally wounded; like the magic has been snuffed out.

—Kevin McCready (1997), director,
San Joaquin Psychotherapy Center, Clovis, California

Ritalin made me withdrawn. Ritalin made me lifeless. My mother noticed a boy who was not her son anymore. She took me off after two weeks.

—A.G.[1]

How do children feel about stimulants and will they tell their doctors the truth about it? Questions like this are almost never examined by advocates of ADHD/Ritalin. With few exceptions, the literature doesn't comment on what the children themselves feel about any aspect of being diagnosed and drugged. One terse exception was provided by Paul Wender (1973) who noted early on, "they never like the medication." This is confirmed by the high rates of "noncompliance"—failure or refusal to take the medication. Noncompliance to Ritalin can vary from 10% in closely monitored research projects to one-third in clinical practice according to Safer and Allen (1989).

If you read the next pages, you'll have more information than, up to now, has been available to mental health professionals. Two of the major studies that look at the thoughts and attitudes of these children have been unpublished, one for reasons about which we can only speculate, and the other because it consists of a recently completed doctoral dissertation.

Many Hate the Drug

The feelings of children in reaction to Ritalin were studied by a project from the Institute of Child Behavior and Development at the University of Illinois.[2] The results—seldom cited in ADHD/Ritalin reviews—were shocking.

Among the 52 children diagnosed hyperactive, many hated the drug but lied to their doctor about it. The researchers checked the actual viewpoints of the children by finding inconsistencies in their interviews, by observing their behavior outside the sessions, and by questioning adults about the children's willingness to take the drugs.

The study concluded, "Above all else, we found a pervasive dislike among hyperactive children for taking stimulants." The authors believe, "The intensity of the dislike of many hyperactive children for taking stimulants is a troubling phenomenon." Forty-two percent "disliked" or "hated" it. Six children reported feelings of "depression" in reaction to the drug, such as "I don't want to play," "It makes me sad…" and "I wouldn't smile or anything." Seven reported a "drugged feeling," including "spaced out," "It numbed me," and "It takes over of me; it takes control." Ten reported negative changes in perception of self, such as "It makes me feel like a baby" and "Don't feel like myself." One reported rebound, stating he was "wild" after the medication wore off.

While only four children said so openly, the researchers felt that 16 of the children felt that "taking medication was a source of embarrassment to them." The children also mentioned adverse physical reactions of insomnia, anorexia, and stomachache.

As the extensive documentation in this book confirms, these children were not exaggerating. These effects are often reported by physicians, sometimes as improvements when the children become more numb or docile.

Telling Doctors What They Want to Hear

The interviewers in the University of Illinois study found many inconsistencies within the interviews, and between the interviews and the child's statements and behavior elsewhere. Their main tendency was to "overstate their enthusiasm for drug treatment and their adherence to the prescribed regimen." Children will almost always tell authority figures such as doctors what they imagine the adults want to hear. They may consciously or unconsciously lie in order to gain approval. They may want to avoid negative responses or punishments for not liking or not taking the drug. They may want to avoid being forced to take more of the drug.

When told what they want to hear by children, adults too often will accept it as the truth. In this study, "Of 23 interviews proven totally or partially unreliable, 21 were coded by raters as having good credibility." The children, while distorting the truth, came across as "sincere and believable" to the doctor and two other raters. This is not so much a criticism of the children who could be expected to play up to doctors who are trying to drug them. It is a commentary on the doctors who ought to know better than to accept "apple polishing" as the truth. The study also raised the possibility that a "great many" children are "thought to be improved because of their medication but are failing to take it."

From Walter Reed: Kids' Ideas on Why They Take Stimulants

Will giving children drugs to control their behavior end up undermining their sense of autonomy and self-control? The only two studies to examine this problem are unpublished.

Peter Jensen, as noted earlier in the book, was chief of the NIMH research branch on children and adolescents and is now a professor at Columbia University. He was on the staff of Walter Reed in Washington, DC at the time that he authored, "Why Johnny Can't Sit Still: Kids' Ideas On Why They Take Stimulants."[3] It is unpublished but briefly summarized in *Science News*.[4]

Using interviews, child psychiatric rating scales, and a projective test entitled "Draw a Person Taking the Pill," Jensen and his team systematically evaluated twenty children given Ritalin by their primary care physicians. Taking Ritalin produced the following negative psychological, moral, and social effects:

(1) "defective superego formation" manifested by "disowning responsibility for their provocative behavior"

(2) "impaired self-esteem development"

(3) "lack of resolution of critical family events which preceded the emergence of the child's hyperactive behavior"

(4) displacement of "family difficulties onto the child."

Many of the children concluded that they were "bad." They believed they were given the pills to "control them." They often ascribed their negative conduct to outside forces, such as eating sugar or failing to take their pill, and not to themselves or their own actions.

Jensen and his colleagues were concerned that the use of stimulant medication "has significant effects on the psychological development of the child." They warned that it distracts parents, teachers, and doctors from paying proper attention to problems in the child's environment. In effect, the act of prescribing Ritalin seemed to relieve everyone involved, child and family, as well as teachers and doctors, from taking responsibility for improving the situation of the child.

The researchers conclude:

> Research investigating children's perceptions of the meanings of stimulant medication, as mediated by the family context, adult and child attributions, and the child's developmental level, are long overdue.

A School Social Worker Asks the Children What They Think

Kate Clarke is a social worker in an Illinois public school. In her research for her unpublished doctoral dissertation in social work, she interviewed twenty children to find out what they thought about their experience being diagnosed and then treated with Ritalin.[5]

Adverse Medical Effects

Most of the children said that the drug was helpful to them, often citing improvement in whatever area they thought the drug would be helpful. For example, one child reported that the drug had no effect except to help him speak better, even though his speech had always been normal. Observations like this led Clarke to believe that many of the children were saying what they were expected to say about the drug's supposed benefits.

The children described a variety of adverse drug effects consistent with the drug's actions on the body, including "stomachaches, headaches, loss of appetite, dizziness, sweating, and difficulty falling asleep." Some worried about not growing as much or as fast as they should. Many of the children feared the unknown long-range effects of the drug: "Sometimes I wonder, I mean I'm still young, and I'm not going to get like totally hurt by swallowing a pill." In this regard, they seemed more realistic than most psychiatrists and other advocates of the drug.

Loss of Stamina and Ability

Many children reported a "decrease in their abilities in several respects." Tiredness and loss of energy were commonly attributed to taking the medication: "On Ritalin it's just like, you're really not in the mood to do anything;" "I'm lazy, and I can't do as much, I mean, I'm more tired," and "At recess I don't like to want to run, like play, because it (the Ritalin) makes you tired." One child felt he "lost power" and another spoke of "getting used to being tired from taking the pills." Another child described her heart beating fast when she took the drug, along with a "hyper" burst of energy, after which "you're tired and you're... lousy...and like lazy...and tired."[6]

When Clarke made these observations, she was unaware of evidence that the drugs work primarily by flattening normal spontaneous behavior in favor of rote, command performance. The reports by the children seem to confirm that Ritalin defuses the child's energy, especially for spontaneous activities. The energetic youngster is then more willing or able to perform required tasks.

Impact on the Child's Sense of Self

Five children expressed fears that taking the medication made others think of them as "stupid," "weird," or "sicko." A few described being teased or ridiculed by peers. According to Clarke, "One youngster admitted, 'I kind of feel weird, because you need a pill to control yourself.'" Clarke observed, "Very few were comfortable with peers knowing about their taking medication."

As in the Walter Reed study, being diagnosed and medicated seemed to undermine many children's sense of being in charge of themselves, their actions, or their lives. One child said, "I think it is a kind of sickness, because it, it kind of takes over, I know it takes over my body... it's like you don't have that much control... I kind of feel weird, because you need a pill to control yourself."

Only one of the students saw the drug in what Clarke describes as a healthy perspective. While receiving support from the drug, he realized he still had to control himself. "However," Clarke concluded, "so healthy a conception of the medication experience was rare." All the other children "felt dependent on their pills." They feared lower grades and less control over their behavior if the medication were no longer available to them. They attributed their failures or difficulties to insufficient medication effect. The Ritalin "wasn't working so well at the time," or "hasn't kicked in all the way."

A number of the children saw their drug use as "very troubling" in a way that reminded Clarke of how youngsters feel about using illegal drugs. They felt it was wrong or bad to be relying on a drug. Drug-taking was in conflict with their values. This of course is a conflict created by a society that conducts a "Just say no to drugs" campaign against stimulants obtained illegally while it conducts a "Just say yes to drugs" campaign for stimulants prescribed by physicians.

While to some extent these children felt empowered by the drug, the power is experienced as coming from an external source. Their responses to the interview indicated to Clarke that "feeling dependent on the drug" also made them feel "helpless" and unable to live without it. Many felt fearful of their future without the drug while remaining fearful as well about taking it for the rest of their lives.

Consistent with feeling dependent on the drug, many of the children thought that their need for the drug made them different in a negative way. Clarke pointed out:

> The often heard expression, "he's ADD" or "I'm ADD" carries with it the impression of defining the person. Add to that an ongoing daily routine of taking pills for the condition, and children's perceptions of being different in a negative way and [their] sense of embarrassment become understandable.

One child admitted, "I kind of feel weird, because you need like a pill to control yourself... It's not something to be proud of." According to Clarke, "Clearly then, children do appear to infer from the medication experience the meaning that they are different in a negative way. This would account for the shame and fear of being perceived that way by peers."

Why Are Experts So Oblivious?

Why are ADHD/Ritalin experts so little aware of the feelings of the children they diagnose and medicate? In part because they don't want to know and therefore don't ask. They then read the silence as if it's a positive communication. Clarke was already counseling two of the children before they became part of the research project. Neither ever brought up any problems with Ritalin during the counseling sessions. Yet they "expressed anxieties and reservations regarding taking medication" during her research interview in which she asked about their attitudes. She concludes, "It would appear that children are unlikely to initiate a discussion about problems associated with having to take medication for ADHD, even in a counseling session with a therapist, but, if invited and given the opportunity to do so, they will talk readily and willingly." A caveat should be added, however. The children might be ready and willing, provided they are talking with a warm, empathic professional like Clarke. It also helps if the professional is not invested in hearing the children praise the drug.

Afterward, a More Concerned Clarke

Clarke's research, and subsequent experiences, have made her more wary about Ritalin. In a personal communication to me (1997b), she described rebound effects:

> In my work as a school social worker, children and parents have informed me of the difficulties they have in coping with the 'rebound effect' some children experience at home in afternoons when the effect of the noon

dose of Ritalin administered at school wears off. These children become so hyperactive that parents administer another dose at home. This then results in difficulty falling asleep. Consequently, some young children stay up until 10:00 PM or later, and for some sleeping pills are routinely prescribed.

Parental Responses
When Their Children Are Diagnosed and Medicated

There are, of course, an infinite number of ways parents can respond to their children being diagnosed and treated with mind-altering drugs. Many parents will feel a myriad of confusing and even contradictory feelings: relief at "having an answer," relief at "having something we can do," gratitude if the child seems to be doing better, concern over stigmatizing their child, worry over the unknown or long-term effects of the drug.

There are also more detrimental responses that parents can undergo. Jensen's group recognized that parents and other adults in a child's life tend to stop offering as much help once the child is diagnosed and medicated, and that family problems tend to become blamed on the child.

William Stableford (1976) and a group from the University of Vermont Department of Psychology addressed the impact of giving drugs on the parents themselves. Their clinical observations were bolstered by two cases in which they substituted placebo for Ritalin and Dexedrine, and found no change in the child's behavior. When they then tried to stop the placebo, one child's behavior drastically deteriorated. They observed what they felt was a strong dependence on the placebo on the part of the two sets of parents:

> A child, his parents, teachers, etc. all become dependent on the ingestion of pills per se, independent of the chemical effects of a drug.

They warn that it's best to try alternative treatments before drugs, because after drugs are given, parents are not likely to want to try anything else:

> Handing a child a pill each day is a simple task, and it allows the parents the comfort of placing the explanation for their child's hyperactive behavior on his physiological makeup. They are thereby absolved of any responsibility.
> Too often, they confirm, parents are unwilling to look at their own contribution to their child's problems. Diagnosing and medicating the child reinforces this tendency.

In another early paper, Schleifer and his colleagues (1975) described the devastating psychological and social effects of Ritalin on preschoolers. They also documented the eagerness of parents to attribute any positive change in their children to medication. They noted that parents "tended to have high expectations that the drug would help their children" and that some mothers reported "dramatic behavioral changes while their children were receiving placebo." The authors had the "clinical impression that mothers preferred to attribute improvements to medication rather than to other variables." They also raised the possibility that the teachers and the children were responding to placebo as well, and that the mothers might be observing genuine changes in their children. Since the children were only three and four years old, it seems that the placebo was more likely affecting their parents than the children themselves who might not have had such grand expectations of the drug.

Nowadays it would be unusual to find papers like these in the professional literature. Professionals and parents have joined in an unfortunate alliance to absolve themselves of any psychological, social, or spiritual responsibility for the child's well-being. Instead, they rely on diagnoses and drugs. This not only harms the child, it robs the professionals and parents alike of the deeper satisfactions that come with understanding the child's situation and reaching out to fulfill the child's needs.

Who Has the Wrong Idea— the Children and Parents, or the "Experts"?

In 1991 Alan Kwasman, Barbara Tinsley and Heidi Lepper published a survey taken of pediatricians that included questions about their use and knowledge of stimulant drugs. Asked to describe parental misunderstandings about medications, they listed several negative ones, "including such responses as parents believe medicine is addicting, dangerous, or damaging to the body, causes zombielike states, and inhibits growth." The authors also seem to think that these are mistaken ideas. They don't want to believe that so many parents hold these views. They suggest that the reports of the pediatricians were an over-reaction to "a vocal minority of parents who are dissatisfied." This is most remarkable. The parents in fact are reporting real problems with these drugs. But the surveyed pediatricians and the authors of the survey dismiss them.

Similarly, the surveyed pediatricians were asked to report the children's misunderstandings about ADHD: "Specifically, pediatricians reported that children believe that drugs make them feel different, drugs take away control of their behavior, they should say no to drugs, drugs make everything better, and that medication harms them." Once again both the surveyed physicians and the authors of the article reject these supposedly mistaken perceptions. Yet with the exception of "drugs make everything better," the children's perceptions are based in reality. And considering the hype they are given about drugs, it's understandable that the children have the idea that "drugs make everything better."

The survey describes a most remarkable situation: Parents and children reported accurately on some of the dangers associated with stimulant drugs; but the doctors and experts didn't agree with them or believe them. The doctors probably tried to talk the parents out of their valid perceptions.

How is it possible that parents and children have better insight into the dangers of Ritalin than the doctors themselves? The parents and children are learning from their own experiences and from the experiences that other parents and children share with them. The doctors habitually reject what they are told by patients and their families and instead spout the medical party line.

Fifty-three percent of the doctors in this survey reported spending an hour or more making their initial evaluation of the child. If it is true that half of them spent an hour or more with their patients (it does seem doubtful to me), then about half were spending *less than an hour*, making life-shaping decisions to diagnose and medicate the children in their practices. From their negative responses to what the parents and children were saying about Ritalin, no matter how much time they spent with their patients and families, they wouldn't really be listening.

Psychologist David Keirsey warns (1988):

> The people who prescribe chemotherapy for inattention and restless action have no idea of how damaging it is.... As for mental effects, such as the child coming to see himself as a damaged person, these prescriptors remain quite oblivious.

Being Stigmatized Has Career Consequences

Not only are children being stigmatized in their own eyes by the ADHD diagnosis and drugs, they may meet rejection in adult life because of their prior history of diagnosis and treatment. Psychiatrist Mortimer Ostow (1997) recently *encouraged* the stigmatization of adults diagnosed with ADHD. In a letter to the *New York Times*, he declared that "the stigmatization of political candidates who have had psychiatric treatment" is in some cases warranted. He cites "adult attention deficit disorder" as a "mental disorder" that is "usually" accompanied by impaired emotional control and judgment. Once again it is psychiatry itself that stigmatizes its own patients.

Most people are not planning to run for political office. But many of the youngsters labeled ADHD may want to enter the armed services. Will their diagnosis be an impediment? At a recent convention, a man with ramrod stature approached me and explained that he was a retired career Army officer. He had a story he wanted to share through my book. His son, Ian, was always lackadaisical about school, always passing but almost never getting good grades. Sometimes he would finish an assignment and then forget to bring it to school. Other times, he would forget to do it altogether. Like a lot of kids who are bored at school, he was a computer whiz. But it didn't translate into academic performance.

In Ian's senior year of high school, his parents took him to a University of Tennessee psychiatrist who recommended Ritalin. Everyone hoped it might salvage some of his school career. Taking the drug during the weekdays only, it was easy to see the effect. Ian became nervous and talkative. He had trouble sleeping and lost weight. At night he had a tendency to become tired and depressed as the drug wore off.

But Ian's grades improved. Dad wasn't sure, though, if the drug was doing it. At the doctor's urging, Dad had changed his own attitude by "staying on Ian's butt" about school. He became more involved than ever before in his son's school efforts.

When Ian went off to college, he decided he didn't like what Ritalin did to him, and he stopped taking it. School still didn't interest him, and after talking it over with his parents, he decided to follow in his dad's footsteps by joining the Army.

Ian aced the Army aptitude test with a 95 out of 100. But the Army wouldn't take him because he'd been honest enough to write on the questionnaire that he'd taken Ritalin the year before. No illegal drugs—just prescription Ritalin. The Army sent him a notice that they could not induct anyone who had taken prescription Ritalin after age twelve.

Dad was horrified and outraged. He got a second opinion from a psychologist who was kind enough to declare Ian "lackadaisical" rather than ADHD. Dad then used his pull as a retired officer to get Ian into the service.

Ian's done well in the service, even earned a humanitarian award. But he's got no future in the Army. While the Army did agree to induct him, it put a ceiling on his level of responsibility. Despite his computer abilities, he can't have assignments of higher responsibility, such as electronic surveillance or radar, or even a military driver's license. Dad knows how unjust this is because he worked with tank drivers who, he's certain, had borderline intelligence.

Ian and his dad are not alone. Gary Kane's 1996 news service story has an even more disappointing outcome. Kane tells about a young man from Georgia named Christopher Gore who was prescribed small doses of Ritalin from 1985 to 1988, and then intermittently until 1991. He was turned down for the Coast Guard in 1994. "It was a disappointment," he said, "And the irony is that I never wanted to take Ritalin in the first place. It wasn't like I was dependent on it."

Because of the young man's outstanding intelligence and personal qualities, his local Coast Guard recruiter appealed his case. Without a military father to back him up, Chris wasn't as lucky as Ian. He was turned down for "Use of Ritalin after age 12 years."

Reporter Kane learned from the Pentagon that "All branches of the armed services reject potential enlistees who use Ritalin or similar behavior-modifying drugs." A long-standing Department of Defense directive also instructs the military to reject those with a "chronic history" of academic skill deficiencies, including ADD, if these have continued after age twelve. Kane was also told that potential enlistees who took Ritalin as teenagers to treat ADHD would also be rejected. A spokesman for the service said that Ritalin was considered a "mind-altering drug." Ironically, as described in chapter 1, the occasional use of small doses of stimulants is encouraged among flyers in the armed forces in order to handle fatigue during combat missions.[7]

The military can be an ideal place for young men to learn to control problems that they have with attention and impulse control. It certainly finds adequate outlets for "hyperactivity." Ironically, the institution that might help these young men the most is now closed to many of them due to the success of the ADHD/Ritalin advocates in promoting Ritalin.

A recent report by Joyce Baldwin in *Psychiatric Times*, titled "Military Policy on Ritalin Use Under Examination," indicates that the military is reviewing its policy. The Department of Defense policy paper quoted in Baldwin's article points to the need for "service members who can be deployed worldwide without the need for specialized medical treatment or prescription medications." It adds, "Equally important, because Ritalin is a controlled drug with considerable abuse potential, we cannot allow it to be possessed by our recruits while in basic or advanced training."

Since the publication of the first edition of *Talking Back to Ritalin* in 1998, the military had changed its policies. Information from recruiting centers indicates that the armed forces now make individual determinations concerning whether or not prior use of prescribed stimulants will prevent induction. However, I was unable to obtain any written regulations clarifying the new standards.

A Sound Warning

While few studies have actually asked children about their responses to being diagnosed and drugged, some professionals have warned that there can be negative effects. Paul Lavin (1991), a psychologist at Towson State in Maryland, states "The aim of school is to educate children to become productive members of a democratic society. We want our children to become self-confident, successful persons who can assume responsibility for their behavior." He concludes that "our current treatment of ADHD" flies in the face of achieving these goals. Children labeled ADHD "come to believe that external events such as luck, fate, or other people are responsible for their success or failure. Such an attitude is hardly conducive to the development of self-confidence and success. Rather, it leads to low self-esteem, depression, and feelings of ineffectiveness."

Mina Dulcan, whose reviews on the treatment of children appear in widely read textbooks, recognizes that there may be adverse moral, psychological, and social effects on children who are prescribed Ritalin. According to Dulcan (1994), these include:[8]

...indirect and inadvertent cognitive and social consequences, such as lower self-esteem and self-efficacy; attribution by child, parents, and teachers of both success and failure to medication, rather than to the child's effort; stigmatization by peers; and dependence by parents and teachers on medication rather than making needed changes in the environment.

"Child, Your Brain Is Broken"

One of the saddest aspects of the ADHD/Ritalin movement is the unbridled willingness to tell children they have "broken brains," even in books written for children.[9] To call this a stigmatization of children is not strong enough. Children can grow up and overcome a stigma if they feel it's unwarranted or unjust. But how can children overcome the idea, taught to them by doctors, that they have defective brains?

Putting on the Brakes (1991) is a book for young children by Patricia O. Quinn, a pediatrician, and Judith M. Stern, a teacher. The book begins by comparing the child to a sports car:

Imagine a slick, hot, red sports car driving around a track. It's flying down the stretches, speeding around the curves, smooth, low to the road, the engine racing...BUT...it has no brakes. It can't stop when the driver wants to stop. It can't slow down to a safer speed. It may get off the track, or even crash! It will certainly have a hard time proving to everyone what it really can do.

If you have attention deficit hyperactivity disorder (ADHD), you may be just like that racing car. You have a good engine (with lots of thinking power) and a good strong body, but NO BRAKES.

Professionals like Patricia Quinn are seemingly so remote from the feelings of children that they don't realize the dreadful implications of telling children that they are like a soul-less automobile.

In their chapter entitled "What Is Going On In The Brain?" Quinn and Stern hammer home to the children that they have a brain disease. The authors display, "courtesy of Alan J. Zametkin, M.D.," misleading photographs of brain scans from Zametkin's 1991 publication.[10] The child will learn from this misinformation that "the decreased brain activity shows up in these pictures in the darker areas" or "the brain may not have enough neu-rotransmitters to relay messages consistently." What a dreadful thing to tell children about themselves. It's not even true! As Zametkin himself admits,[11] the brain scans don't show anything abnormal! There's no way to tell the brain of a child labeled ADHD from the brain of a "normal" child. But even if there were scientific evidence to support such a contention, should PET scans indicating an abnormal brain be put in a book for children to read about themselves?

Putting On The Brakes demonstrates the incredible insensitivity, the utter lack of empathy, of many ADHD/Ritalin advocates. The book has endorse-ments from the big brass of the ADHD/Ritalin movement, including Alan Zametkin, Russell Barkley, and Barbara Ingersoll.

We are raising a generation of children, many of whom are being told they have something wrong in their brains that won't ever go away. Not only are they stigmatized in their own eyes; they are stigmatized in the eyes of others. Many of them understand that they have been given pills instead of love, understanding, or attention. Most, of course, will not realize what they are missing from other people. They will assume that adults are supposed to give pills to children instead of giving them psychological and spiritual support. The children will end up blaming themselves for wanting more love and attention than they have been given.

The biopsychiatric establishment complains self-righteously about the "stigma" attached to "mental illness." But who is responsible for the stigma—who is telling six-year-olds that they have "brain disorders"? It is the ADHD/Ritalin advocates themselves. Psychiatric organizations and drug companies, as well as parent groups like CHADD and NAMI, sponsor cam-paigns for "mental illness recognition week" and for treating "the mentally ill" with drugs and electroshock.[12] These groups cling to and promote the idea of labeling people mentally ill. They continue to expand this horrendous label to cover more and more children. Yet they lament the stigmatizing effects brought about by their own policies.

The issue is not whether individual physicians are kind and thoughtful people. Of course they are! But if they implement the basically destructive ADHD/Ritalin approach to children, they will be doing a great deal of harm. They will not only offend the basic Hippocratic principle, "First, do no harm," they will be doing more harm than good.

The Self-Fulfilling Prophecy: You Can't Control Yourself

Educator Michael Valentine writes books and conducts workshops in which he emphasizes that our belief system about a child will affect our expectations and communications with the child. He makes clear that the ADHD diagnosis limits our expectations and encourages children to give up self-control.

Valentine observes (1987):

Imagine that Mrs. Morgan believes that Jeff, a student in her fifth-grade classroom, has Parkinson's disease because she observed him shaking. Would she tell him to stop shaking? Probably she would not—because of her belief that he could not control his behavior. However, if Jeff always stopped shaking while talking to his best friend but shook during all other interactions, then what would Mrs. Morgan think? Perhaps she would question her belief that it was Parkinson's disease which caused Jeff to shake in all situations and that he thus had no control of his behavior.

Valentine's point is critical to how adults relate to children once they are diagnosed with ADHD. The adults adopt limited expectations. For example, they are likely to assume that the child cannot learn normal self-control. This is one of the most damaging aspects of diagnosing children with behavioral disorders. We encourage the harmful behavior by limiting our expectations for the child.

Valentine is able to examine in detail how an adult's beliefs about a child will govern the kinds of things that are said to the child. In simplest terms, if you believe that an unruly boy is incapable of sitting down, you are not likely to command him to do so in a firm and convincing manner.

Putting a Face on the Child

Paul Wender (1995), the father of ADHD, declared:

I believe that ADHD is a genetically transmitted and biologically mediated group of conditions and that it is virtually certain that the individuals we classify as having ADHD are genetically—and therefore biologically—heterogeneous [varied]. I am here hypothesizing that genetically transmitted psychiatric disorders are no different from other genetically transmitted medical disorders. Thus, I believe that ADHD might be like the disorders of hemoglobin synthesis, such as sickle cell disease, hemoglobin C, and the thalassemias, of which there are at least 300 forms, or the more than 200 variants of glucose-6-phosphate dehydrogenase.

Let's put the face of a living, breathing child on these biological theories. The approach epitomized by Paul Wender has consequences for the children who are diagnosed and treated. Let's indulge a fantasy. Imagine you are a small child, perhaps eight years old, who is feeling fidgety and awkward in the presence of a famous doctor. Your mom has told you that the doctor is one of the greatest child psychiatrists. He holds views similar to those of Wender who declares "Thus, I believe that ADHD might be like the disorders of hemoglobin synthesis, such as sickle cell disease, hemoglobin C, and the thalassemias, of which there are at least 300 forms, or the more than 200 variants of glucose-6-phosphate dehydrogenase."

You already feel like something of a freak because you need to see a shrink, and because you can't seem to get along at school, and because your mom and dad have separated, and it seems like your dad hardly ever tries to visit you. Now you look up at this important doctor, a man with a big face like your dad's, and he looks a little scary. As he looks down at you, you can see he's noticed that your foot is moving nervously. You try to hold it still. You can sense him inspecting you with all the empathy of a man peering at one of "the thalassemias, of which there are at least 300 forms, or the more than 200 variants of glucose-6-phosphate dehydrogenase." You can't explain why, but you want to crawl into a little ball and hide.

Listening to a Fourteen-Year-Old

We do need to listen more to our children. Writing in his junior high newspaper, "The Pyle Print" in Bethesda, Maryland, Matt Scherbel (1995), age 14, declared:

They are dreamers. That doesn't mean they are wrong. They just don't fit the norm, so they are labeled and damned, labeled as ADD. So the doctors dope us up with Ritalin and control our minds with low doses of speed. The teachers pay us no mind until our minds are under control. It screws up our train of thought and makes us one-dimensional.... It takes away that extra imagination and flow of the mind, hence destroying the true, purest ideas of my mind.... The system should shape our education around our idiosyncratic minds, our quaint minds, our quirky minds, our curious minds.... I look forward to the day when Ritalin isn't an answer, and every student is labeled "learner."

Chapter 7

DO STIMULANTS HELP CHILDREN AND WILL DOCTORS TELL YOU THE TRUTH?

What Three Decades of Research Reveal

Sufficient data on safety and efficacy of long-term use of Ritalin in children are not yet available.... Long-term effects of Ritalin in children have not been well established.

—Ciba-Geigy Pharmaceuticals,
manufacturer of Ritalin, 1997

Ritalin calms children, indeed it often turns rambunctious kids into socially inhibited conformers, which, though it may make things easier for teachers and parents, is but suppressing the growing-up problems not solving them.

—Thomas Millar,
child psychiatrist (1997)

As documented in the initial chapters of this book, Ritalin is far more dangerous than parents, teachers, and doctors have been led to believe. Research discloses that Ritalin can produce both gross and subtle malfunctions in the brain and probably permanent brain damage. The amphetamines such as Dexedrine and Adderall are known to cause permanent brain damge and brain cell death. Furthermore, the drugs "work" by crushing spontaneous mental life, constricting awareness, and enforcing conforming compulsive behavior.

This chapter examines the effects of Ritalin from the viewpoint of the advocates themselves. Using their own criteria for improvement, and their own research, what have the ADHD/Ritalin proponents been able to show about the *efficacy* of Ritalin?

The Doctor Says He'll Grow up to Be a Criminal

Recently doctors have begun to warn parents that the long-range outcome for children who have ADHD is not good unless they receive treatment. These doctors mention studies showing that boys diagnosed ADHD will suffer from a higher incidence of criminal behavior and other problems in young adulthood. To any parent of a young boy who displays tendencies toward "inattention, hyperactivity, or impulsivity," this is a very frightening prediction. It's enough to pressure parents to accept long-term Ritalin for their children.

There is a catch to the studies: The children who grew up to have problems were being *treated with Ritalin*. In fact, the treatment was conducted free at an advanced "no-cost research clinic."[1] These reports should *discourage* parents from handing over their children to the doctors. They suggest that being diagnosed ADHD and being treated with stimulants leads to a long-term negative outcome for children.

A very extensive review of the literature by James Swanson of the University of California, Irvine, Attention Deficit Disorder Center addressed the question of long-term stimulant effects on behavior. It came to the unequivocal conclusion that "parents and teachers should not expect long-term improvement in academic achievement or reduced antisocial behavior." This chapter will address these issues in greater detail; but here it is important to underscore the conclusion that long-term stimulant use *will not reduce antisocial behavior.*

A mainstream review in the American Psychiatric Press *Textbook of Psychiatry* similarly states unequivocally:

> Stimulants do not produce lasting improvements in aggressivity, conduct disorder, criminality, educational achievement, job functioning, marital relationships, or long-term adjustment.[2]

A recent review by a prestigious team of stimulant advocates, assembled by the National Institute of Mental Health, came to the same conclusion: "the long-term efficacy of stimulant medication has not been demonstrated for *any* domain of child functioning."[3]

These statements about stimulants' lack of long-term effectiveness should be enlarged onto posters and put up in every clinic and office that dispenses stimulants. There is not a shred of evidence that taking these drugs protects a child from growing up to have serious difficulties!

There's another even more ominous possibility raised by these outcome studies—that diagnosing children ADHD and drugging them with stimulants worsens their chances for a normal childhood and young adulthood. A consensus will be found among researchers that stimulant drugs are of *no long-term help* to children in *any* aspect of their lives, including their psychological, social, family, or academic life. If hundreds of studies prove that stimulants cannot help at all long-term, it takes no great leap of imagination to suspect that being drugged long-term may be having an adverse effect. The potential hazards involved with long-term medication should certainly discourage giving stimulant drugs to children for months and years at a time.

Of course, if our children are having serious problems, we should be concerned about their future. That's common sense. But it's also common sense that some of the kids with the roughest starts become the most remarkable adults. And it doesn't mean an individual child *will* run into continued difficulties. Having an upset or difficult child is reason to feel very concerned—and to seek out caring, rational solutions—but it's no reason to diagnose and to drug the child.

What the Studies Really Show— Ritalin Is Not Effective

James M. Swanson is one of the more widely published researchers in the psychopharmacology of Ritalin and a member of the ADHD/Ritalin establishment. He was an invited presenter at the 1996 annual meeting of CHADD, the biologically-oriented parent's organization that is partly funded by the drug company, Ciba.[4] In the same year, he was elected to CHADD's "ADHD Hall of Fame." Swanson's Attention Deficit Disorder Center at the University of California at Irvine (UCI) is funded as one of a small number of research hubs by the U. S. Department of Education.

Swanson is such a staunch supporter of the ADHD/Ritalin viewpoint that he advocated "increased production of methylphenidate"[5] at a time when the Drug Enforcement Administration[6] (DEA) and the International Narcotics Control Board[7] began warning that America is using too much Ritalin. Because he is such a strong advocate of stimulants for children, Swanson's conclusions about the limited value of Ritalin gain added weight.

Swanson's ADD Center team (1992) has assumed what it calls "the lead role" in organizing and synthesizing the literature on treatments. As Swanson (circa 1993) described in an Executive Summary for the Department of Education, he and his team produced a comprehensive "review of reviews" of the Ritalin literature based on 300 reviews and 9,000 original articles spanning nearly 55 years. Here, verbatim, are the first four conclusions reported by Swanson at a forum sponsored by the Department of Education in 1993:

- Long-term beneficial effects have not been verified by research.

- Short-term effects of stimulants should not be considered a permanent solution to chronic ADD symptoms.

- Stimulant medication may improve learning in some cases but impair learning in others.

- In practice, prescribed doses of stimulants may be too high for optimal effects on learning, and the length of action of most stimulants is viewed as too short to affect academic achievement.

Based on his experience and his "review of reviews" from the ADD Center, Swanson (1993) also concluded about Ritalin:

- No large effects on skills or higher order processes—Teachers and parents should not expect significantly improved reading or athletic skills, positive social skills, or learning of new concepts.

- No improvement in long-term adjustment—Teachers and parents should not expect long-term improvement in academic achievement or reduced antisocial behavior.

How Short Is Short-Term?

Since the definition of short-term is central to understanding the impact of Ritalin, it is important to know that Swanson (1993) defines "short-term" as "7 to 18 weeks." *Even by standards of the ADHD/Ritalin advocates, Ritalin has no proven beneficial effect on behavior beyond 7–18 weeks!*

Amphetamines, if anything, have an even more short-term effect. Judith Rapoport, basing her estimate on thirty controlled double-blind amphetamine studies, found that amphetamine controls behavior for "4–12 weeks" and no more.[8] *Even by the standards of ADHD/Ritalin advocates, amphetamine has no proven beneficial effect beyond 4–12 weeks!*

When the Pill Is Stopped...

In regard to whatever good effect Ritalin is thought to achieve, it disappears when the drug is stopped. This is consistent with the principle that stimulants work by producing sufficient brain malfunction to suppress behavior. When the direct toxic effect is removed, the children usually revert to previous behavior. Whalen and Henker (1997) observe:

It is often disheartening to observe how rapidly behavior deteriorates when medication is discontinued. Apparently, whether a child is medicated for 5 days, 5 months, or 5 years, many problems return the day after the last pill is taken.

Of course, these children may also develop rebound and withdrawal reactions. This will make them much worse off than before they ever took the drug.[9]

NIMH Confirms Lack of Stimulant Efficacy

Swanson's University of California ADD Center is not unique in finding limited short-term benefits and no long-term benefits from Ritalin. In 1992, the National Institute of Mental Health (NIMH) described how it is once again trying to establish the efficacy of Ritalin by spending millions of dollars on research.[10] Chapter 8 will examine the first published reports concerning that research. Here I want to emphasize that in justifying the need for further studies, the NIMH authors confirmed that short-term effects are limited to behavioral control such as reducing "class room disturbance" and improving "compliance and sustained attention." They also confirmed that the drug seems "less reliable in bringing about associated improvements, at least of an enduring nature, in social-emotional and academic problems, such as antisocial behavior, poor peer and teacher relationships, and school failure."

In 1995, NIMH continued to justify pumping more millions of dollars into Ritalin research on the grounds that the drug's efficacy remains unproven.[11] The report was authored by a team made up of some of the biggest names in the ADHD/Ritalin field, including Peter Jensen, C. Keith Conners, Laurence Greenhill, William Pelham, and others. The report concludes that there is no evidence for even a short-term positive effect on academic performance. In longer-term studies, their conclusion—as noted above—is even more bleak: "long-term efficacy of stimulant medication has not been demonstrated for *any* domain of child functioning."[12]

In their recent 1997 review, Whalen and Henker came to the same conclusion as declared in a heading "Unsubstantiated Long-Term Benefits." Their review could document no "long-term advantage" to taking Ritalin.

Ritalin Fails the Grade

Since the goals of improved learning and academic performance often motivate parents to go along with Ritalin and other stimulants, they are worth focusing on. Swanson and his colleagues (1992) declare "even now, despite several more years of extensive research, there is very little objective evidence to support the notion that stimulant medication improves learning in ADHD children." They leave little room for uncertainty:

> The lack of a pervasive favorable response to stimulation medication represents a severe limitation on the educational benefits of stimulation medication to treat ADD students, and often the unfavorable response is in the area of learning.

Stating that they have been "surprised about the consensus expressed in this large literature," Swanson and his team (1992) summarize:[13]

We believe that the most important limitations are that the short-term effects of stimulants on academic performance are minimal compared to the effects on behavior, and that there is no evidence of beneficial effects on learning or academic achievement.

These conclusions should come as no surprise. Many students use "uppers" such as Ritalin and amphetamine to cram for exams; but few educators view this as a positive step toward a liberal education.

In another extensive 1990 review that cites numerous reports, Deborah Jacobovitz and a team from several universities conclude: "To date, there is no evidence that stimulants enhance academic performance." They point out that based on a review of seventeen studies, Russell Barkley himself found that "these drugs have almost no effect on scholastic achievement." Popper and Steingard (1994) come to similar conclusions in their textbook review.

More than a decade ago it was known that "efforts to establish its long-term efficacy have failed repeatedly."[14] In fact, the failure of stimulants to produce any positive long-term effects was well documented by the mid-1970s.[15] The more recent reviews we have been citing merely confirmed what had been known for more than two decades.

Do Stimulants Have a Better Effect in Combination with Other Treatments?

Writing in *The Comprehensive Textbook of Psychiatry*, L. Eugene Arnold and Peter S. Jensen (1995)[16] state it clearly: "Even the expected additive or synergistic effect of combining modalities has not been satisfactorily demonstrated." Jensen, remember, was the head of child and adolescent research at NIMH. Carol Whalen and Barbara Henker (1997), both long-time researchers in the field, recently came to the same conclusion. They find that research has failed to show any advantage in combining stimulants with psychological, family, or school interventions. A team of the most respected ADHD/Ritalin advocates also found that there's no scientific evidence for the efficacy of multimodal treatments.[17] Parents, however, are often led to believe that the dismal results from drug treatment by itself can be improved by combining it with other approaches.

Combining stimulants with other drugs, such as tranquilizers or antidepressants, has not improved the effectiveness of medication for ADHD.[18] It is not FDA-approved and not recommended in most textbooks. Combining medications is, instead, likely to increase the risk of adverse effects and severe toxicity.[19] Nonetheless, clinicians frequently add other medications without explaining to parents the lack of proven efficacy or the inevitable increase in potential hazards.

Learning in the Lab Versus the Classroom

Studies have shown that under laboratory conditions, stimulants can temporarily improve certain kinds of concentration and learning in children and adults regardless of whether or not they are diagnosed ADHD or have any learning difficulties. The beneficial effect is similar to that of caffeine in helping people temporarily to stay alert and focused. These benefits do not transfer to the complexities of classroom and academic learning.

Swanson and his ADD Center colleagues (1992) find that "there are no studies clearly linking drug effects on performance on laboratory tests to drug effects on classroom performance." They also conclude that improvements found in short-term lab studies have not been confirmed in more lengthy ones. Furthermore, the improvements shown in the lab involve tasks that require little effort or thinking, such as the commonly used Continuous Performance Task or CPT. Based on many studies, they also observe that "clinical doses that improve behavior may even impair performance on some learning tests."

These recent observations by Swanson's group are merely reconfirming what was known many years ago. In 1973 Sroufe and Stewart realized that the drugs affect normal adults in the same way as "problem children." They understood that the drugs enhance performance on "repetitive, routinized tasks that require sustained attention" but "reasoning, problem solving and learning do not seem to be [positively] affected in adults or children."

Harmful Stimulant Impact on Learning

In evaluating the potential value of Ritalin and other stimulants, it is important to realize that Ritalin not only fails to improve learning and academic performance, it impairs mental function. Stimulants commonly cause "cognitive toxicity"—drug-induced impairments in higher mental processes including flexible problem-solving and other "higher-order" functions. Stimulants tend to produce obsessive over-focusing on otherwise boring or uninspiring tasks. The drugs limit a child's awareness of his or her surroundings, enabling a more obsessive focusing, but this occurs at the expense of brain function. Normal social desires can be inhibited, making the child less sociable. The drugs can also limit a child's overall enthusiasm and energy level. The robotic effect that makes children temporarily more obedient and compliant is the result of drug-induced brain malfunction.[20]

Do Behavior Modification Techniques
Have a Better Record?

Writing in the *Comprehensive Textbook of Psychiatry*, Arnold and Jensen (1995)[21] also make clear that neither behavioral approaches (behavior modification with rewards and punishments) nor drugs have any proven long-term effect:

The short-term (a few weeks or months) efficacy of both has been established beyond a reasonable doubt in controlled studies. However, the long-term (years) efficacy of each modality remains to be demonstrated satisfactorily.

They also raise doubts about the effectiveness of these treatments in "everyday clinical practice" compared to the more highly selective and controlled research settings in universities.

Most behavior modification techniques used with children involve carefully controlling the child's activities through a pre-determined series of rewards and punishments. For example, as a reward for good behavior in class a child may be given additional privileges, more time to play during recess, or a certificate with which to purchase things from a canteen. Behavioral techniques are the favored psychological approach of many ADHD/Ritalin advocates. They are consistent with controlling the child's behavior, rather than with encouraging the child's autonomy. These techniques focus on changing the child, rather than on improving the child's family and school life.

Behavioral techniques minimize the need for adults to reappraise their own capacity to provide rational limits, a stimulating environment, and loving care. They tend to be most effective when children are restricted to a heavily controlled environment at school or at home where they have no choice but to comply with the "system."

Children readily see through systematic rewards and punishments as one more way of manipulating them. They will go along with the program as long as they are compelled to, or until they rebel. But they are not likely to "internalize" the values that are being imposed upon them. Instead of learning to love learning, they will learn to pursue rewards. Instead of developing genuine respect for the rights of others, they will behave in ways that earn rewards.

Even if children don't consciously realize it, they intuitively know that they are being given rewards in the form of privileges, tokens, smiley faces, or even a kind word, instead of being given genuine attention to their basic needs and unconditional love. Children who eagerly submit to these procedures may be desperately seeking approval. They are willing to settle for superficial tokens of success that don't meet their real needs. Exposure to behavioral techniques can confirm for these youngsters that adults will not treat them as feeling, thinking human beings.

Some of my colleagues believe that they have success with teaching behavioral techniques to parents and teachers. Some adults may improve their approach to children by developing a routine for encouraging good behavior with rewards, especially if they use the opportunity to give up more harsh methods. Any regular contact with adults will help a child if the adult expresses love and concern for the child in the process. To the extent that a behavioral program provides more adult attention to a child, it is likely to be helpful.

However, I prefer methods that approach the child more directly through a caring relationship bolstered by rational expectations and limit-setting. Developing realistic expectations for the child, and communicating with them in a caring, firm manner, will be much more helpful in the long run than trying to shape the child's behavior through rewards. Rational, direct communication treats the child with more respect and focuses the child on the need to develop his or her own personal autonomy.[22]

Is It Mostly Placebo?

The power of placebo—the "sugar pill" with no medicinal value—cannot be over-estimated. People feel better and sometimes get better as a result of believing that they have been given an effective treatment. At the 1997 American Urological Association meetings, it was reported that many men didn't want to give up their placebo pill in a multi-center two-year study of prostate gland hypertrophy.[23] The inactive placebo, made of flour, did not shrink their enlarged prostates. In fact, their prostates continued to grow in size. But the men not only felt better, their urine flow, measured by computerized technology, actually improved!

Studies comparing Ritalin and placebo indicate that Ritalin leads to parent-teacher ratings of short-term behavioral improvement in 75% of children while placebo leads to similar ratings of improvement in 40%[24] or even 70%[25] of children. After a controlled Ritalin trial that demonstrated strong placebo effects, Cotton and Rothberg (1988) concluded, "There is probably a need to repeat this study in other schools where unnecessary treatment may be taking place on a large scale." Melvin Richards (1995), Chief of Pharmacy Services at an Air Force base, describes a study in which children in the clinic were given either placebo or Ritalin. The effects of the placebo were so positive that "Within a year, methylphenidate prescribing at the hospital decreased significantly."

Since stimulants almost always produce obvious side effects, it is usually possible for doctors, parents, and children to tell whether or not the pill is a placebo or "the real thing." If observers can guess that the child is getting the drug rather than the placebo, they are more likely to report positive effects.[26] Some children in controlled studies don't take the medication when it is prescribed for them but may report positive effects to please the adults. Overall, the results of drug studies cannot be uncritically accepted.[27]

I have no doubt that Ritalin has a dramatic effect on children—that it can suppress a child's mental processes and behavior. But the placebo effect contributes to why parents and teachers are so willing to see this drug-induced dysfunction in such a positive light.

But NIMH Says It's 90% Effective...

Psychiatric researchers and experts often say one thing when they communicate among themselves in journals and another when they talk to the public. The data I am using are drawn almost entirely from professional publications and sources such as the National Institute of Mental Health (NIMH), the U.S. Department of Education, and published research in journals. For contrast, let's look at a document intended for public consumption, a 1993 booklet from NIMH entitled *Learning Disabilities: Decade of the Brain*:

> The effects of [stimulant] medication are most dramatic in children with ADHD. Shortly after taking the medication, they become more able to focus their attention. They become more ready to learn. Studies by NIMH scientists and other researchers have shown that at least 90% of hyperactive children can be helped by either Ritalin or Dexedrine.

No wonder teachers and parents are ready to use the drug! NIMH makes promotional claims to the public that are contradicted by its own professional publications, its staff, and its advisors. First, the drugs do not have any different effect on "children with ADHD" than on normal children or even animals. Second, children do not become "more ready to learn." They become more docile and compliant, but their learning ability can be impaired by a drug-induced loss of interest and by toxic effects on cognitive function. Third, it is wrong to say that "at least 90% of hyperactive children can be helped." Helped in what way? As already noted, NIMH itself has admitted that the children won't get any short-term help with learning or academic performance, and no long-term help in "*any* domain of child functioning."

Furthermore, by no stretch of the imagination are stimulants effective 90% of the time. About half the prescriptions written for Ritalin are not renewed.[28] Both lack of efficacy and adverse effects discourage parents from continuing with stimulants, so that 50 percent or more of children won't get beyond the first month or two before stopping the medication. That cuts the 90% figure immediately down to less than 50% at the start. As we have seen, this is well within the range of placebo or sugar pill.

What Does the Most Widely Read ADHD Advocate Tell Parents?

In light of all the evidence reviewed in this chapter, as well as Barkley's own conclusions in the professional literature, the reader may be surprised by what Barkley tells teachers and parents in his popular books.

In his *Attention-Deficit Hyperactivity Disorder: A Clinical Workbook* (1991), Barkley opens by stating "The most substantiated treatment is the use of stimulant medications."[29] There is no mention whatsoever of the limits, leaving parents and teachers to believe that substantial claims can be made for Ritalin and amphetamine. Earlier in the book, we noted that Barkley gives the extremely misleading impression that Ritalin is not related to the amphetamines when he states "Ritalin and Cylert are nonamphetamines."[30] He then speaks of a 70% improvement rate without mentioning that the effects are short-term and situational, with no long-term benefits, and that academic achievement will, at best, be unaffected.

Barkley then goes on to state that drug-treated children "feel better about themselves, and self-esteem rises." To the contrary, there is a consensus that there's no drug-related improvement in any aspect of the child's life.

Finally, as if in passing, Barkley mentions that "At present, however, there is some controversy as to the degree of learning and memory improvement from the treatment of ADHD children with stimulant drugs."[31] This statement is highly misleading. It does not tell the parent and teacher the crucial truth: There is no improvement in academic performance and learning can be impaired. Barkley allows the parent or teacher to imagine that school work itself will be improved.

Having wholly omitted what he knows to be the limitations of the drug, Barkley leaves the parent and teacher impressed with ringing phrases such as "the most substantiated treatment," "treatment of choice," and "drugs are unquestionably successful..."

In the section entitled "How Do Drugs Change Learning and Academic Performance?" in *Taking Charge of ADHD* (1995), Barkley talks around the issue, leaving parents to assume that the drug does something very good.[32] He never tells the simple truth—no improvement, and possible harm, in learning and academic performance. In the section on "What Do the Drugs Do for Behavior and Emotions?" he somehow fails to mention that they do *nothing* positive long-term even by ADHD/Ritalin advocate standards.

There is an astonishing gap between what Barkley should know and what he tells parents and teachers. The gap, however, is endemic in the popular literature written by ADHD/Ritalin advocates. The material on lack of drug efficacy, while readily available in the professional literature, is not presented to the public. The widespread use of stimulants is maintained on the basis of keeping parents and teachers—and most doctors as well—in the dark about the limits of the drugs.

Not Just Barkley

Most of the ADHD/Ritalin community lives in a world of unreality when it comes to stimulant treatment. This is exemplified in a 1997 *Psychology Today* feature article by physician and author Edward M. Hallowell (1997) who claims to suffer from ADHD. Hallowell believes that "Drugs are beneficial in about 80 percent of ADDers, working like a pair of eyeglasses for the brain, enhancing and sharpening the mental focus." The "pair of eyeglasses" metaphor, as already noted in chapter 2, is a favorite one for ADHD advocates.

In what they call a "reasoned and reasonable approach to using medication," Sam and Michael Goldstein (1992) start off by declaring: "Medication, at this time, is the most effective treatment for hyperactivity, and the hyperactive child's response to medication is among the most dramatic in medicine."[33] Writing in Russell Barkley's book, *Taking Charge of ADHD*, DuPaul and Costello (1995) declare, "The stimulants, the drugs most commonly used, have been shown to be effective in improving behavior, academic work, and social adjustment in anywhere from 50 to 95% of children with ADHD."[34] These are remarkably misleading testimonials.

Testimonials from Abroad

There is an explosion of stimulant prescriptions in Canada.[35] This doesn't happen by chance. Primary care physicians must be convinced. In a 1996 Canadian review aimed at primary care physicians, Normand Carrey and his colleagues state, "successful pharmacological treatment can improve the patient's potential for achievement in academic, family, social and recreational activities." Although the primary care physician would have no way of knowing it, this statement is simply false. There is no evidence for improvement in *any* of the arenas they mention: school achievement or family, social and recreational activities. On the basis of articles like this, it's no wonder that Canadian doctors have rushed into prescribing stimulants.

Germany has also begun to show increasing interest in stimulants for ADHD. Walter Eichlseder (1985) reported in *Pediatrics* on 1,000 hyperactive children he treated with stimulants in Germany. He dismisses criticism from parents in his practice who are concerned about the drug making their children depressed. He also ridicules public concern. He then launched into exaggerated claims that had already been proven false by research.

Can Bias Be Confused with Science?

In the field of ADHD and Ritalin, Alan Zametkin (1992) from the National Institute of Mental Health is one of the nation's leading and most frequently quoted experts. He and I were on opposite sides as medical experts in a Ritalin malpractice case.[36] I was testifying on behalf of a parent who believed her son had been injured by Ritalin and he was testifying on behalf of the defense.[37] In deposition testimony under oath for the case, Zametkin made a remarkable admission.

Earlier in the deposition, Zametkin indicated that by short-term he meant two to four months.[38] Then Charles Anna Bennett, the Atlanta attorney for the plaintiff, asked him about the lack of evidence for long-term benefit from Ritalin.[39]

> **Bennett:** So you're saying that the long-term benefit of the drug has not been demonstrated or has not been concluded?
>
> **Zametkin:** In scientific studies, the answer is, that's correct.
>
> **Bennett:** It has not been?
>
> **Zametkin:** That's correct.
>
> **Bennett:** So what would be the use to give the kids medication for six years, three to six years, if you say that there is —.
>
> **Zametkin:** Well, the fact that science has not been able to demonstrate something does not mean that is not an incredibly useful beneficial intervention.

Zametkin explicitly and consciously rejects the scientific evidence in order to promote his biased support for the long-term medicating of children. On the one hand, he acknowledges that science does not support his position; on the other hand, he testifies under oath that science makes no difference in this regard.

Biopsychiatrists like Zametkin try to claim the scientific ground for themselves. They present their views to the public as *the* scientific and hence valid approach. Yet they distort the scientific evidence in favor of their opinions—for example, Zametkin's own PET scan studies of ADHD[40]—while they reject substantial evidence that contradicts them.

A New "Positive Study" Receives Press Coverage

A new Swedish study, covered in the *New York Times* and elsewhere,[41] tried to demonstrate that amphetamine was superior to placebo in a fifteen month trial with children labeled ADHD. The lead author of the new study, psychiatrist Christopher Gillberg (1997), actually warned "It is my firm belief that these drugs are overused in the United States."[42] He added that they were "possibly underused in Europe," where they are hardly used at all.

In an editorial comment in the same issue of the journal that published the Gillberg study, Michael Rutter (1997) of London's Medical Research Council voiced trenchant criticisms:

> The clinical implications of this finding [the study results] are severely constrained by the heterogeneity of the sample,[43] by the exclusion of children with major psychosocial problems, and most of all, by 1 curious feature. The withdrawal of active drug at 15 months did not lead to any significant deterioration in behavior during the subsequent three months

(unfortunately no details of this crucial finding are provided). Also, because the children received no nonpharmacological treatment, it is not known how the benefits of the drug compares with those of psychological intervention.

There were other problems as well. The statistical validity of the study was weakened when ten of the original 72 children dropped out within the first month mostly due to a combination of adverse effects and no drug effect. Only 32 children completed the study: 8 in the placebo group and 24 in the treatment group. In order to come out positive, the statistical analysis had to include patients who were no longer in the study at the time of completion.

In Pursuit of the Holy Grail: Proof of Long-Term Improvement

Judith L. Rapoport, head of child psychiatry at the National Institute of Mental Health, has for years been an ardent supporter of diagnosing and drugging children. She recently declared,[44] "The Holy Grail is to show whether stimulant drugs taken long-term do anything." With so many knights of biological psychiatry failing in their pursuit of this elusive goal over so many decades, we might conclude that this Holy Grail is a myth. Such persistently negative results over so many years are almost unheard of in psychiatric research. As I've described in earlier books,[45] psychiatric drug studies are so easily subject to manipulation and subjective interpretation that efficacy can usually be demonstrated in research studies despite a treatment's utter lack of any real value.

Even if the current vast expenditures of money on stimulant research are able to produce a few positive studies, the real results are already in. Three decades of failed attempts to show long-term results cannot be overcome by current desperate attempts to produce a few positive studies.

Still Useless after All These Years

Thirty years of scientific literature generated by ADHD/Ritalin advocates affirms that Ritalin and other stimulants have, at best, a very short-lived "positive" effect on children. The effect lasts no more than four to eighteen weeks. During that brief time, stimulants control or subdue the child's behavior without improving learning or academic performance. Mental abilities may be impaired. Longer-term, there is no positive effect on any aspect of a child's life. The child's behavior, feelings and attitudes, academic performance, family relationships and social life will be unimproved or worse after several months on stimulants. This is true whether or not other therapeutic approaches are included with the stimulants.

Parents should be vigilant about exaggerated claims in popular books or doctor testimonials. They should clearly understand that stimulant medication has very limited short-term effects of questionable benefit and no positive long-term effects whatsoever even in research conducted by ADHD advocates.

At the conclusion of its conference on ADHD and Ritalin in December 1996, the Drug Enforcement Administration (DEA) declared:

> [T]he use of stimulants for the short-term improvement of behavior and underachievement may be thwarting efforts to address the children's real issues, both on an individual and societal level. The lack of long-term positive results with the use of stimulants and the specter of previous and potential stimulant abuse epidemics, give cause to worry about the future. The dramatic increase in the use of methylphenidate in the 1990s should be viewed as a marker or warning to society about the problems children are having and how we view and address them.

The public has been sold a completely unrealistic picture of Ritalin's value as a treatment. The many professional testimonials about the effectiveness and safety of stimulants are as unreliable as sales pitches for other industrial products that are pushed on consumers.

What about the Violent Child?

Although the vast majority of children labeled ADHD and medicated with stimulants are not violent, I am frequently asked "What can you do about the violent child?" Since serious violence is rare, especially among children diagnosed ADHD, usually this question is raised more as a challenge than a real-life problem. The question implies that "being loving" might be good for easy kids but not for the toughest ones.

A very violent child is a very angry child, and a very angry child is a very hurt child. That's all there is to it. As much or more than most children, the very hurt and angry child needs unconditional love in a safe relationship with a wise adult. Regardless of how badly a child has been emotionally hurt, or how disturbed or violent the child has become, the help remains the same—to offer the child a relationship that is safe, secure, predictable, disciplined, and loving.

There are no drugs that can help children learn to overcome their violent feelings or actions. No drugs have ever been approved for this purpose. Even if they are someday, it would remain the wrong approach. Anger springs from hurt, especially from feelings of worthlessness and humiliation.[46] The way to ease a child's anger is to ease the child's feelings of worthlessness and humiliation. That means treating the child with love and respect.

When a little boy, for example, will physically resist or attack adults at the risk of getting hurt, that little boy especially needs gentleness and kindness. An enraged child is a child especially in need of adults schooled in the art of nonviolence. Diagnosing and drugging a child is a violent response. It's meeting violence with violence. In the long run, it will breed more reactive violence on the child's part. If the child does become submissive, it's out of fear—with smoldering resentment cooking dangerously beneath the surface.

Yes, we can subdue most children, temporarily at least, with large doses of toxic agents. But I believe it is abusive and I think it should be illegal. It harms the brain of the child and undermines any hope of a peaceful, loving resolution of the conflicts the child is having with other people.

When I give workshops or write about how to help violent children, I emphasize the importance of the adult caregivers becoming nonviolent. This is not always an easy task. It involves paying more attention to how we feel and act.[47] It requires us to find the resources to project a caring, nurturing, safe presence in the face of the child's fear and aggression. A child will often become more peaceful when in the presence of an adult who is devoted to being firm, gentle, and nonviolent, even in the face of physical threats. However, helping a very upset, angry child is no easy matter.[48] The subject will be further addressed in later chapters in this book.

Can Drugs Ever Help?

Many people want to believe that there are drugs that can be used as a last resort. They want to have faith in something outside themselves and beyond the usual human resources.

How can drugs *ever* truly help a child when they interfere with the child's mental ability to feel and to care about relationships? How can drugs *ever* help when they flatten the child's spirit rather than meeting the child's basic needs?

It is sometimes claimed that drugs make a child "more available" or "more amenable" to communication and a therapeutic relationship. This depends on the definition of communication and therapy. Drugs can make a child more easy to be *around* but not more easy to be *with*. Drugs enforce submissiveness rather than frank communication or a genuine relationship. Drugs can make a child more obedient by making the child's brain malfunction. It is tragic that we often seem to prefer an impaired child to a child with a normal brain.

Drugs are only useful when we are focused on our needs as adults rather than on the needs of the child. Every time we drug a child we are choosing our convenience and our peace of mind over the child's real needs. This is another reason *never* to use drugs. It is unethical to drug a child for our own convenience. It is wrong to distort the function of a child's brain with drugs in order to "improve" the child's behavior.

How is it possible that such a dangerous, useless drug has become so widely used? How have so many parents and teachers—and even doctors—become convinced that it's valuable and even indispensable? We turn now to the main justification for prescribing Ritalin—the ADHD diagnosis. Then we will examine the promotion of Ritalin by interest groups that benefit from its sale and use.

In today's society, the drugging of children to control their behavior is viewed as a medical activity, but it has little or nothing to do with the genuine practice of medicine. It is the technological control or suppression of behavior. The fact that medical doctors implement the control does not make it a legitimate medical enterprise. The drugging of children for behavior control should raise profound spiritual, philosophical, and ethical questions about ourselves as adults and about how we view the children in our care. Society ignores these critical questions at great peril to itself, to its values, and to the well-being of its children.

Since the publication of the first edition of this book, the National Institute of Mental Health (NIMH) has once again failed to demonstrate the effectiveness of stimulant medication, despite the expenditure of millions of dollars of the taxpayers' money. We turn now to this latest attempt to convince Americans to medicate their children for behavioral control.

Chapter 8

DEFINITIVE STUDY OR SCIENTIFIC HOAX?

NIMH Funds Research on Ritalin

The National Institute of Mental Health (NIMH) is a government agency. It is mandated to pursue the interests of the people of the United States. But in recent years, NIMH has vigorously promoted the interests of the giant corporations that peddle psychiatric drugs to the people. It has become a political hotbed of dedicated advocates for the increased diagnosing and drugging of America's children.

Many of the most ardent drug advocates in this nation are past or present full-time employees of NIMH. Most of the others regularly benefit from large NIMH grants and other government perks. Much of the flawed research purporting to show a biological basis for ADHD has been carried out or funded by NIMH.

NIMH employees like Alan Zametkin, F. Xavier Castellanos, and Judith Rapoport continue to push the biological model and drugs for children from their positions at NIMH. Peter Jensen in the recent past and Paul Wender in earlier years used their full-time NIMH positions to foster the current avalanche of child drugging.

In the early 1990s, when psychiatrist Fred Goodwin was at the helm, NIMH attempted to organize and fund the proposed federal violence initiative. This racist multi-agency initiative intended to explain violence in the inner city on the basis of biological and genetic defects in African-American infants and children. It planned intrusive, biological research on infants and children, including blood tests, spinal taps, and brain studies. Working with our International Center for the Study of Psychiatry and Psychology and African-Americans in the U. S. Congress, Ginger Breggin and I organized a campaign against the violence initiative that effectively shut it down and resulted in the forced resignation of Fred Goodwin from the government. We describe this political and scientific conflict in *The War Against Children of Color* (1998.)

In recent years, NIMH has taken a new and more dangerous road by directly funding clinical drug trials for children. The institute is now doing the job that the drug industry used to have to pay for out of its own profits. These government-sponsored clinical trials are even more biased and scientifically flawed than those conducted by the drug companies. The drug companies are answerable to some extent at least to the FDA; NIMH appears to be answerable to no one except the drug companies.

NIMH recently published a multi-center study of stimulants for children. Criticism of the study became more essential when NIMH announced its intention to carry out a similar project in which hundreds of four-to-six year old children will be subjected to stimulant drug experiments (chapter 1).

Much Ado about Nothing:
The Multi-Center NIMH Study

Amid a media blitz orchestrated by NIMH, the multi-center study was published in December 1999. The stated aim was to "resolve controversies and clinical quandaries about the relative value of medication and behavioral treatments."[1] TV news programs and other media received advanced press releases and began asking for my response to the new "proof" that stimulant drugs are both effective and safe for children.

Regardless of the study's quality, there was no lack of expenditure of time or the taxpayer's money. The NIMH-sponsored research was conducted at six separate medical centers in North America.[2] At each site, four treatment groups or conditions were compared: (1) stimulant medication alone, (2) a combination of medication and behavior therapy, (3) behavior therapy alone, and (4) community care. Medication therapy consisted of stimulant drugs. Behavior therapy consisted of group training sessions for parents, as well as some classroom and individual interventions. The children who remained in the community care group were treated by their own doctors and usually received stimulant drugs.

The study's first phase lasted fourteen months. The average age of the children was eight and 80% were boys.

Omitting the Best Treatment

Unfortunately, the NIMH study failed to examine the kind of interventions that, in actual clinical practice, prove very effective in helping children labeled with ADHD. These interventions include family counseling aimed at improving relationships and childcare practices in the family, and individualized educational approaches that inspire children in school. The study also ignored the causes of behaviors that get labeled "ADHD," such as inadequate educational background, boredom in the classroom, peer abuse in the school, or inconsistent parenting in the home.

This failure to utilize the best methods for helping children turned out to be the tip of the iceberg.

No Placebo Controls

In well-conducted clinical trials, a drug is compared to a placebo or "sugar pill." This is because patients or experimental subjects taking medication often experience the "placebo effect:" they feel better whether or not the drug has any physical effect on them. They are responding to the belief or the hope that they are receiving a good treatment. Similarly, observers will also rate the subjects as improved because they are biased toward a good outcome on the drugs. Therefore, clinical drug trials usually compare the effects of the drug to the effects of a placebo pill.

As one major textbook remarked, "Placebo effects, which occur in a large percentage of patients, can confound many studies—particularly those that involve subject responses; controls must take this into account."[3] The use of placebos is so important that, for FDA approval, a psychiatric drug must prove superior to placebo in two or more studies.

The NIMH study had no placebo control group, making it impossible to tell if the stimulant drugs were having a real effect or not.

No Double-Blind

As a further attempt to assure a degree of scientific objectivity in drug studies, the observers and the subjects must be kept in the dark about which patients are taking the drug and which are taking the placebo. This is called the "double-blind."[4]

Readers may recall the Pepsi commercials in which a consumer was offered sips from two cups, one with Pepsi, the other with Coke. Playing at being scientific, the participants in the commercial were blindfolded to prevent them from knowing which drink was being tasted.

Simple principles, simply omitted: There were no placebo controls and no double-blind in the NIMH clinical trials. The parents and teachers who rated the children knew whether or not they were receiving medication that everyone expected would work. But wait; it gets worse.

Finding Subjects Who Already Favored Drugs

When selecting a group of patients for a clinical trial, it is important to avoid pre-selecting a group that will be highly biased in favor of the drug. But 32% of the children in the NIMH study were already taking stimulant drugs![5] This indicates that many of these parents, as well as the teachers, were already convinced of the usefulness of stimulants.

Building in Bias in the Untrained Observers

Remarkably, NIMH chose not to use trained observers. Experience and training, as well as objectivity, are required to properly evaluate the impact of psychoactive agents. In nearly all published scientific studies in the field, professionals use rating scales and other tools for evaluating a drug's efficacy and adverse effects. Not here! NIMH relied upon the observations of the parents and teachers who were given preprinted checklists to record both improvement and adverse drug effects.

We have already seen that many adverse effects of stimulants—such as loss of spontaneity and increased obsessive behavior—are easily mistaken for improvements by parents and teachers. The use of aware, experienced professionals, rather than parents and teachers by themselves, was absolutely necessary in order to determine the frequency and severity of adverse drug effects.[6]

There is no evidence that the parents and teachers received training about how to evaluate drug effects. To the contrary, they were reassured in writing in advance that the drug was safe and that the side effects were not serious. The "Teacher Information" handout informed them that the children would be treated with a **safe and effective** dose of medication…" (bold in original).[7] Yet the study was to help determine, *for the first time ever*, if stimulation medication would be safe and effective over a several weeks or months period of time.

Since the teachers knew which children were receiving the drugs, this built-in bias invalidated their subjective evaluations of drug safety and efficacy. The teacher information handouts also demonstrate the bias of the NIMH researchers who had pre-determined to their own satisfaction that the stimulants would prove safe and effective over the lengthy study period. But if the safety and efficacy of Ritalin over many weeks had already been proven, there would have been no need for the study in the first place.

The "Information for Parents" handout had similar built-in biases, including a reference to biochemical imbalances and genetic factors in "ADHD."[8] Based on the information handouts given out by Columbia and the NYSPI for the NIMH study, the parents were not provided informed consent. They were not given sufficient information about the potential harmful effects of stimulants to make an informed decision before submitting their children to weeks and months of drug exposure.

What the Study Got Right—and Buried

The NIMH study did utilize one group of observers who carried out "blinded ratings of school-based ADHD and oppositional/aggressive symptoms…"[9] This group observed the children in the classroom without knowing which of them had been placed on drugs.

The blind raters did not find any positive drug effect. Since this was the only objective rating process in the study, these negative results should have been emphasized as indicating a lack of stimulant effectiveness. Instead, the finding was buried in a table and was not even mentioned in the study conclusions.

NIMH left out other information that didn't fit the agenda behind the study.

The Children Did Not Rate Themselves Improved

The study asked the children to rate themselves on an anxiety scale.[10] Those taking the drugs did not rate themselves as more improved than any of the other children. This result supports the use of safer non-drug treatments.

Furthermore, I received inside information from an anonymous source associated with the studies that the children were also asked to rate themselves on a depression scale. This information was confirmed when I obtained a handout provided by the Columbia University project.[11] It, too, mentions that the children were going to rate themselves on a depression scale. However, the published study failed to mention that the children had taken a self-rating depression scale.

Why did the investigators fail to report the results of the depression self-rating scale? Stimulants commonly cause or worsen depression in children, and that finding may have shown up on the self-ratings. Out of scientific integrity, and especially out of compassion for the millions of children on stimulants, the authors of the NIMH study should publish any data they possess on this issue.

NIMH did not interview any of the children concerning their reactions to the drug. In clinical practice, asking children about any potential adverse drug reactions is central to an effective assessment. A child having drug-related problems, such as twitches, headaches, or "blah" feelings, usually does not understand their source or tell anyone about them until specifically questioned. Typical of studies conducted by drug advocates, no interest was shown in how the children experienced or viewed the treatment.

Most Children Suffered from Drug Side Effects

Despite the strong pro-drug bias built into the study, 64% of children were reported by their parents or teachers to have some negative drug effects. Of these, 11.4% of the adverse drug effects were rated as moderate and 2.9% as severe.

The authors of the study dismiss the severe reactions because more than half of them involved "depression, worrying, irritability." They explain that this suffering "could have been due to nonmedication factors."[12]

However, as discussed in chapters 2 and 3, depression, worrying, and irritability are common adverse effects of stimulants. The dismissal of known stimulant-induced side effects, like many of the flaws in this study, points to the strong biases of the investigators. It also shows their callousness not only toward the suffering of the children in the study, but to *all* children. Their biased study will be used to justify drugging even greater numbers of children.

No Scientific Measures of Adverse Effects

This relatively long-term study could have provided an all-important opportunity to examine the potentially harmful effects of Ritalin and other stimulants on the physical growth and functioning of children. This opportunity was lost. No measurements of height or weight were taken, so no assessment could be made of growth suppression.

In addition, no measurements of heart rate or blood pressure were taken, and no electrocardiograms were administered, so that potentially harmful cardiovascular effects were not evaluated. There were no neurological examinations for tics or other abnormal movements and no objective tests of mental function, such as memory or attention.

From the opening statement in the study to its conclusion, the investigators made no serious attempt to evaluate the single most important issue surrounding the long-term use of stimulant drugs—the risks it poses to the children.

No Improvement in Academic Performance

Although the data is once again hidden within a table,[13] the study records no improvement or difference in academic performance in spelling or math. The table seems to indicate marginal improvement in reading. However, according to Bertram Karon, Professor of Psychology at Michigan State University,[14] the statistical analysis was flawed. Overall, no academic improvement was found as a result of any treatment. This was an important finding that received no attention from the authors.

It confirms many previous studies that have failed to show any real improvement in academic performance while taking stimulants.

Little or No Effect on Social Skills

The peer group ratings by other children did not rate the medicated children as improved in their social relationships. This is consistent with the majority of published studies that show no improvement in social skills in medicated children. The youngsters simply become more docile and isolated.

Most of the Subjects Were Boys

Stimulants are known to be temporarily effective in suppressing *normal* spontaneous activity and mental life in children and animals. As documented in chapter 4, this drug-induced effect includes the suppression or obliteration of activities such as socialization, play, autonomous choice making, and spontaneity. By chemically subduing children, stimulant drugs make normal boys easier to manage under certain circumstances, such as a home or classroom setting that does not meet their needs for enjoyable physical activity or fails to provide them adequate supervision, discipline, and engaging education.

In part to counter the argument that stimulants are used for the behavioral or social control of normal boys, attempts were made to include a greater number of girls in the NIMH clinical trials. Despite these efforts to recruit more girls, 80% of the subjects were boys. This reconfirms that stimulants are used to suppress the relatively greater activity of normal boys compared to girls.

How Could This Study Have Taken Place?

This highly touted study was fatally marred by scientific flaws, by data that undermine its cheery conclusions, by revelations of adverse effects that were overlooked, and by missed opportunities for important research left by the wayside. And when it did provide useful data about the limits of stimulant medication, those results were ignored.

How did well-known scientists produce a study with so many basic design flaws? And why did they pay so little attention to the information of value that they did unearth?

Examining the biographies of the researchers involved in a study can sometimes shed light on the origin of strong biases. Peter Jensen, who originated and monitored the studies while at NIMH, has already been identified on several occasions in this book as a staunch drug advocate. He's even come out in favor of parents being forced to give stimulants to their children.

The six principal investigators of the individual projects in North America were Laurence Greenhill, C. K. Conners, William Pelham, Howard Abikoff, James Swanson, and Stephen Hinshaw.[15] Each one of them has devoted his career to promoting the concept of ADHD and the drugging of children. Conners has been doing so for four decades.

Laurence Greenhill of Columbia University and the New York State Psychiatric Institute exemplifies the conflicts of interest that exist among many researchers in the field. Before the biographical data were removed during a controversy over their funding of dangerous research on children, the New York State Psychiatric Institute and Columbia University web site listed the funding of its researchers.[16] As of December 21, 1998 Greenhill was listed as having research funding or other financial associations with six different drug companies: Richwood, Bristol-Myers, Solvay, Wyeth-Ayerst, Glaxo, and Eli Lilly.

Greenhill, like all scientific presenters at the NIMH Consensus Conference on ADHD and its treatment, was required to report to the conference organizers any financial conflicts of interest. Through Freedom of Information I obtained the financial disclosure forms for all of the participants. Earlier in the same year on May 8, Greenhill signed Part A of the "Full

Disclosure Statement" which reads, "I, the undersigned, declare that I do *not* have a financial interest or other relationship with any manufacturer(s) of any commercial product(s)."[17] He then left blank the portion of the form where he should have listed the drug company affiliations noted on his medical center's web site. He signed this apparently false statement. Greenhill is in charge of NIMH's stimulant experiments on preschoolers.

In summary, the NIMH Ritalin study was a scientific fiasco, even a hoax, conducted by highly biased advocates of medication. It failed to adhere to the most important, essential scientific standards for clinical drug trials, including double-blind procedures and placebo controls. Therefore, it cannot be used to draw favorable conclusions about stimulant efficacy or adverse effects. Furthermore, despite the multiple built-in biases, the data it generated tends to confirm that stimulant medication produces no better results than any other intervention and that it causes many adverse effects.

Instead of demonstrating the safety and efficacy of stimulant treatment, the NIMH study exemplifies the extremes to which the institute and its handpicked stimulant advocates will go in promoting the drugging of America's children. Most tragically, it displays a callous disregard toward the children and families in the clinical trials and to all the millions of children who are being subjected to stimulant drugs throughout North America.

Remember that NIMH has now begun to conduct similar clinical drug trials on preschoolers. Our society doesn't need more drug experiments on very young children. Our most vulnerable children should be protected from this technological abuse. We need a national moratorium on prescribing psychoactive agents to young children and an end to psychiatric drug experimentation on preschoolers.

PART TWO

ATTENTION DEFICIT HYPERACTIVITY DISORDER
(ADHD)

Chapter 9

THE "SCIENCE" BEHIND MAKING AN ADHD DIAGNOSIS

The driving force behind the over-diagnosis is a system that is out of control. Teachers want compliant, well-behaved children. Parents eager to see children succeed take them to mental health professionals who are quick to diagnose ADHD and seek drug treatment. Under an insurance system that favors drugs over therapy, ADHD is an easy label to apply to undesired behavior; drugs are a quick fix....

Children who are creative, having a different learning style or are oppositional, angry, or depressive all have been diagnosed as having ADHD. Many of these problems can be found only by talking with patients at length.

—Sharon Collins, pediatrician (1997)

According to the American Psychiatric Assn.'s *Diagnostic and Statistical Manual of Mental Disorders (DSM-IV)*, a child has symptoms—which must appear before age seven—if he or she is easily distracted, often interrupts, and fidgets or squirms. Sounds like your basic kid.

—Kate Murphy, journalist, *Business Week* (1997)

Too much contemporary treatment by mental health professionals, including treatment influenced by the *DSM*, maintains this almost exclusive focus on individuals' psyches, as if the major source of their troubles came from within them.

—Paula Caplan, *They Say You're Crazy* (1995)

It would be difficult to convince parents and teachers to drug a child without first making a diagnosis. Attention Deficit Hyperactivity Disorder (ADHD) has one over-riding purpose—to put a medical veneer on the use of medication to control the behavior of children. But does the diagnosis have any independent validity? Is it "real" in the sense that pneumonia, diabetes or head injury is real? Do these children really have "broken brains"?

How Many Children Can We Diagnose?

ADHD advocates vary widely in their estimates of the percentage of children who suffer from the disorder but a range of 9–10 percent of boys and 3 percent of girls is somewhat representative.[1] With increasing emphasis on "inattention" as a central feature, the ratio of boys to girls is dropping.[2] More and more girls are being medicated for "ADHD."

The International Narcotics Control Board figure of 10–12% of boys in the United States receiving Ritalin already surpasses the usual upper limits of boys estimated to have the disorder.[3] In March 1997 the International Narcotics Control Board[4] repeated its concerns about over-prescription of stimulants in the United States: "the Board reiterates its request to all Governments to exercise the utmost care to prevent overdiagnosing of ADD in children and medically unjustified treatment."

Variability from Place to Place, Doctor to Doctor

Physicians vary widely in how many children they diagnose and medicate. A recent study in Michigan[5] found a ten-fold difference in prescription rates from county to county. It concluded that "Relatively few pediatricians account for the largest proportion of prescriptions."

States also vary widely in Ritalin use and they often undergo dramatic shifts over time. My home state, Maryland, went from third among states in 1987 to 47th in 1994. Between 1991 and 1994, my wife Ginger and I were very active in the media as critics of drugging of children. Our media efforts began in 1991 with the publication of my book, *Toxic Psychiatry*. It culminated in 1992–1994 with the publication of our *War Against Children* as a part of our successful campaign to stop a federal biopsychiatric program aimed at conducting intrusive biological research and treatment with inner city children.[6] We probably bear partial responsibility for the drop off in Ritalin prescription but there were undoubtedly other factors as well.[7]

The DSM: Cookbook Diagnosing?

Periodically the American Psychiatric Association empowers committees of professionals to revise and update its *Diagnostic and Statistical Manual of Mental Disorders* (*DSM*). The book provides an official imprimatur to psychiatric labels. Its title suggests a scientific work based on statistical analysis, which it is not.

The *DSM* series has been subjected to criticism dismissing it as something more akin to science fiction than to science.[8] Its enormous growth in size, with the addition of many new diagnoses with each edition, reflects psychiatry's need to broaden insurance coverage and to bring the whole spectrum of human variability under psychiatric authority.

Before we begin to examine the official APA standards for diagnosing ADHD, the following critique by Kirk and Kutchins (1992) provides an important context:

> The language used to present these criteria and procedures exudes the spirit of technical rationality. The diagnosis comes with its unique code number; references to other complex concepts, e.g., mental age; specifications about precise duration (six months) and the number of symptoms needed; vague references to unspecified research about "discriminating power" and national field trials; and defined levels of severity. Through these criteria, describing common, everyday behaviors of children, the rhetoric of science transforms them into what are purported to be objective symptoms of mental disorder.[9]

On closer inspection, however, there is little that is objective about the diagnostic criteria.

ADHD and the DSM

The concept of "hyperkinetic reaction of childhood" first appeared in 1968 in the *Diagnostic and Statistical Manual of Mental Disorders, 2nd Edition* (*DSM-II*). The term "reaction" indicated a behavioral rather than a biological cause. In the 1980 edition of the manual, *DSM-III*, Attention Deficit Disorder made its appearance. The manual was revised in 1987 with the now familiar ADHD. We will focus on the most recent edition, *DSM-IV*, which came out in 1994.

The *DSM-IV* divides ADHD into two types—inattention and hyperactivity-impulsivity. As Kirk and Kutchins describe, the diagnostic items are taken from the everyday behavior of children.

Table III reproduces the criteria for ADHD as they appear in the official diagnostic manual. Within each category, the items are listed in descending order of diagnostic power or importance. Thus "often fidgets with hands or feet or squirms in seat" is considered the most significant sign of the hyperactivity form of ADHD.

Six items from either list qualify a child for the diagnosis. There is no scientific validity or clinical reality to this particular number. In clinical practice, children are routinely diagnosed with ADHD and treated with Ritalin if they display one, two, or three of these characteristics, or even a few behaviors that resemble these traits. While the 1994 edition of the diagnostic manual added the requirement that the symptoms appear in two or more settings, children are commonly diagnosed on the basis of their behavior in school or a single classroom.

Wender's Sign, or How to Diagnose Society's Misfidgets

There are no objective diagnostic criteria for ADHD—no physical symptoms, no neurological signs, and no blood tests. Despite claims to the contrary, there are no brain scan findings and no biochemical imbalances.[10] No physical tests can be done to verify that a child has "ADHD." Advocates of ADHD have sought ways around this embarrassment.

Psychiatrist Paul Wender (1995), Distinguished Professor of Psychiatry at the University of Utah School of Medicine, claims to have located an objective, diagnostic sign for ADHD—foot tapping. According to Wender, foot tapping or fidgeting, in and of itself, is sufficient to make the diagnosis:

> Fidgeting and foot movements (known to our research setting as "Wender's sign") are common signs of hyperactivity in adult ADHD patients—so much so that such patients can usually be diagnosed in the waiting room by a knowledgeable receptionist.... I seriously entertain the possibility that this foot movement may be a biological marker for ADHD.[11]

In an endnote[12] Wender explains that "restless feet are readily observed— in cafeterias, waiting rooms, and group meetings." He believes the "diagnostic sensitivity and specificity" of the sign could be scientifically proven by taking a medical history of foot tappers randomly selected from these groups. However, Wender sees barriers in the way of his cafeteria research, observing that "its execution poses practical ethical problems."

Wender is no fringe advocate of the diagnosis—he is a founding father of the ADHD/Ritalin movement. He wrote the most influential early book, worked to make the diagnosis popular through his former post at NIMH, and remains among the most prominent psychiatrists in the field.

The diagnosis of ADHD, however cavalierly made, carries enormous consequences for the child. Wender reminds the reader that "Wender's foot sign" is "the rapidly flexing knee or foot." He then goes on to say, "The reduction of the foot sign in ADHD patients may also be an indicator of stimulant [drug] response."[13] Thus, Wender first diagnoses the child by the increased rate of foot tapping and then determines the medicine is working when the rate declines. It's as if there's no one attached to the foot.

From Foot Tapping to Jiggle Counters

When animal researchers perform very simplified studies of drug effects on rats or mice, they sometimes use a jiggle box that automatically records the number of times the rodent moves or jumps about. Lucinda Miller and Irvin Kraft (1994) have gone one step further than Wender by trying to quantify a child's restless arm movements with a strapped on "jiggle counter." Officially known as an actigraph, it's a motion detector and recorder packed into a minicomputer worn like a wristwatch. Miller and Kraft hope the Orwellian device will add to the *objective* assessment of hyperactive children. They don't ask how it will affect the *subjective* feelings of the children who must wear it.

ADHD is a "rat in a jiggle box" diagnosis that treats children as if they have no feelings, reasons, or motives behind their actions. As carried to an extreme by Wender, the diagnosis merely counts the number of unwanted, undesirable, or irritating behaviors displayed by a child. It doesn't ask, "Why is this particular child acting so jittery or nervous? What is the child thinking or feeling? What's the child's inner experience? What's the child responding to?" In fact, the diagnostic process rejects any concern with the child's feelings. There isn't a single item among the ADHD criteria that would require asking a child, "How do *you* feel?"

Is There Anything Objective about ADHD Ratings?

In clinical practice physicians often base their assessment of drug effects "on the parents' and sometimes teachers' impressions as to whether the children seemed better, the same, or worse on medication." These remarks were made by Mayes and Bixler (1993) who created a double blind ADHD study to test how much agreement there would be among people making assessments of children as "better, same, or worse." They compared the ratings given by parents and by teachers, as well as by staff.

The results? They found no agreement among raters. In fact, raters were "more likely to disagree than agree." Mayes and Bixler question using global impressions from parents, teachers, or professionals as a basis for diagnosing and drugging children.

The situation in real life clinical practice is even worse than in the study by Mayes and Bixler. In the doctor's office, the parent—usually the mother— isn't even given a simple checklist where she must choose between "better, same, or worse." Instead, the parent chats with the doctor for a few minutes in the office about how she feels the child is doing. Later chats typically take place on the telephone. The physician makes a determination about continuing medication based on a few casual words from the mom on the phone every few months or so. In most of the medical records I've examined, there isn't even an attempt to quantify the drug effect in rough terms such as "better, same, or worse."

How Much Time Does It Take?

Most physicians seem to spend only a few minutes making the initial diagnosis of ADHD. Given the criteria they are using—a mental checklist of behaviors—it's no surprise that so little time is required. Many insurance companies provide an economic incentive for quickie diagnoses by allocating only 15 minutes for evaluating ADHD.[14] Given the superficiality with which physicians are viewing these problems, spending more time might not improve their decision-making.

Children are being diagnosed and medicated on the basis of personal, subjective impressions offered to physicians who then make their own personal, subjective impressions. The entire process is too subjective and imprecise to have objective validity. Yet the drugging of the child is being justified on the basis of medical science.

Seeing What We Expect to See

Therapists, teachers, and non-professionals will evaluate children to a great extent on the basis of what they are told in advance about them. In other words, they see what they expect to see. Years ago, a team led by John Neisworth (1974) from Pennsylvania State University studied the effect of knowing a child's diagnosis on how raters evaluate the child's hyperactivity. In explaining the need for the study, they note that research has shown that teachers and therapists will *rate* and *relate* to people in part depending on their given diagnosis.[15] Neisworth and his colleagues found that "prior knowledge of a child's being diagnosed as hyperkinetic significantly increased the likelihood that the child would be perceived as more hyperkinetic" by the raters.

Hocus Pocus: Now You See It, Now You Don't

The ADHD child, the literature repeatedly observes, may look entirely normal in the office. As a 1995 symposium on ADHD observed, the problem is "the kids are often asymptomatic in your office."[16]

Why don't observations in the doctor's office tell us whether a child has ADHD? When receiving attention in a one-to-one relationship with any adult, including an examining doctor, the youngster is likely to seem normal, or even especially bright and competent. Perhaps because they are so hungry for attention, they may seem especially attentive to any doctor who spends a few minutes showing interest in them.

The *DSM-IV* actually warns diagnosticians that children may not show signs of the "disorder" when they are doing something interesting, when they are involved in a novel situation, when they receive rewards for a job well done, or when they are getting almost any kind of one-to-one attention from an adult. The children may also seem normally attentive and focused when discipline is being maintained. These are such startling admissions by the "official authority" on a presumed disease or disorder that it's worth quoting the official diagnostic manual:

> Symptoms typically worsen in situations that require sustained attention or mental effort or that lack intrinsic appeal or novelty (e.g., listening to classroom teachers, doing class assignments, listening to or reading

lengthy materials, or working on monotonous, repetitive tasks). Signs of the disorder may be minimal or absent when the person is under strict control, is in a novel setting, is engaged in especially interesting activities, is in a one-to-one situation (e.g., the clinician's office), or while the person experiences frequent rewards for appropriate behavior.[17]

Does "ADHD" have more to do with the child's *situation* than with the child's personal *condition*? The checklist of ADHD behavior tells us more about the child's situation than the child's "condition." When the ADHD/Ritalin movement was still a fledgling, J. Larry Brown and Stephen R. Bing (1976) warned, "Considering the joylessness of many schools with their authoritarian structures, it is fair to speculate that hyperactivity may be a 'normal' response—indeed, even a healthy reaction—to an intolerable situation."

A Cruel and Unusual Diagnosis

ADHD scales are frequently given to parents and teachers to use for rating their children and pupils. One of the most popular, the Revised Conners Questionnaire, is basically a variation on the traits listed in the *DSM*. A parent came to me for a consultation because a teacher was using the inventory to prove that her child needed Ritalin. The parent was appalled. The forty-eight items include "daydreams," "sassy," wanting to "run things," "shy," pouting, "feelings easily hurt," "childish... clings, needs constant reassurance," not getting along with siblings, bragging, and getting pushed around—or pushing around—other kids.

One of the items of the Conners scale simply states "cruel." Two of its other items are "Basically an unhappy child" and "Feels cheated in the family circle." Isn't it cruel and unjust to label a child without asking what kind of family and school environment leads the child "to feel cheated in the family circle" and to be "basically unhappy."

Almost any child in almost any family—no matter how ideally the parents conduct themselves—is likely at times to feel "cheated" and "basically unhappy." Being a child is tough; painful feelings are a part of growing up.[18] The aim is to help the child outgrow feeling cheated and feeling basically unhappy, but singling out the youngster for a diagnosis and drugs will only make the child feel more cheated and more unhappy.

The Conners Abbreviated Teacher Questionnaire, with only ten items, is even more simplistic and potentially abusive. The criteria include restlessness, overactivity, failing to finish things, fidgeting, and so on. It's an inventory of the ways children can annoy and frustrate their over-taxed teachers, especially by requiring their increased attention and consideration. Without losing sympathy for the teachers—who are themselves too frequently confined to the same boring, rigid classrooms—we should not diagnose the children who cannot or will not quietly submit to our nation's classrooms.

Daring to Daydream

Daydreaming and looking out the window in class are not mentioned in the official APA list of symptoms but they come up frequently as cardinal signs of inattention in diagnosing ADHD. I have been consulted by parents who were told to seek a "medical evaluation" (that is, medication) for their children because the youngsters were daydreaming in class and "not living up to their academic potential" (that is, not getting high enough grades). Fortunately, I have been able to help these parents fight the pressure to drug their children. Sometimes through consulting with the schools, I have enabled teachers to be more tolerant of children whose imaginations distract them from the humdrum routine of the classroom. At other times, I've helped parents find alternative schools that could capture the imagination of their children. In most cases, there's been little or nothing the matter in the home life of these imaginative children, so their parents haven't needed lengthier therapy to improve their parenting skills.

Daydreaming is risky, concludes reporter Zachary. He quotes therapist and author, Michael Gurian, "The country is making the argument without often realizing it, that boyhood is defective." With the new emphasis on daydreaming, we're making "girlhood" equally defective.

A report in *Pediatric News* summarized symposium remarks by a neuropsychologist:[19]

> Research has shown that children with attention-deficit hyperactivity disorder have "an attentional bias toward novelty and stimulation," whether they find the new stimuli through daydreaming or physical activity...

Consider the implications of "An attentional bias toward novelty and stimulation." It is a prime example of pseudoscientific phraseology—how to make something potentially wonderful into something ugly and threatening by a mere twist of language. It is tragic that loving novelty, and expressing it through daydreaming and physical activity, can result in a child being diagnosed ADHD.

Stimulants, as already documented, will inhibit an animal's aspirations for "novelty and stimulation."[20] They will do the same thing to the child with "an attentional bias toward novelty." But if the child escapes being diagnosed and drugged, these same traits can inspire a wonderful, productive life. Many in my generation have become creative adults because our teachers and parents didn't have the opportunity to drug us as children.

An Infant King Kong: More Extreme Behaviors

The behaviors called ADHD can sometimes become very extreme. Children can be so over-active that they become seemingly impossible to deal with. They may cause harm to themselves and to property, if not to other people. They can turn every venture outside the house into chaos and humiliation for the parents. Impulsivity and inattentiveness can make it almost impossible for a youngster to carry out routine activities and can even lead to dangerous behavior.

Paul Wender described the kind of child who in his opinion requires medication:

> [A]fter an active and restless infancy, the child stood and walked at an early age, and then, like an infant King Kong, burst the bars of his crib and marched forth to destroy the house. He was always on the go, always into everything, always touching (and hence, usually by mistake, breaking) every object in sight. When unwatched for a moment he somehow got to the top of the refrigerator or appeared in the middle of the street. In a twinkling pots and pans were whisked from cupboards, ashtrays knocked off tables, and lamps overturned. The mother usually felt—with good cause—that to take her eyes off him for one moment was to invite disaster: the moment her back was turned, something was broken or the toddler's life was in danger.[21]

From Wender's viewpoint, this is a child who is genetically and biologically defective and in need of medication. When I read this description, I see a child who is endowed with marvelous energy—a child who needs his parents to find a better balance of unconditional love and rational discipline. Given the description of how much "trouble" the child gets in, he probably needs a lot more supervision.

When we see children acting in very irrational and destructive ways, it's tempting to diagnose them. But a behavior can be extreme without being caused by a defect within the child. Extreme behaviors almost always indicate equally extreme conditions in the child's life. If children are very upset or frustrated and out of control, they are in special need of adult attention aimed at recognizing their unmet needs and fulfilling them.

Questions about ADHD-like symptoms are sometimes posed as if they are a matter of degree: "When do these behaviors or attitudes become abnormal, unacceptable, or a problem? At what age? In what numbers? For how long?" But it's better to ask, "What does it *mean* when a child displays an unusually large number of these traits or behaviors? Does it reflect on the child's *condition* or on the child's *situation* and *life experiences?*" In my own experience, extreme behaviors in children are always matched by extreme deprivations, provocations, or confusions in their lives.

When Children Run Amok

Some frantic children can drive their teachers and parents to distraction:[22]

Marty entered third grade, a scrawny brown-haired boy with a quizzical look and a feverish imagination. He annoyed fellow students by following them, pad and pen in hand, jotting down their every word. ... He led a class strike over a math assignment, persuading 25 other kids to repeatedly shout "No pay, No work!" ... [Marty] could drive [his mother] to distraction as well. He had a habit of waking her up in the middle of the night to share his latest tall tale. She had only stopped the practice by giving Marty a tape recorder and promising to listen to his recordings the next morning.

Marty was repeatedly diagnosed as ADHD by teachers and medical professionals who pressured his parents to medicate him with Ritalin. But who is this child? Not someone who lacks the ability to focus his attention. He can focus with compulsive determination on his projects. But he does seem like a child who is desperate *for* attention as he flails about seeking appreciation, recognition, and a place in the world for himself.

Marty follows students around, organizes students in defiance of teachers, wakes his mother up in the middle of the night. These are desperate pleas for attention. Beneath this compulsion to be the center of attention must lie a feeling of despair over not getting the attention he needs. Notice how he marshals enormous imagination and energy toward overcoming his anguish. Here we have the makings of a very creative adult. With a more secure sense of self that comes from receiving love and rational discipline, he could become a future journalist, author, or political leader. With his energy and imagination, he might become all three and more!

When Marty's mother finally gave in to drugging him, she couldn't bear the changes that she witnessed: "He wasn't there. He did everything he was supposed to do. But his personality was gone." She missed him.

Marty's mom stopped the medication and recommitted herself to doing everything in her power to help her son without drugging him. She went to his classes to help him learn discipline, she met with his teachers, she encouraged the school to create more interesting assignments for him, she resolved conflicts with her husband about how to raise him, and she made necessary changes in herself to deal better with her son's lack of self-control.

Now Marty is having a fine year in the 11th grade, still as energetic as ever, getting good grades in courses that interest him, writing screenplays as a hobby, working 20 hours a week at a Pizza Hut, and getting himself to school on time.

There's an unspoken theme in Marty's story that comes up time and again—a seeming lack of involvement on the part of the father. This can make it much harder for Marty to master his unusual abilities and energy. Fortunately, his mother was willing to go to great lengths to help him.

Extraordinary children can make extraordinary demands on their parents—but the rewards can be extraordinary as well.

Still Fighting Despite the Drugs

In my own practice, I sometimes see children who have remained at war with their parents despite being drugged with enough psychoactive substances to knock down an adult. While sedated into near unconsciousness, they find the energy to awaken themselves to respond vigorously to real or imagined insults and humiliations at home or in school. They are like heroes in their own life, fighting both the effects of the drugs and the adults whom they perceive as threatening them.

Tragically, the medications given to these children almost always retard their ability to learn self-discipline and self-control, or to improve their relationships with their peers, parents, and teachers. These children need toxin-free brains before they can adequately exercise their minds toward greater self-determination. As a result, the children do much better as they come off their medications. Although their parents thought the drugs were helping, they were actually impeding progress.

Many of these mothers and fathers were misled by doctors into believing that drugs, rather than improved parenting or improved schooling, were the solution. As a result, they never fully applied themselves to improving the child's home and school life. Instead, they got into a vicious cycle of ever-increasing amounts and numbers of medications.

I have described my treatment of these children and their families in *Reclaiming Our Children* (2000) and I will review some of the basic principles in the later chapters of this book. Here I want to confirm that well-meaning parents can almost always be helped to regain control over their angry, violent children.

Usually it's possible to understand how the child got out of control by spending an hour or two in the office with the parents while they interact with their offspring. Often there are obvious conflicts between the parents concerning how to mete out discipline. Often one or both parents seem to ignore very destructive behavior while over-reacting to rather harmless behavior. Typically, the parents already have a glimmer of what they are doing wrong, but they haven't been able to formulate it clearly or to come up with a better alternative. In these situations, it's possible to give a guarantee that if the parents will work on developing the right balance between rational discipline and unconditional love, the child will develop self-control. Often the therapy only requires a few months of hard work by the family.

Sabrina's Story

The more tragic end of the continuum of "ADHD children" is illustrated by the short, tortured life of Sabrina Green who died at age nine suffering from untreated burns, blows to her head, and gangrene that destroyed her hands.[23] Sabrina was supposed to be taking "medication that stabilized her hyperactivity." Ritalin had been prescribed "for her hyperactivity and attention deficit disorder."

Sabrina's story raises many unanswered questions. Who diagnosed her ADHD without taking notice of the abuse and neglect in her life? Who prescribed Ritalin to subdue her behavior when she needed adult intervention to prevent further abuse? How could she be described as suffering from ADHD in a story that details her horrendous history of abuse?

At best, the ADHD diagnosis obscures a child's real needs. At worst, the diagnosis covers up severe child abuse. It accomplishes these tragic aims first by diagnosing the child rather than the child's situation and second by suppressing the child's distressed behavior with drugs.

Rejecting the Feelings of Children

As already described, the child's feelings are almost always ignored in making the ADHD diagnosis and then in determining the effect of the medication.[24] There is almost nothing in the professional literature about the viewpoint of children labeled ADHD and treated with Ritalin. The diagnostic criteria in the ADHD diagnosis are consistent with this rejection of the feelings of children. Specifically intended to justify the use of medication to control behavior, they focus on behavior to the complete exclusion of the child's feelings.

This point cannot be over-emphasized: The ADHD diagnosis does not concern itself with how the child feels. A child gets diagnosed ADHD without any regard for his or her emotions, thoughts, inner experience, attitudes, or viewpoint.

ADHD/Ritalin advocates Dulcan and Popper (1991) note: "ADHD children show distractibility (especially when bored)...." But words such as "bored" or "frustrated" do not appear in the official diagnosis, and they are left out of most ADHD discussions, because they reflect the child's feelings or attitudes toward the environment. To be "bored" or "frustrated" indicates that the child is reacting to the world rather than being driven like a machine by an internal disorder.

Getting To Know The Child

A few ADHD/Ritalin advocates recognize some of the problems involved in making the diagnosis. Dulcan and Popper (1991) observe:

> Clinical expertise is necessary to differentiate ADHD from *normal high activity level*, which may be causing complaints from parents or teachers. Problems of recent onset and brief duration may represent an *adjustment disorder*. In addition, *situational anxiety, child abuse and neglect*, or simply

boredom can clinically present as inattention, hyperactivity, or impulsivity.[25]

From the heart of the ADHD/Ritalin community comes this open admission that almost anything—from normal behavior through boredom, anxiety, and child abuse—can be mistaken for supposedly genuine ADHD. In reality, there is no "genuine ADHD" that emerges without provocation from the child's brain.

Children can meet the ADHD criteria for an infinite number of reasons. As I've already suggested, many are average or normal children who are being evaluated by standards of behavior that are too narrow. It is ironic that we tolerate an increasingly narrow band of behavior from our children at the very moment that we have lost our authority over them. This combination of narrow standards and weakened adult authority creates constant conflict.

Some "ADHD children" are especially creative or energetic and cannot bear the confines of their classrooms or homes. A few are physically ill or injured. Some lack the intellectual tools to cope with ordinary classrooms. Others are emotionally traumatized or disturbed. A number need more time to grow up. Some need more rational and consistent discipline but others have undergone too much harsh discipline. Some have had their whims overindulged by their parents but others haven't received enough unconditional love. Nearly all of them—like most children in America—could benefit from more individual time with their parents, especially their fathers who are frequently uninvolved with them.

Knowing that a child fits perfectly into the category called ADHD tells us little or nothing about the child's mental or physical state, or about the child's situation at home or in school. It tells us very little, if anything, about the child's unique needs. It takes time and effort to identify each child's unique needs, and even more time, effort, and patience to respond to them.

Cutting out the Cookie-Cutter

Stamping children with cookie-cutter diagnoses may seem "scientific" but in reality it is ill conceived and harmful. Making believe that these children have a mental disorder is dreadfully stigmatizing and leads to unfounded medical treatments.

My own experience confirms that many children who get diagnosed ADHD are especially energetic, creative, and independent youngsters struggling within the confines of inattentive, conflicted, or stressed environments. We end up drugging those children who display the most potential to live a zestful, inspired life—those otherwise destined to make an outstanding creative contribution to society.

Lynne Azepeitia and Mary Rocamora (1997) in the "Misdiagnosis of the Gifted" report similar findings in their work:

It's well-known among researchers of the gifted, talented and creative that these individuals exhibit greater intensity and increased levels of emotional, imaginational, intellectual, sensual and psychomotor excitability and that this is a normal pattern of development.

These characteristics, however, are frequently perceived by psychotherapists and others as evidence of a mental disturbance... ADHD and ADD are a few of the diagnostic labels mistakenly used...

When working with the gifted, a therapist must address the following intrapersonal issues: the internal stress of being gifted; the emotional trauma of rapid development; the effects of introversion, intensity, perfectionism and extraordinary sensitivity to self and others...[26]

Hallowell (1997) is an exception among ADHD/Ritalin advocates in recognizing that his own ADHD "condition" has a positive side, in his case "the high bursts of energy and creativity and an indefinable, zany sense of life." Similarly, Dulcan and Popper (1991) point out the potentially positive aspects of childhood disorders, including ADHD:

Certain individuals may even learn to turn childhood deficits such as excessive sensitivity (separation anxiety), unrelenting stubbornness (oppositional defiant disorder), or uncontrolled activity and enthusiasm (attention-deficit hyperactivity disorder) into strengths in adulthood.[27]

Dulcan and Popper further suggest that, as a result of "compensatory abilities and an enhancing environment," many of these children will achieve even beyond the apparent limits of their IQ scores. But neither Hallowell nor Dulcan and Popper cast doubt on the basic concept of ADHD as a "disorder." They do not consider the possibility that many or most of these children in fact have nothing wrong with them, and that their vitality and individuality brings them into conflict with individual adults and particular environments.

In his early work, biological psychiatrist Paul Wender (1973) indirectly recognized redeeming features in the "ADHD child." Most of these children, he stated, display "increased independence" and can be "excessively independent."[28] But the tone and context does not suggest that Wender values these tendencies.

It is difficult to distinguish between a child who has an attentional problem and a child who isn't getting enough attention, or between a child who has a discipline problem and a child who isn't getting appropriate discipline. Often they are one and the same. It's best if we take responsibility as adults and decide that it's our job to provide more attention or better discipline rather than to assume the problem lies in the child.

As I've already indicated, there's no real way for a psychiatrist, pediatrician, primary care physician, or other clinician to differentiate between a child who is especially sensitive, physically precocious, daring, independent, energetic, or creative, and a child who supposedly has a disorder. It's best for the children when we assume that they are in fact unique and wonderful, and when we decide that it's our job as adults to help them bring out and to master their special qualities.

Once again it comes down to identifying a child's real needs, to finding better methods of resolving conflict between adults and children, and to helping children develop their unique talents and qualities. Anyone who has raised or taught children knows that the most interesting and exciting children can be the most trying. In the words of Themistocles, the ancient Greek philosopher, "The wildest colts make the best horses."

Can Doctors Tell What's Going on in a Child's Family?

ADHD/Ritalin doctors believe that their clinical expertise enables them to separate the "ADHD child" from one who is suffering from a conflicted family or stressful classroom, or even from one who has been abused. This is nonsense; no one can be sure about what goes on behind the closed doors of a family.

Even in intensive and lengthy psychotherapy with experienced professionals, parents and children can easily hide the truth about their family life. If the parents want to present the child as the problem, then they will very likely withhold evidence to the contrary. If the doctor also wants to see the child as having a disorder, then there's almost no possibility that underlying family problems will surface. I've evaluated families who have taken their children to multiple doctors, including specialists at leading universities, without ever being asked about conflicts and stresses in the family. Often obvious conflicts were overlooked by the evaluators.

Studies show that clinicians and researchers have no special ability to know when they are being told the truth by children. They cannot discern whether children are telling the truth about such simple matters as how they feel about medication and whether they are really taking it.[29] Without obvious signs, such as bruises or abject terror, they often cannot tell if the child is being abused.

ADHD and Control

Gerald Golden (1991), an ADHD/Ritalin advocate, observes: "The behavior is seen as being disruptive and unacceptable by parents and teachers, and the child is socially handicapped as a result." Russell Barkley (1981)[30] put it this way: "Although inattention, overactivity, and poor impulse control are the most common symptoms cited by others as primary in hyperactive children, my own work with these children suggests that noncompliance is also a primary problem."

Is it surprising that children would be noncompliant—resistive, defensive, or even rebellious—with Barkley? He sees the child as entirely the source of the problem: "there is, in fact, something 'wrong' with these children."[31] As for the teachers and parents, he continually makes clear there's nothing wrong with them.

What Is a Syndrome and Why Does It Matter?

ADHD is sometimes defined as a syndrome. What does it mean when a syndrome does not exist? The English word syndrome comes from the Greek word meaning concurrence—coming together. A syndrome is "a set of symptoms which occur together; the sum of signs of any morbid state; a symptom complex."[32]

There are dozens of syndromes listed in any medical dictionary or textbook. An example that many people have experienced is "The Chinese Restaurant Syndrome"—a symptom complex of head throbbing and lightheadedness, sometimes accompanied by tightness of the jaw, neck, and shoulders, as well as backache. I have seen cases associated with anxiety as well. It is caused by monosodium glutamate, a seasoning in Chinese food that produces dilation of the arteries.[33]

A syndrome, then, is a group of symptoms that have a meaningful relationship to each other and presumably to an underlying cause, such as the ingestion of monosodium glutamate. The point made by many critics is that ADHD does not represent a rationally related group of symptoms, nor does it reflect an underlying disorder. In other words, it is not a valid syndrome. According to Armstrong (1995):

> While there are thousands of studies that have been done in the past three decades using some version of the A.D.D. myth as a governing paradigm, once we begin to peel away the artifice, layer by layer, we discover that— as with the disappearing Cheshire cat in Lewis Carroll's classic children's tale—all we're really left with in the end is the smile, if that.[34]

Calling Children Lots of Names at Once

One of the major purposes of a diagnosis is to name a syndrome or disorder that can be evaluated as a separate, specific, or unique entity. If the diagnosis always overlaps with several other diagnoses, the value of the diagnosis itself can be called into question. Let us suppose, for example, you were trying to describe a new type of personality disorder. However, your research discloses that it almost always overlaps with several other personality types, even with normal personalities. Or suppose you want to describe a new kind of skin rash but your research indicates that it shares qualities with several other skin rashes, even with normal skin. After a while, you would begin to wonder if you were describing anything meaningful or useful in your new personality disorder or your new rash.

In psychiatry, the term comorbidity indicates the presence of more than one independent or separate mental disorder in the same person at the same time. Every expert acknowledges that the ADHD diagnosis is usually comorbid with other disorders.

John Richters (1995) and a large team assembled by the National Institute of Mental Health cite studies indicating that 30–50% of children diagnosed ADHD are also diagnosed oppositional defiant disorder or conduct disorder, syndromes that include negative or destructive behaviors. Another 15–75% are found to have mood disorders, such as depression; yet another 25% have anxiety disorders, and a remarkable 10–92% have learning disorders. There are other comorbid disorders that they don't even mention, in particular, post-traumatic stress disorder, a common problem that mimics many of the so-called ADHD symptoms.[35] Of course, these huge numbers are only intelligible in terms of many of the individual children having many overlapping disorders.

Another summary declared of children with ADHD:

> Roughly 30% of these children will have major depression. Approximately 30% of boys and 40% of girls have anxiety disorders. Between 10% and 25% have juvenile mania, and roughly 30% have language processing problems or other non-attention deficit hyperactivity disorder learning disabilities.[36]

We have already seen how the collection of symptoms described as ADHD also occurs in normal children when they are exposed to a boring or stressful environment, as well as children who are especially creative. It can also occur in medically ill children. Now we discover that ADHD commonly appears in children who are suffering from almost every conceivable childhood psychiatric or educational diagnosis, from learning problems to mania. Furthermore, it begins to look like a case of "pure ADHD" is rather rare. All this confirms that ADHD is a relatively meaningless list of behaviors that can pop up almost anywhere, that can mean almost anything, and that can occur in almost anyone, including even normal or especially bright and creative children.

Given these facts, there seems no likelihood that ADHD could turn out to be a biochemical or genetic entity. It simply isn't an identifiable entity, so how could it have a specific physical cause? Of course, many children—for an infinite number of reasons—do show signs of being distractible, overactive, or impulsive, often depending on their circumstances or physical condition at the time; but that doesn't mean they have a disease, disorder, or syndrome suitable to treatment with stimulant drugs.

The Learning Mystique

In discussing the overlapping of diagnoses, we found an estimate that 10–92% of children diagnosed ADHD will also be diagnosed with Learning Disorders (LD). Obviously, many children diagnosed ADHD are also diagnosed LD. This overlap is so extensive that it becomes difficult at times to distinguish between the two diagnoses. To the extent that children have difficulty with paying attention in school, they are also likely to have trouble learning.

The term "LD child" is probably as commonplace as "ADHD child." According the *Diagnostic and Statistical Manual of Mental Disorders, IV* (1994), learning disorders are divided into three main categories: "Reading Disorder" (previously called dyslexia), "Mathematics Disorder," and "Disorder of Written Expression." The disorders are diagnosed "when the individual's achievement on individually administered, standardized tests in reading, mathematics, or written expression is substantially below that expected for age, schooling, and level of intelligence." In other words, the child isn't performing up to expectation. The everyday concept of the "underachiever" has been turned into a disorder.[37]

The concept of learning disabilities grew out of the same hope as ADHD—that the failure of children to meet adult expectations could be explained by minimal neurological dysfunctions within the brains of the child. As psychologist Gerald Coles observed, "After decades of research, it has still not been demonstrated that disabling neurological dysfunctions exist in more than a minuscule number of these children."[38]

Much like ADHD, LD takes a problem that can result from innumerable causes and reduces it to a simple-minded medical-sounding diagnosis. Again, like ADHD, the diagnosis overlaps with many others in the manual.

The *DSM-IV* specifies that learning disorders must be differentiated from normal variations in academic attainment. But it provides no guideline except that a learning disorder is relatively severe and interferes with school or life performance. The definition doesn't allow for a rational way to distinguish it from underachievement with its multiple causes.

The *DSM-IV* also tries to differentiate learning disorders from lack of opportunity, poor teaching, cultural and language differences, mental retardation, and poor vision or hearing. But that is only the beginning. Learning disorders, if they are specific mental or neurological dysfunctions, must be differentiated from *anything else* that can interfere with learning, including anxiety, lack of confidence, fears associated with success, and family problems that inhibit a child's development.

Given the definition—that the child isn't learning or achieving up to expectation—it's no surprise that these diagnoses are as controversial as ADHD. They have never been found to have a neurological basis. They cannot be detected or diagnosed by specific tests.[39]

In 1987 psychologist Gerald Coles wrote *The Learning Mystique: A Critical Look At "Learning Disabilities."* Parents who feel pressured to believe that their children have learning disorders ought to read his book. The concept of LD, like ADHD, blames the child's brain. This discourages adults from looking at the true sources of the problem, such as normal developmental delays, lack of interest in the subject, sexist attitudes that suppress the abilities of girls, poor schooling that leaves children unable to read and write, and family or school expectations that intimidate children into failure.

Educator Michael Valentine (1988) put it succinctly:

> My initial assumptions are that most reading difficulties are the result of an instructional disability, a curriculum disability, a teacher disability, a school-philosophy disability, and/or a specific family interaction or structure disability, rather than a specific physiological, perceptual, or neurological disability… I suspect the incidence of "learning disabilities" in this country would be greatly reduced if we could rule out these other possibilities for poor reading.[40]

Lately there has been growing recognition that a large portion of America's children cannot read because they have never been properly taught.[41] They are also falling behind in math.[42] Fake learning disorder diagnoses such as "Reading Disorder" and "Mathematics Disorder" delayed our recognition of the failings of our educational system by blaming it on individual children.

When children are not achieving according to their innate abilities, labeling them with a disorder is among the worst possible approaches. If parents feel that an intervention is warranted, it should begin with a self-assessment of parental attitudes toward the child's school work. If a child is falling too far behind in a subject such as reading, an experienced tutor can be very helpful. Meanwhile, a parent reading with a child can be one of the most important bonding and learning experiences of the child's life.[43] It can also inspire a lifelong love of books and education.

Overall, parents need to be empowered to assess the needs of their children without handing then over to "the professionals."

But What If a Brain Disorder Is Discovered?

Even if it turns out that some children routinely labeled ADHD have a physical disorder, it doesn't mean that Ritalin or any other psychiatric drug is the answer. Chapter 13 will review a vast array of potential physical causes for ADHD-like symptoms, including the toxic effects of psychiatric drugs, lead poisoning, head injury, and thyroid disease. While few children diagnosed ADHD suffer from any physical illnesses, it is important to remember that ADHD-like behaviors can have a biological origin in *real* diseases rather than in mythological biochemical imbalances. Two points need to be made in regard to the possibility of finding medical causes for individual children who display ADHD-like behaviors. First, when a medical cause is found, the disorder is no longer diagnosed ADHD. It is called by the name of the genuine disorder, such as hypothyroid disease, closed head injury, or drug intoxication. Second, as a real disease, it is almost never treated with Ritalin or other stimulants.

Since the stimulant drugs, one and all, impair brain function, they should be avoided when there's a known physical disorder at the root of a child's problems. Ritalin, for example, is not helpful to people with known brain injuries.[44]

These drugs, as amply demonstrated, have no beneficial effect on the brain. Instead, the stimulants produce brain malfunction and will worsen the condition of an already impaired brain.

Adult ADHD

The criticisms made of the ADHD diagnosis throughout this book, including the next few chapters, apply to the adult form as well. Adult ADHD is also not a valid syndrome or disorder.

The promotion of adult ADHD in the United States has disastrous implications for children. It encourages parents and doctors to keep children on the drug indefinitely, anticipating they will need it in their adult years as well. With overwhelming evidence that long-term use has no positive effects and many potentially irreversible hazards, this is a prescription for countless tragedies.

What keeps this harmful nonsense going? A combination of ADHD/Ritalin promotional efforts and positive media coverage. After pointing out estimates that 729,000 adults will receive prescriptions for Ritalin this year, a front page *New York Times* report describes the drug as nothing short of miraculous:[45]

> For some adults, a remedy cannot come too soon. Left untreated, people with the disorder are often inattentive, impulsive and hyperactive.... Therapy can be so successful, though, that it is often impossible to pick out a person with the disorder who is undergoing treatment.

The newspaper story uncritically repeats the usual speculations about causation as if they are established facts, declaring "the disorder stems from a genetic dysfunction, probably a short circuit in the brain." Later it suggests that Ritalin "is thought to increase levels of dopamine, a chemical that appears to be in short supply in A.D.D. sufferers." Although toxic exposures are also mentioned as potential causes of ADHD-like symptoms, there's no hint that inattention could be generated by environmental factors in the family and school. Undoubtedly drawing on ADHD/Ritalin advocates, the report states:

While, virtually all psychiatrists frown on recreational use of Ritalin, many point out that it is preferable to speed or cocaine. Because Ritalin stays in the body only four hours, overdosing is difficult, they say.

It's worth re-emphasizing that while Ritalin's half-life ranges from 1–3 hours (or 2–4 hours in some estimates), a considerable amount of the drug will remain active in the body over many hours as the blood level continues to halve. Furthermore, drug effects can long outlast the presence of the drug, even producing a lifetime of damage.[46] Nor does a short half-life make a drug safe. A short half-life makes a stimulant more toxic and more likely to produce the acute euphoria that encourages drug abuse. This is why addicts inject or snort stimulants—to shorten and heighten the impact. This is also why crack cocaine is so dangerous—it has a very brief half-life.

Journal editors often seem even less critical than the media in publishing nonsensical, unfounded pronouncements by "experts." The August 1997 *Psychiatric Annals* devotes an entire issue to adult ADHD. Consider Paul Wender's report on adult ADHD, subtitled "A Wide View of a Widespread Condition." With even more certitude than the newspaper reporter, Wender announces his mythology as truth:

In conclusion, the syndrome of ADHD is common in adults. In most cases, ADHD is genetically transmitted and mediated by decreased dopaminergic activity in the brain.

As we'll confirm in the following chapter, there's no scientific evidence for these assertions.

Marvelously, the media sometimes transcend what they are spoon fed by the experts. Writing in the *Wall Street Journal*, journalist John McGinnis (1997) observes:[47]

That the line between cure and disease should be so blurry is no surprise, since there is no objective test for ADD or ADHD. In fact, despite countless attempts, no one has ever demonstrated that either disorder exists. But harried teachers and counselors have learned to recommend an ADD diagnosis to parents in order to get their more rambunctious students on Ritalin, an easy way to quiet them down.

Never a Useful Diagnosis

Whether children are "normal," mildly upset and impaired, or severely disturbed—they all need the same thing. Whether they come from families and communities that are thriving or those that are suffering poverty and oppression, all children need the attention of mature, informed adults who know how to identify and take care of their basic needs in the home, at school, and in the community.

Diagnosing a child ADHD is basically harmful and should never be done. It declares the child to be the sole source of the problem. In effect, it labels the child incorrigible—unreachable by the best adult efforts. This is an extremely negative viewpoint to bring to a child. Its main purpose is to justify the use of drugs.

When adults take stimulant drugs to improve their mood or mental function, it is misguided. It can be viewed as self-abuse. When children are given stimulant drugs, it should be viewed as a form of pseudo-scientific child abuse. We should not blame the many well-intentioned parents and teachers who have been grossly misinformed about the real effects of stimulant drugs. Instead, we should hold responsible the pharmaceutical companies, government agencies, professional organizations and advocacy groups that promote these dangerous drugs. We should also hold responsible the cadre of professionals who have devoted their careers to pushing these drugs on the nation's children.

Diagnosing children ADHD and drugging them would be considered unethical and illegal in a society that truly valued its children.

Chapter 10

SCIENTIFIC EVIDENCE FOR A
BIOLOGICAL CAUSE OF ADHD

You Can't Argue with a Brain Scan, Can You?

The notion that human beings are nothing more than complicated machines dies hard. It is the primary if not sole notion advanced by biopsychiatrists to account for diverse and complex human behaviors such as violence and "attention deficit disorder." It is also a notion that gives us a false sense of security and certainty. With it we can imagine that much of life's challenge is predictable and controllable.

—Ronald David, pediatrician and chief medical officer,
D.C. General Hospital (1997)

Johnny was not lazy, nor was the school failing to educate him decently: He had a learning disorder. Or he had an attention disorder. And the root of these disorders was a biological or neurological or genetic glitch. Poverty was let off the hook. Social injustices were let off the hook. Parents were let off the hook. Lousy schools and dysfunctional teachers were let off the hook. There was simply something biologically wrong with these children that accounted for all the things that teachers, parents, and Boy Scout leaders did not like about a whole panoply of childhood behaviors: not sitting still, not paying attention, not learning to read correctly (on time), butting in...

—Louise Armstrong, author, *And They Call It Help* (1995)

God is not a malevolent neurochemist who has fallen asleep on the assembly line.

—Denis Donovan, child psychiatrist (1997)

The previous chapter demonstrated that the ADHD diagnosis is not based on objective signs or criteria—that it is not a specific disorder, disease, or condition. ADHD/Ritalin advocates nonetheless claim there is evidence that the behaviors are caused by genetic and biological factors. Pediatricians, psychiatrists, neurologists, psychologists—an endless variety of health professionals—tell parents that ADHD is a proven "neurological" or "neurobiological" disorder. What is their evidence?

Making Something out of Nothing

As we look at the argument that ADHD is biological, we should begin armed with skepticism. How can something be biological when the something has no basis in reality? Nonetheless, media coverage and pronouncements by experts have left the public with the impression that there is a genetic, biochemical, or biological basis to the diagnosis.

Recently a TV producer responded to my skepticism by telling me about two "completely out of control ADHD children" whom she had filmed jumping around like crazy on the couch in their home. There was no doubt in her mind that these children were so hyperactive that they could have a brain disease just like cerebral palsy or multiple sclerosis.

"What are they like as kids?" I asked.

"Oh, they were delightful children. I took one of them out for a walk and lunch."

"Was he hyperactive when you were alone with him?"

"Yes…" she said hesitantly. And then, more hesitantly, "No, in fact, no, he was quite calm when we were alone. He was *easy* to be with."

"Do you think," I asked, "that a child's cerebral palsy goes away when he's having a nice time with a friendly, attentive adult?"

She was stunned. "No, of course not.…"

The Politics of the Brain Scan Scam

Chapter 1 and especially Chapter 3 documented that that there is no evidence for brain scan abnormalities, or any brain abnormalities, in children labeled ADHD. These scientific conclusions have been confirmed by both the November 1998 NIH Consensus Development Conference panel and the 2000 American Academy of Pediatrics official guidelines. To the extent that brain scan studies do show abnormalities in these children, the scans are detecting damage and dysfunction caused by stimulants and other psychiatric drugs.

Why return once again to debunking brain scans? Because so many people continue to be influenced by these false claims. The next sections will focus on some of the unscientific political manipulations behind the brain scan scam, in particular the fake science and media blitz behind the most highly publicized study of all.

Measuring Level of Activity—Not Abnormality

Earlier brain scan studies used single photon emission computed tomography (SPECT) to measure the perfusion or blood flow in various parts of the brain. More recent studies involve positron emission tomography (PET), a similar scanning procedure that can measure the rate of glucose uptake in parts of the brain. Glucose is the brain's only food source, so its rate of utilization is a measure of metabolism or energy utilization. The basic aim of both the SPECT and PET studies is to find areas of the brain that are comparatively hypoactive or hyperactive in children or adults diagnosed with ADHD. This is a limited measurement of brain function that addresses nothing more than the relative level of brain activity. It's roughly equivalent to taking the normal variations in temperature of various parts of the body.

If you happen to be using particular muscles, for example, their energy utilization will go up compared to other muscles that have not been active. The active muscles may even feel warm to the touch. These rough measures of energy utilization in no way indicate an abnormality in the underlying biochemical or neurological processes of the muscles. They only indicate that these muscles were recently exercised more than the colder muscles. Similarly, if you are visually active at a given moment, the visual cortex of your brain may consume relatively more glucose during that time. Or if the right side of your brain is especially active, then it may show a comparative increase in energy utilization compared to the left side. These relative degrees of activity say nothing about whether the activity is abnormal or normal. In fact, these differences can and do occur from moment to moment all day long in perfectly normal brains.

Pictures of multi-colored brain scans in newsmagazines and presentations can be an especially seductive touch. Brain scans are in fact two-tone—black and white with shades of gray. The different colors give the impression that specific areas are abnormal in some fashion, but the colors merely represent degrees of intensity. These colored brain scans are similar to newspaper weather maps in which 75–80 degrees is indicated by orange and 80–85 degrees is represented by red. The use of several different colors to highlight degrees of intensity adds an aura of science to brain scan maps, and makes them look much more complex than they are.

It seems unlikely that anything as simple as level of energy consumption will tell us much about the complex mental processes routinely diagnosed and treated by psychiatrists. Neurologist John Friedberg (1997) has described the PET as a "fuzzygram looking for a use. Like other such hinterland tests it has been overly applied to non-existent mental illnesses."

Timing Science with Politics

A team lead by NIMH's Alan Zametkin received national media acclaim for finding decreased brain metabolism in PET scans of adults with a retrospective history of ADHD in childhood.[1] The study has become the mainstay for "proving" that ADHD is a "neurobiological" disorder. It was timed to come out during critical debates in Congress over the reauthorization of the Education of the Handicapped Act, renamed the Individuals with Disabilities Act (IDEA).[2] The powerful ADHD/Ritalin lobby, led by the drug company funded parents' group, CHADD, was attempting to get ADHD included as a disability under the act. Zametkin is on CHADD's Professional Advisory Board.

The famous Zametkin research turned out to be a smoke and mirrors show. Despite all the ballyhoo about implications for children, the Zametkin study did not involve any children. The subjects were adults who were thought, in hindsight, to have suffered from ADHD as children. While the researchers were able to show some statistical differences between their scans of "ADHD" adults and "normal" controls, the effort required considerable statistical manipulation. When the sexes were compared separately, there were no statistically significant differences between the controls and ADHD adults. That should have ended the show right there, but it didn't. In order to get a significant result, the data was lumped together to include a disproportionate number of women in the controls.

When individual areas of the brain were compared between controls and ADHD adults, no differences were found. For example, a comparison of the frontal lobes of the ADHD brains and the controls showed no differences—yet the frontal lobes are alleged to be the critical areas in ADHD. There were no differences between any specific parts of the brain. Yet Zametkin told *Washington Post* reporter Sally Squires (1990), "Not only is brain metabolism abnormally low in this disorder, but it is low in the parts of the brain that we have known for years and years to be important for attention, handwriting, motor control and inhibiting responses."

It is almost always possible to shake up numbers like dice in a bowl enough times to produce some sort of statistical result, however worthless or misleading. Zametkin's study exemplifies this.

Making Political Hay
out of the Zametkin Study

Despite the flimsy quality of the results, Zametkin made repeated claims that his study supported the use of medication. He also claimed that it disproved environmental causes in the family or school. In November 1990, Zametkin told reporter Robert Engelman, "There are people who say you should not use medications, that it is a matter of upbringing. We're hoping that this [study] will put an end to that kind of thinking." Nor was Zametkin alone in making much out of nothing. ADHD/Ritalin advocate Joseph Biederman told Sally Squires that this "substantiates the notion that this is a biological condition." All of this is pernicious nonsense.

Of course, even if Zametkin is right about his study—that there is reduced energy utilization in some areas of the brains of individuals labeled ADHD—it would not justify giving them toxic stimulants. Many people have problems caused by brain disorders, from stroke to brain tumors, but responsible physicians do not recommend psychiatric drugs as a solution. Furthermore, even if Zametkin's study did show differences between the brains, it wouldn't necessarily indicate an abnormality. For example, the brains of the children might be more active but entirely normal, or they might reflect normal responses to unusual stress.

In reality, there was nothing whatsoever wrong with the brains of any of the people in the Zametkin study. The differences between brains generated in Zametkin's studies—and all other such research—appear only as the end result of mathematical formulae used to analyze data that have been grouped together from comparisons among many brains. The results are expressed as statistical variations between groups of brains. To repeat, the individual brain scans in Zametkin's studies—or in any other similar studies—cannot distinguish between the supposedly normal and the supposedly abnormal individual. *None of the brains of the subjects in Zametkin's PET scan studies looked abnormal and none of them were known to be abnormal!*

When a scan picture is shown in a magazine or flashed on a screen to show "differences" in the "ADD brain," the viewers are encouraged to believe that they are seeing the abnormal brain of an adult or child with ADHD. They will assume that Alan Zametkin or some other researcher could actually look at the particular brain scan and determine, "This one is from a child or an adult with ADHD." Nothing could be further from the truth.

In December 1996 the Drug Enforcement Administration (DEA) held a two-day conference on ADHD and Ritalin. One of the sections dealt with studies of the biological basis of the disorder and included several ADHD/Ritalin advocates, including Alan Zametkin. The conference concluded that no "specific neurological lesion or deficit" had been found in people diagnosed ADHD. As we found in regard to drug efficacy, the behind-the-scenes consensus is much different from the public image promoted by advocates.

Misleading Everybody—the Public and the Profession Alike

The Zametkin PET scans are frequently used to mislead the public and the profession into believing that abnormalities can be seen in the brains of children or adults diagnosed ADHD. The National Institute of Mental Health (1994), which has become a public relations agent for biopsychiatry, stoops to this deception in its booklet on ADHD. It shows PET scans of adults that allegedly demonstrate a difference between normal and ADHD brains. Perhaps more surprising, even textbooks of psychiatry fail to mention the flaws of the Zametkin study and show paired "normal" and "ADHD" brains as if there is a way to tell them apart.[3]

Few psychiatrists will have the time, interest, or background to critically evaluate the original research. They will accept what they read in newspapers, magazines, or books. An endless chain of misinformation is created.

The press has often leaped at Zametkin's studies, claiming, for example, "Such data helped pin down a biological basis for ADHD."[4] But can the press be blamed for responding with enthusiasm to the hoopla from Zametkin and NIMH?

As Richard E. Vatz and Lee S. Weinberg, professionals who are Associate Psychology Editors for *U.S.A. Today Magazine* (1995), observe:

> Periodically, there are "discoveries" that are trumpeted as the Rosetta stone for those seeking to define ADHD as a disease. Such was the case of the "landmark" 1990 study on hyperactivity and cerebral glucose metabolism in adults, published in the *New England Journal of Medicine*, that was—and is—heralded widely as demonstrating the biological basis for hyperactivity. However, it does not demonstrate that ADHD is caused by "abnormal brain chemistry," a misrepresentation regularly made by journalists and even researchers.

Even Zametkin Agrees

On one occasion since the publication of his study, Zametkin has admitted that he cannot tell the difference between a so-called "ADHD" brain and a normal one (1991):

> One commonly asked question of our brain imaging studies is whether PET scanning can be used to diagnose ADHD. Unfortunately, this is not currently possible because there is considerable overlap in our study between normal and ADHD brain metabolism.

In this particular interview, Zametkin further states that no specific defect has been found in the brains of people diagnosed with ADHD:

> Could it be that a dysfunction of the central nervous system is the key to our understanding of the etiology of Attention Deficit Disorder? Individually each finding is insufficient to prove that ADHD has a neurobiological basis. Indeed, it may still be a long time until the underlying cause of ADHD is established.

These are most remarkable admissions for a man whose work is flashed around the country in the media and at conferences as evidence that a difference can be seen between the "normal" brain and the "ADHD" brain. These are startling disclosures from a man who has repeatedly claimed that his studies show that ADHD children have flawed brains requiring stimulant medication.

Zametkin Fails to Confirm His Own Study

In the end, there's no great need to discredit Zametkin's 1990 study. When he actually got around to scanning the brains of adolescents diagnosed ADHD, the findings were not consistent with his original, much-publicized study.[5] The 1993 study is far more relevant because the subjects were not adults diagnosed in retrospect with childhood ADHD, but teenagers diagnosed at the time.

Once again, Zametkin and his team managed to produce some statistical correlations. However, the results are so weak that the researchers do not attribute much importance to them. In the 1990 study they had obtained no significant differences between individual areas of the brain but some global ones. This time they got the opposite—some individual differences but no global ones. The "Conclusions" section to their article does not bother to mention the few statistical correlations they managed to generate. Instead, it states unequivocally that "global or absolute measures of metabolism" showed no statistical differences. The study not only came out negative, it contradicted their earlier one. Although they don't discuss it, any possible findings could have been attributed to drug exposure, since 75% of the youngsters had been prescribed stimulants.[6]

Stretching Ethics

Did Zametkin and his colleagues publicize their negative findings in 1993 as fervently as they publicized their supposedly positive ones in 1990? Not even close. They did not hold any press conferences and interviews to point out that their new findings contradicted their earlier study. Instead, they developed another kind of smoke screen. Having stretched statistical manipulation to the limit, now they stretched the limits of ethics.

Having failed to prove their point about differences in the brains of children labeled ADHD, Zametkin now made much of proving that it's possible to get the parents of normal teenagers—used as controls in the study—to submit to tests involving radiation. This dubious claim is given more space in the summary than the negative results of the study:

> Positron emission tomography scans can be performed and are well tolerated by normal teenagers and teenagers with ADHD. The feasibility of normal minors participating in research involving radiation was established.

They further boast:

To our knowledge, ours is the first study … to use radiopharmaceuticals in normal minors in the United States for research purposes only.

Is this something to brag about? Or is this another example of what Ginger Breggin and I have called "technological child abuse?"[7]

In their 1990 PET scan study, Zametkin and his colleagues stated that they were using adults with ADHD instead of children "because of ethical concerns about exposing children to a radioactive tracer." It took only three years for their viewpoint to mature from one of ethical concern about exposing children to radiation to pride in having been the first to do it to *normal* children!

Several years later, writing in the *Archives of General Psychiatry*, C. T. Morton raised ethical concerns about Zametkin exposing normal children to radiation for research purposes.[8] He questioned whether there is sufficient information to determine "the maximum safe radiation dose in healthy research subjects of adolescent or younger ages." He also cast doubt on whether or not standards of consent for children were adequate to the complexity of this kind of research.

An "Alternative" Biological Extreme

Even "alternative" physicians who promote non-traditional physical treatments too often end up arguing that ADHD symptoms are caused by biological factors. *No More Ritalin* by Mary Ann Block (1996), an osteopathic physician, can be commended for its criticism of the use of Ritalin. Yet the book remains, in Block's words, a "physician's approach." In this vein, she declares, "In fact, I have found that children with ADHD symptoms usually do have an underlying health problem that has gone undiagnosed and untreated."

Block believes that "Low blood sugar, or hypoglycemia, is the most significant underlying problem I find in children who exhibit behavioral problems."[9] This is a most remarkable statement that seems to fly in the face of scientific, educational, and psychological evidence, as well as common sense. Even if some children with behavior problems may have periods of low blood sugar, it is absurd to claim that most do or that it is the primary cause.

Block is so convinced that hypoglycemia is the most common cause of childhood behavior problems like ADHD that she does not bother to give each patient a glucose tolerance test to make sure before she institutes her diets.

At least Block does not give toxic medications. But as a physician, she continues to locate the problem in the child's biology. As a result, she cannot ask why so many children are being diagnosed ADHD, and she cannot focus sufficiently on the stresses placed on children in modern schools and families. Nor can she advocate psychological and social approaches. Instead, she proposes an unproven fad-like explanation, low blood sugar, plus a hodgepodge of other alternative approaches. Once again, the most fundamental issue is ignored—the role of adults in failing to meet the basic needs of children in the family and the school. The child is betrayed by being told that the problem lies in his or her body. Parents, teachers, and other adults are absolved of responsibility for the child and lulled into hoping for quick and easy physical interventions.

On the other hand, there may be indirect benefits to imposing a diet on the child. In order to implement such a rigorous dietary schedule, the parent will have to provide the psychological ingredients missing in many children's lives—adult attention, rational discipline, and a set of principles to follow.

Ironically—and sometimes tragically—physicians with their own idiosyncratic versions of "what's the matter with children" are also likely to miss genuine medical problems that can contribute to a child's emotional difficulties (chapter 11). Block, for example, focuses only on hypothyroidism among the multiple *known* medical causes that can contribute to disrupting a child's emotions and conduct. Psychiatrist Paul Wender (1973, 1987, 1995) falls into the same trap. He so heavily emphasizes the mythical genetic and biochemical causes that he does not provide a comprehensive review of real medical disorders that can affect the child's mental functioning. The same is true of most books by ADHD/Ritalin advocates,[10] even though they claim to provide an extensive evaluation of the disorder. Goldstein and Goldstein (1992) are a refreshing exception in that they do review a number of medical causes. Michael Goldstein is a neurologist, rather than a psychologist or psychiatrist, and that may account for the greater emphasis on genuine medical causes.

Biochemically Driven Out of Control

When talking to parents who have no medical or scientific background, ADHD/Ritalin advocates frequently claim that ADHD is known to be caused by a biochemical imbalance. Statements to this effect have so little foundation that they could, at times, be considered outright lies. In their professional writings, not even staunch ADHD advocates try to claim there is a proven biochemical imbalance in the brains of children labeled ADHD.

As stated in the 1997 edition of the *American Psychiatric Press Textbook of Neuropsychiatry*:[11] "Efforts to identify a selective neurochemical imbalance have been disappointing." In regard to the two most frequently discussed neurotransmitters in ADHD, they find there are "no reliable differences on blood, urine, or cerebrospinal fluid (CSF) measures of dopamine or norepinephrine metabolites." Like true believers, the authors then march off briskly into yet another hoped for biochemical cause of the most speculative nature.

The notion of a biochemical imbalance in the brain of children diagnosed with ADHD is wild speculation. Meanwhile, we know with certainty that every child treated with a stimulant will suffer from multiple drug-induced biochemical imbalances.

They Say It's Genetic

Biopsychiatrists and ADHD/Ritalin advocates constantly remark that there is evidence that ADHD is genetic. Three basic concepts are worth repeating from my earlier works:

First, since the inception of psychiatry, psychiatrists as medical doctors have always claimed that almost everything they treat is biological and genetic. The claims, in other words, are nothing new. They are not scientifically based. They are inherent in the medical viewpoint. In reality, not a single psychiatric diagnosis, including schizophrenia and manic-depressive disorder, has been proven to have a genetic or biochemical origin.

Second, it is extremely unlikely that "ADHD" can be genetic, since ADHD is not a disease or disorder but a collection of behaviors displayed by a range of children from those who are bored to those who are abused.

Third, there have been many previous analyses of the false hopes and political motives behind attempts to link behavior with genetics.[12] Ideology and bias run riot in scientific studies of human behavior, especially when the studies aim at justifying a biological model and social control. This is nowhere more true than in the field of behavioral genetics whose entire history is dominated by political concerns, economic and racial agendas, and outright fraud.

Harvard professor of biology Ruth Hubbard and Elijah Wald (1993) observe, "The myth of the all-powerful gene is based on flawed science that discounts the environmental context in which we and our genes exist. It has many dangers, as it can lead to genetic discrimination and hazardous medical manipulations."

Even advocates of genetic explanations admit, in the privacy of their professional newspapers and conferences, that they haven't as yet proven that any psychiatric diagnosis has a genetic basis. Gene researcher Kenneth S. Kendler was quoted in *Psychiatric Times*, a newspaper for psychiatrists:[13]

> There is no area of psychiatry where the ratio of heat to light is greater than in the area of how genes and environment interact. Everybody speculates about this and waves their hands about that, but the amount of actual, rigorous data that we have is really very modest and is limited mostly to a couple of adoption studies.

As much as the media has tended to give enthusiastic headlines to every false start that links genetics and behavior, there appears to be a growing skepticism. In the April 21, 1997 issue of *U. S. News & World Report*, journalist Wray Herbert reviewed the evidence for genetic factors in everything from personality differences and homosexuality to alcoholism, mental disorders, and criminality. He summarized the multiple failed claims for genes that affect behavior. He concludes:

> If there's a refrain among geneticists working today, it's this: The harder we work to demonstrate the power of heredity, the harder it is to escape the potency of experience…. Yes, the way to intervene in human lives and improve them, to ameliorate mental illness, addictions and criminal behavior, is to enrich impoverished environments, to improve conditions in the family and society.

There have, of course, been repeated *claims* that one or another psychiatric disorder is genetic in origin; but the claims concerning ADHD are among the weakest. The leading biological psychiatrist in promoting the concept of ADHD now claims that the disorder may have 200–300 genetic variations, which reduces to absurdity any claims he might make for a proven genetic link.[14]

Nonetheless, ADHD/Ritalin advocates often claim genetic causes for "ADHD children." Zametkin has been quoted as saying "These kids really are born to be wild."[15] ADHD/Ritalin advocates are wedded to the genetic viewpoint because it bolsters their research funding and their careers, as well as their ideology. Note, however, that they do not look for genetic causes in the parents or the teachers, but in the children. In this case, claiming that the children can't control themselves exonerates the parents and teachers of the same obligation. The result is the escalating authority of biologically-oriented professionals and the simultaneous escalation in the drugging of children.

ADHD/Ritalin advocates commonly claim that ADHD runs in families. This may be true. Virtually every kind of attitude and behavior runs in families. To state the obvious, a boy is likely to speak the same language as his parents, adopt the same religion, and even root for the same sports team. If instead he were adopted at birth into a different family in a different part of the world, he would grow up with a different religion, different language, and a different sports team. None of it is genetic. The process is entirely learned. Yet it runs in families in a highly predictable fashion.

Similarly, if the boy's father is a known criminal, the odds increase that the boy will also get into trouble with the law. If his father lives by solid ethics, he is likely to adopt those as well. If he watches his father abuse his mother, the odds are increased that he too will become an abuser. Conversely, if he observes his father treating his mother and all women with respect, he is likely to follow that path.

Even medical problems can run in families without being genetic. It was thought for a time that pellagra was a genetic disease because it appeared in so many poor families. It turned out to be a vitamin deficiency disease caused by inadequate diet among the poor.

There is another serious flaw in genetic studies of ADHD that bears repeating. The genetic connection doesn't make rational sense. Children are diagnosed ADHD because they pose management problems, usually in the schoolroom. Factors having nothing to do with the child can and frequently do lead to a diagnosis of ADHD. Since there is no indication that ADHD is a real syndrome, let alone a biological entity, the search for a genetic cause is as likely to be fruitful as searching for the genetic cause for speaking English or rooting for the New York Yankees. If a study claims to show a genetic connection between an entity that doesn't exist and a possible genetic cause, it should be greeted with skepticism.

Thyroid Disorder or ADHD?

If a rare genetic abnormality is found in a tiny fraction of children who are labeled ADHD, it should not be used to justify the ADHD diagnosis or giving psychiatric drugs, such as Ritalin, to the afflicted children. When a gene was supposedly found in association with a rare form of inherited hypothyroidism, behavioral geneticists and psychiatrists claimed that it showed a genetic basis to some cases of ADHD.[16] The National Institutes of Health made a public announcement.

Guess who was second author of the study. Alan Zametkin! Once again on the basis of nothing, he declared "It's not bad parenting, overcrowded schools or unmotivated kids. ADHD is a neuropsychiatric problem based on brain physiology."[17] Once again, this is nonsense.

It's no revelation that hypothyroidism can cause ADHD-like symptoms. This has been known for a long time. So can many other disorders, everything from adverse drug reactions to Ritalin to head injury and lead poisoning.[18] But if a child does have a hypothyroid disorder, an adverse drug reaction, head injury, or lead poisoning, it's no longer even considered to be ADHD. Instead the disorder is properly diagnosed as hypothyroid disease, an adverse drug reaction, etc. It's treated with thyroid replacement, or other appropriate therapy, and not with Ritalin.

It was also admitted from the start that the finding could, at best, account for only a "fraction" of the cases of ADHD.[19] In fact, the research turned out to be useless in regard to children labeled ADHD. By 1995, textbooks were already dismissing the study. Arnold and Jensen wrote:

> However, screens of ADHD samples have not yielded a significant portion of mutant [thyroid] receptors. One screen of several hundred ADHD subjects found no mutant receptor but did find a 2 to 3 percent incidence of other thyroid abnormalities.

What this means is that some children mistakenly diagnosed ADHD may in fact have hormonal disorders which may or may not be causing ADHD-like symptoms. Tragically, these real physical problems are likely to be missed by doctors in their preoccupation with finding the fake disorder, ADHD.

Once again, psychiatrists like NIMH's Zametkin made much ado about nothing. These failures are the theme song of thirty plus years of searching for a biological justification for drugging difficult or disappointing children, or children who are in conflict with the adults in their lives. It should be the swan song.

Hope, however, springs eternal. ADHD/Ritalin advocate Dennis Cantwell declared (1996), "At this point, no gene has been described or found, but this is an active area of research and is likely to bear fruit in the foreseeable future."

Being Genetic without Being Abnormal

The fact that a trait is genetic doesn't mean that it's abnormal. It's worth remembering that the normal physical structure of the human being is largely genetic in origin.

ADHD/Ritalin advocates usually assume that any physical or genetic difference found in an "ADHD" child is an indication of an abnormality. This is by no means the only logical possibility. A recent genetic study from Australia led by Florence Levy (1997) claims to find a genetic tendency toward ADHD that may simply represent a deviation from acceptable norms rather than a disorder, much as being short or tall usually indicates nothing more than a deviation from a norm.

The Australian study has sufficient flaws to land it on a mountainous discard heap with nearly every other genetic psychiatric study. In the study, for example, identical twins have the same rate of inheriting the problem as nonidentical twins. Siblings also have the trait. It turns out that the supposed genetic tendency is spread throughout the entire population without regard for familial genetic lines.

The study discusses an alternative interpretation to the pathology model. It suggests that there is no gene for an "ADHD" disorder but rather a normal genetic continuum that on the extreme end gets *called a disorder*. The authors put it this way, "The findings suggest that ADHD is best viewed as the extreme of a behavior that varies genetically throughout the entire population rather than as a disorder with discrete determinants." In other words, it's like skin color or height, a trait that varies along a normal continuum.[20]

The authors of the Australian study observe, "the problem is one of deviance from an acceptable norm." When put that way, it becomes more clear that the "acceptable norm" may be the problem rather than the children themselves. The acceptable norm may be at fault in expecting energetic, curious children to sit still and shut up for hours at a time in group classrooms. If it ever is proven to be genetic, the "it" may in fact be a constellation of genes for a very positive trait, such as high energy, independence, or creativity. These qualities can put children in conflict with many schools and families.

A Sensitive Child

Psychologist and author Ty C. Colbert used a personal illustration to make his point:

> I remember when I took my first typing class in high school. I was quite sensitive at the time and prone to embarrassment. I remember dreading the times when the teacher started to walk over to see how I was doing. As she approached, my mind started spending more and more energy keeping track of her, hoping she would bypass me, trying to suppress my own feelings of failure, and wondering if she would say something that would embarrass me in front of my peers.
> Consequently my ability to focus and concentrate—at the time I needed to do so the most—was drastically hampered.
> If it was possible to put a brain scan instrument on my head at the time, I am sure it would have measured a difference in how I was metabolizing glucose. Furthermore, if the brain scan instrument was put on others who suffered from the same anxiety, researchers could perhaps come up with consistent patterns at times.
> But even if persistent patterns could be found, that does not indicate a disease or defect. It just means that, as human beings, some individuals may deal with the fear of rejection in a consistent way.

Every child is a sensitive child. All of us had experiences like Ty's in childhood. If we remain aware of how it was to be a child, we are much less likely to grow impatient with the children in our care. We will try harder to understand their feelings and their responses, and to find ways to help them improve their lives without resorting to diagnoses and to drugs.

Chapter 11

BACK TO THE FUTURE

Psychiatry's Long History of Perpetuating False Biological Ideas about "ADHD"

The past 25 years has led to a phenomenon almost unique in medical history. Methodologically rigorous research indicates that ADHD and hyperactivity as "syndromes" simply do not exist. We have invented a disease, given it medical sanction, and must now disown it. The major question is how we go about destroying the monster we have created. It is not easy to do this and to save face, another reason why physicians and many researchers with years of funding and an academic reputation to protect are reluctant to believe the data.

—Diane McGuinness, professor of psychology (1989)

The concept that "ADHD" is a biological or neurobiological disorder is entirely fabricated. Thousands of studies have failed to demonstrate a physical defect in these children who have been variously diagnosed over the years with Organic Drivenness, Restlessness Syndrome, Brain Injured Child, Minimal Brain Damage, Minimal Brain Disorder, Hyperkinetic Impulsive Disorder, Hyperkinetic Child Syndrome, Hyperkinetic Reaction, Attention Deficit Disorder, and finally Attention Deficit-Hyperactivity Disorder.[1]

How is it that such a patently false idea can be perpetuated as the truth by the medical and mental health professions?

History of the Controversy

Physicians, by natural bent and by training, as well as by self-interest, are motivated to believe that they are dealing with biological disorders suitable for medical treatment. Throughout the history of medicine and psychiatry, physicians have claimed that nearly everything that falls under their authority is genetic and biological in origin, and is best treated with their limited array of medical tools. G. F. Still, who is generally credited with being the first to identify ADHD-like symptoms in 1902, believed from the beginning that he was diagnosing an inherited neurological disorder.[2]

The biological cause of ADHD is an article of faith—a faith bolstered by strong professional interests. But the public is misled into believing that ADHD advocates base their biological viewpoint on recent scientific break-throughs. To the contrary, it's a matter of back to the future: Most of the major figures in the ADHD/Ritalin movement have been making the same biological claims from the start of their careers in the 1960s or early 1970s.

C. Keith Conners, whose simplistic tests have justified the medicating of millions of children, was writing in favor of Ritalin for behavioral control thirty-five years ago.[3] He was already formulating his commonly used teacher rating scales in the 1960s.[4]

Judith Rapoport two decades ago was studying the urine of hyperactive children for abnormalities.[5] Now she's moved on to more dangerous and intrusive technology. Under her direction at NIMH hundreds of children have been subjected to spinal taps and brain scan radiation in order to find her self-proclaimed "holy grail"—the elusive biological causes of their con-flicts with parents, teachers, and other authorities.[6]

Paul Wender, one of the leading psychiatrists in the field, was already pub-lishing a book in 1971 to justify the diagnosis and medicating of children with "Minimal Brain Dysfunction," whether or not the children had any objective signs of brain dysfunction. He was convinced that the presumed genetic and biological problem should be dealt with as speedily as possible with drugs. By then, these views were commonplace in the field.[7]

Dennis Cantwell (1972), who published a biologically oriented review of ADHD in 1996, was also among the old-time ADHD/Ritalin pioneers.[8] Russell Barkley (1977), perhaps the most frequently cited contemporary ADHD/Ritalin advocate, was writing extensively on Ritalin more than twenty years ago. Then, as now, he was emphasizing "compliance"—med-icating children to force them to conform to authority.

Instead of being based on new findings, the resurgence of ADHD/Ritalin is a matter of politics. Biological psychiatry and related interest groups have been pressing for decades to capture the child market for drugs and for their professional services.[9]

Challenging the Basic Concepts from the Beginning

Since the 1970s, clinicians, scientists, and other thoughtful critics have criticized the idea that there is a specific disorder behind the collection of behaviors described as hyperactivity, inattention, or impulsivity. At each stage of development, from "hyperactivity" and "minimal brain disease" to "ADD" and "ADHD," the concept has been challenged. Three excellent books mark the three decades of criticism: Peter Schrag and Diane Divoky's *The Myth of the Hyperactive Child* (1975), Gerald Coles' *The Learning Mystique* (1987), and Thomas Armstrong's (1995) *The Myth of the A.D.D. Child.*

Ritalin Controversy in the 1970s

Some of the most basic issues were raised very early in the ADHD/Ritalin movement. On September 29, 1970, a Subcommittee of the Committee on Government Operations of the U.S. House of Representatives held hearings entitled "Federal Involvement in the Use of Behavior Modification Drugs on Grammar School Children." With an estimated 200,000 to 300,000 children on Ritalin at the time, the subcommittee was concerned that its use might "zoom" even higher in the future. An FDA official, Ronald Lipman, said that as many as 4 million children might have "minimal brain dysfunction" (MBD), making them subject to treatment with stimulants.[10] Ciba advertising materials were estimating that 5% of America's children might suffer from the disorder.[11]

The subcommittee chair remarked on the irony that "each and every school child is told that 'speed kills,'" while many other children are being forced to take speed in the form of Ritalin.[12] The committee warned that the Ritalin movement could undermine "our extensive national campaign against drug abuse" and condemned "a certain glibness about the experimentation on young children in this country, used as guinea pigs." It noted that the federal government had been sponsoring research on medication for behavior control since 1961.

Testifying before the committee, author and educator John Holt asked how can we determine that a child's energy level should be considered a "disease":

> The answer is simple. We consider it a disease because it makes it difficult to run our schools as we do, like maximum security prisons, for the comfort and the convenience of the teachers and administrators who work in them. The energy of children is "bad" because it is a nuisance to the exhausted and overburdened adults who do not want to or know how to and are not able to keep up with it.
>
> Given the fact that some children are more energetic and active than others, might it not be easier, more healthy, and more humane to deal with this fact by giving them more time and scope to make use of and work off their energy?... Everyone is taken care of, except, of course, the child himself, who wears a label which to him reads clearly enough "freak," and who is denied from those closest to him, however much sympathy he may get, what he and all children most need—respect, faith, hope, and trust.[13]

Concerns were already being expressed to the congressional subcommittee about "coercion of parents by harassing techniques used by teachers and administrators, along with threats of expulsion of children from public schools," as well as "rejection of any diagnosis that did not result in a prescription for some medication."[14] Three decades later, I would testify before yet another congressional committee concerned about the same kind of coercion of parents (Chapter 1).

Writing in *Psychology Today* in 1974, Carole Wade Offir proclaimed a warning that is more true today than when she wrote it over twenty years ago:

> Undoubtedly the slavish reliance on chemical solutions is due to a general impatience with complex situations, and a need for easy, push-button answers. Sometimes technology can provide such answers. Often it cannot.

In 1975 Peter Schrag and Diane Divoky wrote in *The Myth of the Hyperactive Child*, "There is nothing new about teachers and parents complaining that children are difficult to teach or control." "What is new, however," they explain, "is the increasingly fashionable attribution of common problems to neurological abnormalities, and the increasingly common description of 'these affected children' as victims of a clearly defined medical syndrome."[15] They called it "inventing a disease." Schrag and Divoky were also aware of many of the serious adverse effects of Ritalin, including psychosis and addiction, and they cite research indicating that the drug has no positive long-term effects.

Ritalin Controversy in the Late 1980s

The next wave of criticism of Ritalin broke in the late 1980s. By then, an estimated 800,000 children were on the drug. There were stories in the *New York Times*,[16] *Wall Street Journal*,[17] *Washington Post*,[18] and *Los Angeles Times*[19] as well as on television with Ted Koppel's June 10, 1988 "Nightline."

The late 1980s also saw a rise in malpractice suits about ADHD and Ritalin against doctors who injured children by prescribing Ritalin; product liability suits against Ciba for a variety of alleged failures in promoting the drug; suits against school districts for pushing Ritalin; and even one lawsuit against the American Psychiatric Association for manufacturing the diagnosis.[20] However, this earlier legal assault on the ADHD/Ritalin interest groups was far less potent and potentially effective than the current Ritalin class action suits (Chapter 1).

In a scientific review, Diane McGuinness (1989) referred to ADD as "the emperor's new clothes." She observed, "It is currently fashionable to treat approximately one third of all elementary school boys as an abnormal population because they are fidgety, inattentive, and unamenable to adult control." Nonetheless, "two decades of research have not provided any support for the validity of ADD" or hyperactivity. Neither clinical studies nor psychological testing have been able to identify such a group.

Frank Putnam (1990), a director of one of NIMH's research units, applauded "the growing number of clinicians and researchers condemning the tyranny of our psychiatric and educational classification systems." Putnam found that it is "exceedingly difficult to assign valid classifications" to children, and yet "children are by far the most classified and labeled group in our society." He warned against "the institutional prescriptions of a system that seeks to pigeonhole them." In 1991 I wrote a detailed critique of ADHD and stimulant treatment in my book *Toxic Psychiatry*.

The Controversy Continues

The controversy over Ritalin is once again heating up in the media with dozens of articles in major newspapers, including the *New York Times*, *Wall Street Journal*, and *USA Today*.[21,22]

Michael R. Valentine (1997) is an educator who presents workshops that are critical of ADHD. He offers alternatives for teachers in helping children who seem inattentive or out-of-control in their classes. Valentine points out that ADHD is found coupled (covariant) with every other childhood disorder and therefore cannot be a separate or valid syndrome. He reminds us that there is no medical evidence for a physical cause and no physical, educational, or psychological test that can diagnose "this supposed medical condition." Furthermore, the use of the diagnosis runs counter to more enlightened trends: "Most professionals and parents are moving away from labeling students and towards providing services for all students."

Fred A. Baughman, Jr. (1993, 1996) is a neurologist who has analyzed how ADHD lacks the criteria for a genuine medical disorder or syndrome. In correspondence with him, officials of two federal agencies have confirmed his critique.

On October 25, 1995, Gene R. Haislip, at the time a Deputy Assistant in the DEA's Office of Diversion Control, wrote to Baughman:

> Some materials provided by advocacy groups refer to ADHD as a neurobiological disorder. The American Psychiatric Association classifies ADHD as a behavioral disorder. We are also unaware that ADHD has been validated as a biologic/organic syndrome.

Psychiatrist Paul Leber is the head of the Division of Neuropharmacological Drug Products of the Food and Drug Administration (FDA). He is in charge of the approval process for all psychiatric drugs and an advocate of biological psychiatry. On December 22, 1995, Leber wrote to Baughman: "We acknowledge that the condition known as ADHD has been historically controversial, and that as yet no distinct pathophysiology for the disorder has been delineated."

These are extraordinary admissions for government officials enmeshed in the ADHD/Ritalin controversy.

In response to renewed research spending on ADHD by the National Institute of Mental Health, Baughman (1996) himself writes:

> Invented by a committee of the American Psychiatric Association, ADHD has yet to be validated as a disease, syndrome, or anything biological or organic.
>
> Nowhere in the voluminous literature on ADHD is there proof of a biological link. Positron emission tomography (PET), MRI, and biochemical assays have yielded nothing. Initial excitement over PET scan findings in 1990 proved to be baseless, as did a reported association of ADHD with an inherited resistance to thyroid hormone.

Baughman makes clear that the NIMH research study might do more harm than good by labeling the children with a fake disorder:

> Given the lack of proof of any effective therapy and, more fundamentally, the lack of validation of ADHD as a disease, the diagnosis of ADHD in and of itself might have adverse effects....

Writing in the *Journal of the American Academy of Child and Adolescent Psychiatry*, Deborah Jacobovitz and her colleagues (1990) reviewed the literature on stimulant treatment for ADHD and concluded, "The authors would urge greater caution and a much more restricted use of stimulant treatment pending more research on long-term effects, both concerning positive and negative consequences...."

The DEA Takes a Stand

One federal agency, the Drug Enforcement Administration (DEA) (1995a,b&c, 1996), has issued warnings about the escalating rates of Ritalin prescription in this country. In an extraordinarily frank and detailed analysis, the DEA (1995b&c) questions the tactics of Ritalin's manufacturer, Ciba, as well as some of the drug's advocates. It also raises serious questions about the drug's safety and efficacy.

The DEA (1995b) points to research indicating "that a small percentage of primary care physicians are writing nearly half of all methylphenidate prescriptions for children" and "that children under the age of six are being treated with methylphenidate contrary to labeling guidelines in the absence of controlled studies suggesting that this is appropriate." The DEA warns that Ritalin use "may be a risk factor for substance abuse"—that is, prescribed Ritalin may encourage the child to become a drug abuser. It provides a fairly comprehensive list of adverse effects.

The DEA (1996) also makes clear that there is no known biological cause for ADHD: "Studies that have tried to find a specific neurological lesion or deficit have not been successful."

An International Eye on America

The International Narcotics Control Board (1995, 1996a&b, 1997) of the United Nations has also expressed concern to the U.S. government about the escalating prescription of Ritalin.[23] The Board's report asks "all governments to exercise the utmost vigilance in order to prevent the 'over-diagnosing' of ADD in children and medically unjustified treatment with methylphenidate and other stimulants."[24] It shows particular concern about the United States, not only because of its vastly greater use of Ritalin but also because of the tendency to place children on the medication for longer periods of time than in other countries.

In 1995, the International Narcotics Control Board[25] issued a statement of concern over "the unprecedented sharp increase" in Ritalin consumption in the United States due to "its controversially extensive use in the treatment of 'attention deficit disorder (ADD)' in children." The Board stated it "shares the concern of the United States Drug Enforcement Agency (DEA) about the increased use of methylphenidate." The Board continues to express concern to government agencies with a recent warning about the "easy" solution approach that involves "highly subjective" judgments about behaviors such as inattention and impulsivity (1997).

The Impact of Public and Professional Criticism

In the early 1990s concerns were voiced by ADHD/Ritalin stalwarts, such as Alan Zametkin of the National Institute of Mental Health, that the use of Ritalin was declining due to adverse media.[26] Ritalin prescription may have briefly declined between 1987 and 1990, especially in Baltimore and other regions where the media took up the issue.[27] Malpractice and product liability litigation also added to the controversy.[28] Our own reform efforts aimed at publicizing and stopping the psychiatric abuse of children were also at a peak in our home state of Maryland during this period of time.[29] But at the moment that advocates were publicly lamenting a decline in Ritalin prescription, they had already created a renewed escalation of it in 1990–93.[30]

In the year 2,000, the controversy surrounding the ADHD diagnosis and the use of stimulants has heated up again. The public, the media, and a segment of the health professions are becoming increasingly outraged at the widespread use of drugs to subdue the behavior of children. Yet the leaders of the ADHD/Ritalin movement remain impervious and unresponsive to criticism, and the drugging continues to escalate.

Are Medical Doctors the Answer?

If ADHD is not a real disease or disorder, and if drugs don't provide genuine help, should parents take their children to medical doctors for help with behavior problems? Should parents expose their children to any specialists who believe in ADHD/Ritalin?

In a society that wants "doctors" and "specialists" to provide answers to every sort of difficulty, it may seem strange to question "going to the doctor." But the idea that doctors know how to raise or to educate children is relatively new. And it isn't based on reality. ADHD/Ritalin advocates don't have any special wisdom, insight, or understanding about parenting or teaching. Instead, their ideas interfere with adults doing as good a job as possible in taking responsibility for the children in their care. It is hazardous to your child's health to take the youngster to a doctor who believes in diagnosing ADHD and prescribing drugs to modify behavior.

Ultimately, it will be up to parents, teachers, and other caregivers to take their children back from the health professionals who are pushing drugs on America's children.

Chapter 12

PARENTS, CAREGIVERS, AND TEACHERS MAKE THE DIFFERENCE

Scientific Evidence that ADHD/Ritalin Advocates Ignore

Terrified helpless youngsters are too often silent witnesses or survivors of violence in homes, schools, streets, and war zones all over the world. In the United States alone, based on conservative estimates of the incidence of sexual and physical abuse and exposure to community and domestic violence, more than 3 million children were exposed to traumatic events last year...

—Eitan D. Schwarz and Bruce D. Perry,
Psychiatric Clinics of North America (1994)

What distinguishes effective from ineffective caregiving? Scientists have identified two fundamental aspects of caregiving that are particularly important for children's adjustment. The first concerns how much warmth, nurturance, and acceptance (versus hostility and rejection) caregivers convey to children. The second concerns how much control, structure, and involvement (versus permissiveness and detachment) caregivers display toward children.

—National Advisory Mental Health Council (1995)

Contrary to the claims of ADHD/Ritalin advocates, there is no convincing evidence that "ADHD" is caused by biological or genetic factors. The real breakthroughs in science are about the environmental factors that produce ADHD-like problems and about the caring, non-coercive approaches that help children to develop their full potential.

Deprivation and Trauma Impair a Child's Mental Development

The National Advisory Mental Health Council (NAMHC) (1995), an NIMH advisory committee, summarized research on the potentially negative effects of disrupted family life and misguided caregiving:

Not surprisingly, extreme coldness, open hostility, or rejection by caregivers often contributes to children's emotional distress, aggression, and delinquency....

Research indicates that caregivers who are excessively controlling undermine children's persistence, competence, self-regulation, and overall ability to cope with life's problems.... In families in which adults consistently escalate their hostility and intensity of conflict, both parents and children are at high risk for distress and psychopathology. Across many social classes and ethnic groups, marital dissolution and childrearing outside of marriage often have long-term negative effects on children, including lowered achievement and intellectual test scores, increased school dropout, early motherhood, and antisocial behavior.[1]

Recent research has also confirmed that spanking increases antisocial behavior.[2] In other words, how we raise our children really matters!

Trauma Causes ADHD-Like Symptoms

Alan Green's (1989) extensive review in *The Comprehensive Textbook of Psychiatry* describes how most childhood problems—from autism to hyperactivity—can result from environmental trauma and stress. He further confirms that adults can provide harmful or healing alternatives to children. Mina Dulcan (1994) in her table on causes of ADHD or ADHD-like symptoms lists "physical or sexual abuse, neglect, boredom, overstimulation, sociocultural deprivation," as well as "normal behavior."

Eitan Schwarz and Bruce Perry (1994) estimate that 3,000,000 children are exposed yearly to severe trauma in the United States. Traumatized children can end up meeting the official criteria for ADHD. Stress and trauma can affect the basic ADHD-like functions, including "behavioral irritability, locomotion, attention." Severe trauma can adversely affect all the functions mediated by "this complex organ [the brain]," including "emotional, cognitive, behavioral, and psychological."[3]

According to Martin Teicher and his Harvard research team (1997), "Children abused early in life who develop symptoms of post traumatic stress disorder (PTSD) also frequently meet criteria for ADHD," including cognitive problems and hyperactivity. One study found that almost one-quarter of children with PTSD also met the criteria for ADHD and another found that 38% of hospitalized abused children fit the category of ADHD.[4]

Negative caregiving can impede cognitive development.[5] Bridget Murray (1997) confirmed that the intellectual development of children is negatively affected by mothers who use more coercive approaches to getting them to perform. Conversely, she found that "research underscores that parents' involvement shapes children's academic success... Cognitive guidance from parents is also crucial during the children's first three years." Gentle parental guidance in problem solving resulted in children with higher intelligence scores and fewer learning problems.

Charlotte Johnston (1996) found that parents of ADHD children use more "negative-reactive" and fewer "positive parenting" strategies. In children labeled ADHD who displayed oppositional or rebellious kinds of behavior, "parenting self-esteem" was lowest and the fathers displayed more "psychological disturbance."

Family Life and the Economic Factor

A study of caregivers in poor inner-city families[6] found that stress correlated much more with family income and other financial factors than with the behavior of the children. They also found that younger caregivers reported more delinquent behavior in their children, indicating that youthful parents may have more impaired children.

The authors conclude, "These stressors serve to intensify the problems with parent-child interactions, particularly problems with compliance, thereby increasing symptom display in their ADHD youngsters." They urge that the children be helped by "identifying appropriate sources of support for these at-risk families."

Overcoming Negative Effects of Upbringing

Thus far we have emphasized the potentially negative impact of parenting and caregiving in causing ADHD-like symptoms. The NIMH's National Advisory Mental Health Council report also confirms that parenting and caregiving are key to the positive development of children: "high levels of caregiver warmth are associated with children's elevated self-esteem, compliance with caregiver demands, internalized moral standards, cognitive competence, and social adjustment."[7]

NIMH's advisory council concludes:

Research with both animals and humans has shown that caregiving behavior provides a rich mixture of stimuli to the offspring that often affects both physical and psychological development. For example, holding and touching infants not only provides the sensory stimulation and protection essential for physical growth and survival, but also conveys the comfort and security necessary for early social and emotional development.

Animals and Infants

Animal research confirms the importance of early nurturing.[8] Rats develop better methods of handling stress later in life when they are not exposed to unpredictable, intense stress in infancy. It should be no surprise that human infants and children are at least as sensitive to their emotional environment.

Infants are exquisitely sensitive to the emotional states of their caregivers. When they sense negative emotions, they "may respond with symptomatic disturbances of global functioning, excessive crying, eating, sleeping, psychophysiological lability, overstimulated states, or apathy and failure to thrive."[9]

Even the Most Disturbed Children Can Respond

Psychoanalytically oriented research demonstrated many years ago that early childhood experiences of abandonment in institutions can profoundly affect a child's emotional development and that the return of the small child to the family can eventually restore emotional health.[10] Kim Chisholm's recent research on Rumanian orphans demonstrate that the longer the children were institutionalized, the more difficulty they had developing normal attachments with foster parents.[11] Fortunately, negative effects could be overcome through unconditional love. Formerly institutionalized children developed the most secure attachments when their foster parents responded to them with unconditional love—nurturing them under any and all conditions, even when the children avoided them or threw tantrums.

Working with the family is the key even in the most severe problems in children and young adults. Julian Leff's well-known research has shown that teaching families positive communication can greatly improve the outcome for grown children labeled schizophrenic.[12] Conducting research for the World Health Organization (WHO), Giovanni de Girolamo (1996) found that patients labeled schizophrenic frequently fully recover in cultures in which they have the support of their extended families. According to de Girolamo, these very disturbed patients tend to do much better with family support but worse with modern psychiatric treatment.

Finnish adoption studies by Pekka Tienari (1987) and his colleagues tracked the development of children raised outside their families of origin. The Finnish research found that regardless of their genetic background, none of the adoptive children became seriously disturbed unless they were *raised* in seriously disturbed families. Conversely, "no seriously disturbed offspring is found in a healthy or mildly disturbed adoptive family." Environment was more powerful than any possible genetic influence even in regard to the development of that supposedly biological and genetic disorder, schizophrenia.

Family environment plays a determining role—for better or worse—in the most severe problems that are thought by many psychiatrists to be genetic and biological in origin. Family can play an even stronger role in healing the relatively less severe problems of children labeled ADHD.

The Brain Is "Enormously Malleable"

A report from the NIMH and the National Institutes of Health emphasizes the "plasticity" of the brain in response to environment:[13]

The developing brain appears to be enormously malleable with regard to the organism's experience. To the extent that the environment presents stimulation and events that are characteristic of the organism, more or less normal patterns of development will result. But when the environment presents unusual events or conditions, development may be abnormal.

The brain creates new brain cell synapses (connections) and prunes old ones in response to experience.[14] Each infant and child's brain is formed in part by each child's unique environment. Although the science is in its infancy, it is becoming possible to study microscopic structural and chemical changes in brain cells that accompany learning.[15]

The brain is not nearly as pre-programmed as biopsychiatrists would have us believe. Instead, the brain grows in response to the quality of the nurturing present around the infant or child. Some of the newest and most elegant research confirms that the development of infants and children depends on good caregiving from parents and teachers.

Poor caregiving does not "hard wire" the brain into fixed negative reactions. The brain does not seem to possess "hard wires" comparable to those in a computer or television. Instead, the brain is a plastic, even stew-like, organ that grows new pathways and connections in response to changes in its environment. This can go on throughout life.

The brain and mind of the growing child responds well to positive changes in the environment. When nurturing has gone awry earlier in the child's life, there's still time for parents, teachers, and other caring adults to make a big difference in the child's future progress.

Schools That Build Brain Synapses

New educational systems are being designed that more closely resemble a creative workplace. Writing in the *Wall Street Journal*, Ann Carrns vividly describes the old approach: "Forget dreary rows of desks, dusty chalkboards and pea-green halls lined with lockers." The new idea is to "fit the school into a structure that already exists," such as businesses, libraries, museums, and zoos. According to Carrns:

Almost by definition, the new school buildings also provide a stimulating environment that dovetails with the growing "active learning" movement, and the neurological research underpinning it.... Researchers now know that while people are born with a fixed number of brain cells, the synapses—or connections—between those neurons multiply in response to new experiences, particularly in childhood. Learning occurs when fresh synapses sprout, or when existing connections are modified in response to new information.... Learning by doing—rather than merely by listening to lectures or watching demonstrations—appears to build these synapse networks most effectively because it engages all the senses.

In *Reclaiming Our Children* (2000), I describe several model school environments that can enhance the lives of all children, including those who have been labeled hyperactive, impulsive, or inattentive in less child friendly classrooms.

Proving the Obvious: Parents Matter

While most of us would agree that parents have a lot to do with how a child behaves at home and achieves at school, ADHD advocates continually deny it. They claim instead that biology and biochemistry are the determining factors.

You may not need to be convinced that parenting matters; but you might want to have some "proof" available the next time you hear ADHD/Ritalin "experts" claiming that there's no proof that parenting and care-giving in general affects how a child does at home and at school.

At Last, Love Makes Headlines

I used to say there were never any headlines in the major media about the healing value of love. It's no longer true. A recent front page headline in the *Washington Post* declared "Love conquers what ails teens, study finds."[16] The ambiguous headline refers to *parental* love. The research led by Michael D. Resnick (1997), and published in the *Journal of the American Medical Association*, was based on more than 12,000 adolescents in grades 7 through 12 in dozens of schools. It found that "parent-family connectedness" and "perceived school connectedness" were protective against every "health risk" they measured except pregnancy. Children who felt closer to their parents and teachers were less likely to feel emotional distress or have suicidal thoughts and behaviors. They were less likely to be involved in violence or to use cigarettes, alcohol or marijuana. They also began to have sex at a later age.

One of the investigators, J. Richard Udry, professor of maternal and child health at UNC-Chapel Hill, told the *Washington Post*, "Many people think of adolescence as a stage where there is so much peer influence that parents become both irrelevant and powerless. It's not so that parents aren't important. Parents are just as important to adolescents as they are to smaller children."

The study cites a mountain of other research pointing in the same direction: "With notable consistency across the domains of risk, the role of parents and family in shaping the health of adolescents is evident." Parental connectedness—"feelings of warmth, love, and caring from parents"—is the essential feature.

Yes, Dads Matter

A carefully conducted survey by the U. S. Department of Education discovered a major factor in academic performance among America's children—parental involvement, including fathers, in the child's school.[17] Involvement was measured by participation in school meetings, scheduled parent-teacher conferences, attending a school or class event, or volunteering at the school.[18]

When fathers were highly involved, nearly half of their children obtained mostly A's for their grades. Children with highly involved fathers also tended to stay out of trouble and to enjoy school more. Whether a father lived in the home with the mother, raised a family on his own, or lived outside the home—his involvement was critical to a child's development in school. A mother's involvement was important, too, but it was insufficient to make up for a relatively uninvolved father. The study confirmed "the already large body of literature that suggests that parental involvement in their children's schools is beneficial for children's school success."

Why didn't this study make headlines throughout the nation? Why wasn't it featured on national TV? Perhaps we would rather hear about a quick fix pill than about parental responsibility.

Psychologist Peter Oas has extensive clinical experience with children labeled ADHD. Working in the military and then in private practice, Oas (1997b) evaluated at least 2,000 children. Often the mother came by herself, and often the child would display ADHD-like symptoms during this first session. When the father would show up for a later interview, the child would almost always act normally.

Positive Effects of Good Care-Giving on Emotional, Cognitive, and Academic Development

The June 1997 issue of *The Monitor*, the newspaper of the American Psychological Association, focused on child development. Fast-breaking research in the field demonstrated the importance of parenting and caregiving in the cognitive and emotional development of children. Here are some of the main findings:

Caregiving affects the development of cognitive skills:

The quality of interaction between the day-care providers and the children in their care is the most important aspect of day care for fostering children's cognitive skills...

Children whose care-givers asked them questions, engaged them in conversations and responded to them when they spoke, scored highest on measures of cognitive and language skills.[19]

Both verbal and mathematical skills are affected by factors such as small day care groups, a small ratio of children to adults, and a narrow range of ages in the group. Better day care improves overall development in toddlers and preschoolers and, in particular, "high quality care results in better cognitive and language development."[20]

Impulse control can be taught by parents. Consistent parenting helps children learn to regulate their emotions. Up to about 18 months of age, soothing support matters most. For older children, impulse control is enhanced through a combination of encouragement in novelty-seeking and a safe secure home base.[21]

Talking, Reading and Loving Go Together

Writing in the *New York Times*, Sandra Blakeslee (1997) reviewed current research on how early language environment affects the child's brain.[22] Unlike electronic wiring, infant learning requires a loving adult presence:

> Furthermore, new studies are showing that spoken language has an astonishing impact on an infant's brain development. In fact, some researchers say that the number of words an infant hears each day is the single most important predictor of later intelligence, school success and social competence. There is one catch—the words have to come from an attentive, engaged human being. As far as anyone has been able to determine, radio and television do not work.

Reading together is another loving activity that greatly enhances cognitive development. One researcher, Betty Heart, declared, "It's as simple as spending more time talking and reading with your children."[23]

Training Parents—It Works

Training parents how to relate better to their children improves the behavior of children, as well as the emotional health and well-being of everyone in the family.[24] Parent training programs are effective not only for those parents with hard-to-handle children, but for all parents.[25]

Most approaches focus on helping parents to observe the behavior of their children and then to respond with positive reinforcement, mild punishment (or no punishment at all), negotiation, and making agreements or contracts. A variety of excellent books are available concerning how to use non-coercive methods for working out differences and plans with children.[26]

Parent management training has consistently proven successful in improving parent self-esteem, in reducing parent stress, and in ameliorating ADHD-like symptoms, especially negative attitudes toward parental authority and aggression. Interventions that also teach self-control to the children themselves are more helpful in controlling hyperactivity.

Strayhorn and Weidman (1989) demonstrated the positive effects of parent training Estrada and Pinsof, 1995, reviewed the literature on parent management training (PMT). Also see Greenfield and Senecal, 1995, for an interesting approach involving teaching parents to play with their children. A parent-training group based on Barkley's methods was effective for children most of whom were not taking any medication (Anastopoulos et al., 1993).

Strayhorn and Weidman (1989) demonstrated the positive effects of parent training on "hyperactivity." They taught parents to have fun with their children instead of emphasizing submission to authority. Their families, including 96 children age 2–5 years, were instructed by trainers whose cultural backgrounds matched the low-income high-risk parents. Four or five 2-hour small group meetings of parents were used to teach improved approaches to their children. Parents then participated in half-a-dozen supervised play sessions with their children. They also watched video tapes on parent-child relating.

The Encouraging News about Parenting

What has happened to our society when we need proof that our parenting really matters? This transformation in basic values—this abrogation of parental responsibility—has not occurred by chance. As later chapters will document, it has required the concerted efforts of powerful special interest groups to convince parents and teachers that they are not responsible for the behavior of the children in their care.

While some parents may be blessed with the opportunity to enroll their children in schools that truly help students to develop basic academic and human skills, parents themselves are likely to remain the child's main source of emotional growth and educational inspiration. In my clinical experience—confirmed by research—families contribute to both the suffering and the healing of their children.[27] When mothers and fathers resolve their more severe conflicts between themselves and improve their parenting, their young children almost invariably respond in a very positive manner.

However, many of a child's problems and stresses are not related to parenting. Chapter 17 will take a systematic look at the kinds of stressors that can affect our children. As parents, we may not cause all the stress that our children inevitably experience, but we are in the best position to identify these stressors and to help our children in dealing with them.

In my psychiatric practice, I avoid blaming parents, and in particular, I try to help them overcome their feelings of guilt. Guilt is a painful, debilitating emotion that rarely motivates us to be more loving or concerned.

It can be useful to point out to parents how they may be contributing to their child's problems, but it's always more useful to provide new directions in how to discipline, care for, and educate the child. Often the problems don't especially lie in the family. Nonetheless, the parents remain most responsible for discovering and correcting the source of the problem. Especially with young children, I encourage as many family members as possible to become involved in the therapy. Siblings and grandparents alike often have a great deal of insight into what's gone wrong, as well as good ideas about how to set them right. As communication and relationship improves in the overall family, the labeled child also improves.

The next chapter looks at possible medical causes for ADHD-like behavior. Although the vast majority of children diagnosed ADHD have nothing physically wrong with them, a few do have identifiable medical disorders that can be treated—not with stimulant drugs but with treatments that address the real physical problem.

Chapter 13

PHYSICAL CAUSES OF
ADHD-LIKE SYMPTOMS

Medical Disorders, Drugs, Food Additives, and Other Factors That Do and Don't Affect a Child's Behavior

As many as 3 to 4 million American children may have unsafe [lead] levels according to current standards, and even lower levels of chronic exposure to lead may be associated with neurobiological disturbances that can affect intelligence and academic performance.

—David S. Younger (1995)

Persistent intellectual, academic, language, and memory problems are encountered by children after severe head injury.... Preschoolers typically exhibit generalized cognitive impairment, including attentional, motor, intellectual, linguistic, and visuospatial disturbances. In school-age children and adolescents, memory, visuomotor, and attentional difficulties are predominant.

—William Miller and Frank Miller (1992)

Over a period of several weeks, seven-year-old Billy became increasingly inattentive at school. His teacher noticed that he had trouble focusing on any kind of paper work. At home he seemed irritable and stubborn. He had trouble falling asleep at night and then resented being awakened for school in the morning. At first his parents blamed the problem on a worsening of his allergies in the fall. They took him to their pediatrician who concluded that Billy was showing early signs of ADHD. Why now? Billy was at the right age and it was the start of the school year when ADHD usually surfaces, the doctor explained.

Billy's parents took their son for a second opinion to another pediatrician who immediately asked what medicine the boy was taking for his allergies. It was an antihistamine in combination with a common nasal drying agent, pseudoephedrine (Sudafed). The physician suspected that the combination was making Billy at times sedated (the antihistamine) and at times over-stimulated (the Sudafed). He recommended stopping the allergy medication. Billy's behavior problems cleared up in a week.

At the start of the first grade, Joan had trouble even concentrating on drawing which she used to love. She seemed to forget instructions and became easily frustrated. Sometimes she cried for no reason at all. The teacher recommended an evaluation for ADHD and suggested a "well-known specialist." Instead, the parents feared that there might be "something really the matter with Joan" and they took her to a child neurologist.

During the lengthy history taking by the neurologist, the family auto accident was mentioned. It happened that past summer, a few weeks before school. They had been hit from behind while waiting at a stop light. No one had been hurt. The car had sustained only slight damage. Joan's head had been "jerked around" by the impact. She had been in her father's lap, and when her head snapped back, it cut his lip. But that was all. She hadn't even cried.

Further careful history taking led to the conclusion that Joan had been fine until the accident. The parents felt guilty about failing to recognize the importance of the accident but the neurologist reassured them that it's easy to overlook the significance of closed head injuries when the patient is seemingly unhurt.

The neurologist found possible abnormalities on brain wave studies. Specialized neuropsychological testing documented a mild cognitive deficit consistent with head injury. The doctor recommended patience with Joan. He referred them to a cognitive rehabilitation center where Joan received the benefit of learning to play with computers while exercising her mildly impaired cognitive abilities. Within a year she was fully recovered—and precocious with the computer.

There Are Genuine Diseases

Are there genuine diseases that can cause ADHD-like symptoms? As the clinical vignettes indicate, the answer is yes. But psychiatrists, pediatricians, family practitioners and others who accept the ADHD/Ritalin approach are likely to overlook real physical causes, such as mild closed-head injury or an adverse drug reaction. Why? Because in order to accept the irrational mythology behind ADHD/Ritalin, they must suspend their medical judgment. They must become dumb about science and medicine, and even simple logic, in order to believe the nonsense. As a result, they lose their genuine medical acuity. Even professional review articles and textbooks of psychiatry fail to review all of the possible genuine medical causes for ADHD-like symptoms.[1] If they did review them all, it would become apparent that ADHD is a meaningless diagnosis.

Similarly, doctors who believe in fad diagnoses are also likely to miss genuine medical disorders. Parents who are concerned about their children's health should have them examined by a physician who is not invested in the ADHD/Ritalin movement or in unusual alternatives, even if the parents are considering an alternative approach. ADHD/Ritalin advocates may be too blinded by mythical biochemical imbalances and "crossed wires" to notice a potentially real physical disorder.

"ADHD" Around The World

The vast majority of children diagnosed with ADHD and treated with Ritalin in the western world do not have a genuine underlying physical disorder that can be medically identified and treated. In some places in the world, however, most of the children who display ADHD-like symptoms may be suffering from inadequate prenatal care and birth injuries, maternal drug addiction, malnutrition, lead poisoning and air pollution, or other physical injuries and diseases. Many others will be suffering from the psychological and social impact of poverty, racism, and other forms of deprivation and oppression. Within areas of poverty in the United States, this array of physical and psychosocial trauma may also play a prominent role in producing ADHD-like behaviors, including hyperactivity, impulsivity, and inattention.

Martin Teicher (1997) and his team suggest, "Worldwide, the leading cause of ADHD may be severe early malnutrition through the first year of life." They believe that "In the United States, low birth weight, fetal alcohol exposure, and prenatal or postnatal lead exposure may be more common etiological factors." While relatively few of the children diagnosed ADHD in the United States will turn out to have an identifiable physical disorder, many different medical disorders can cause or worsen inattention, hyperactivity, and impulsivity. For parents with a persistently disturbed or disturbing child, or for parents who wish to entertain a diagnosis of ADHD and the possibility of medication, a complete medical evaluation for their child is an absolute pre-requisite. The medical evaluation should be much more thorough than many doctors routinely offer.

As the American Academy of Pediatrics[2] notes, any disease that affects brain function can produce the whole array of symptoms listed under ADHD. This includes various traumatic, toxic, infectious, immune, hormonal and neoplastic (cancer) disorders.

The academy list is more comprehensive than most but this chapter adds many additional ones. Ultimately, an experienced physician—or several physicians—is needed to evaluate each suspected cause of physical disorder.

Medications That Can Cause ADHD-Like Symptoms

Many drugs can cause ADHD-like symptoms. Notice that this listing starts out with the stimulants. The very drugs supposed to ameliorate the disorder can produce the entire range of hyperactivity, impulsivity, and inattention.[3] An extensive review of adverse behavioral and mental effects of psychiatric medications can be found in my book, *Your Drug May Be Your Problem* (1999), co-authored by David Cohen.

Most psychiatric and neurological medications:

- Stimulants (Ritalin, Metadate ER, Concerta, Dexedrine and DextroStat, Adderall, Desoxyn and Gradumet, and Cylert, as well as caffeine)

- Antidepressants (including the SSRIs, such as Prozac, Paxil, Luvox, Celexa, and Zoloft)

- Neuroleptics or antipsychotics (Mellaril, Haldol, Thorazine, Navane, Prolixin, Risperdal, Seroquel, and Zyprexa). Also, some drugs used for nausea, especially the neuroleptic Compazine

- Minor tranquilizers, sedatives, or sleeping medications (Halcion, Dalmane, Valium, Librium, Xanax, Klonopin, and Ativan)

- Antiepileptic medications (Dilantin, Depakote, Tegretol, and Neurontin)

- Barbiturates (phenobarbital, amobarbital or Amytal, butabarbital or Butisol, pentobarbital or Nembutal, and secobarbital or Seconal)

- Mood stabilizers (lithium, Depakote, Verapamil)

Asthma medications

- Ephedrine and pseudoephedrine

- Theophylline

- Antihistamines

Over-the-counter cold, allergy and sinus medications

- Most contain antihistamines or mild stimulants that can cause ADHD-like symptoms

Over-the-counter sleeping medications

- Any drug that can make you sleepy can impair alertness and concentration

Steroids
- Prednisone
- Anabolic steroids (used to build muscle mass)

Some antibiotics
- Antibiotics frequently cause fatigue. A number have been associated with mental abnormalities, including various penicillins and cephalosporins (e.g. Ceclor)

All drugs that are abused
- Amphetamine, methamphetamine, Ritalin, and cocaine
- Phencyclidine (PCP)
- d-Lysergic acid (LSD)
- Marijuana
- Glues and aerosols (sniffing)
- All sedatives, hypnotics, and minor tranquilizers, including Halcion, Xanax, Dalmane, Valium, Ativan, and Klonopin
- Alcohol

Medical Disorders That Can Cause ADHD-Like Symptoms

Like the list of medications, the list of physical disorders that can cause ADHD is probably infinite.

Prenatal factors
- Poor maternal health care
- Maternal use of cigarettes, alcohol, and prescription, recreational or illegal drugs
- Maternal malnutrition

Birth and perinatal complications
- Birth injury
- Hypoxia (blue baby)

- Toxemia, eclampsia (hypertensive disorder in pregnancy)

- Prolonged labor

- Low birth weight

- Postmaturity

Inborn errors of metabolism
- Phenylketonuria (PKU)

Stresses in infancy
- Malnutrition

- Abandonment

Trauma and anoxia (absence of oxygen)
- Any head injury, including mild closed head injury

- Shaking (when parents shake their babies in anger)

- Anoxia from any cause, such as drowning, smothering, choking, and strangulation

Toxic exposures
- Lead (often in paint chips and dust; can be in the dirt)

- Mercury (floors of houses and apartments)[4]

- Carbon monoxide poisoning (heating systems)

- Air pollutants

Infection
- Meningitis

- Encephalitis

- Almost any febrile illness (elevated temperature)

Neurological disorders
- Seizures (especially petit mal)

- Sydenham's chorea

- Mental retardation from any cause

- Drug-induced akathisia (inner tension with hyperactivity)

Other specific diseases and disorders
- Insulin-dependent diabetes
- Cerebral vascular accident
- Brain tumor
- Chemotherapy for cancer
- Chronic renal disease
- Lupus with CNS inflammation
- Iron-deficiency anemia
- Hormonal disorders (most commonly, thyroid)
- Vitamin deficiencies

Physical disabilities
- Visual impairment from any cause
- Hearing impairment from any cause, including ear infections

Fatigue and insomnia
- Any cause of chronic tiredness or lack of sleep

Hunger
- Many children, even from affluent families, do not eat properly and may be hungry in school. Sometimes these children suffer from eating disorders

Pain
- Any source of pain, including hidden infections (e.g., ears), stomach and intestinal cramps (constipation), headache

Psychological Problems That Can Cause ADHD-Like Symptoms

Almost any psychological problem can cause some ADHD-like symptoms. The American Academy of Pediatrics,[5] for example, lists autistic disorder, major depressive disorder, generalized anxiety disorder, post traumatic stress disorder, avoidant personality disorder, dysthymic disorder, separation anxiety disorder, and social phobia as possible causes. Dulcan (1994) lists more than a dozen psychiatric disorders that can cause ADHD or "ADHD-like" symptoms.

Without going into the validity of these particular diagnoses or their causes, it is apparent that a range of emotional disturbances can manifest in part, at least, as symptoms listed under ADHD.

Nutritional Causes of ADHD-Like Symptoms
Food Additives and Other Dietary Factors

Many alternative physicians and healers, and some more mainstream experts, believe that dietary factors can contribute to or cause ADHD-like symptoms. Without a great deal of scientific evidence, Feingold (1975) hypothesized in the early 1970s that dyes, preservatives, and salicylates can cause hyperactivity. Since then many experiments have been conducted, some that seem to meet scientific standards.

The main evidence for dietary factors is the observation of beneficial effects during the removal of specific substances from the diet. Improvements associated with dietary changes have not usually been large in rigorous studies.

Bonnie J. Kaplan (1989) and a team from University of Calgary tried to maximize the impact by using an experimental diet that eliminates artificial colors and flavors, preservatives, monosodium glutamate, chocolate, caffeine, and "any substance that families reported might affect their specific child," including milk products if the family reported any difficulties with them.[6] The diet was also low in simple sugars. The authors comment, "it is safe to say that not a single parent believed that participation in this study had transformed their child into an easy to manage person."

Boris and Mandel (1994) reviewed the literature and again conducted an experiment that aimed to maximize effects by removing all additives. The subjects were tested for two weeks to eliminate specific foods to which they showed intolerance, such as dairy products or peanuts. Nineteen of 26 ADHD children responded positively to the initial elimination trial. There was no placebo control, however. Some of the subjects were then tested in several double-blind one day exposures to challenge substances over a week period. The authors found that symptoms worsened on days that the children were exposed to additives.

The prestigious British journal Lancet published a report that tested the effect of injecting enzymes thought to reduce food allergies.[7] The authors believe that their results confirm that many cases of hyperactivity are caused by food intolerance but the treatment itself is controversial.

There is also evidence from controlled studies that the removal of artificial food coloring alone can improve a child's ADHD-like symptoms.[8]

Some mainstream sources now note the possibility that food additives may cause behavioral and cognitive problems. Writing in *American Pharmacy*, pharmacist Gary Levin (1995) observes that "some children may experience a worsening of ADHD symptoms that is related to food additives and dyes." He cites tartrazine (yellow dye number 5) as a potential cause of respiratory distress and hyperactivity. Tartrazine is found in many foods and drugs.

Evaluating the Food Allergy Studies

It is obviously important to make sure that a child is not deprived of a balanced diet with all the necessary nutrients. However, nutritional and food allergy studies seem insufficient in number and quality to draw firm conclusions. There is also the problem of finding the proverbial needle in the haystack: the rare child whose problem may be mainly dietary. By contrast, the vast majority of children are clearly suffering from unmet psychosocial and educational needs, especially informed, caring adult attention.

While there is sufficient evidence to encourage further research, I remain skeptical about proving the impact of nutrition on behavior. It is very difficult to create a controlled study. Almost any therapeutic program is likely to seem helpful if it requires parents to be more hopeful and more involved and if it requires children to be more disciplined in response to an understandable set of rules, such as dietary restrictions.

My own clinical experience contradicts the notion that these children commonly have anything physically wrong with them. Approaches that focus on defects in a child's body, including food allergies, reinforce the mistaken idea that the problem lies in the child. These approaches stigmatize the child and distract from real causes within the family and school.

Low Blood Sugar (Hypoglycemia)

There is no doubt that low blood sugar (hypoglycemia) can impair mental and emotional functioning. Many people become jittery, irritable, and lose their focus when becoming abruptly hungry, probably as a result of a rapidly dropping level of blood sugar. When diabetic individuals accidentally overdose with insulin, causing an abrupt drop in blood sugar, they may feel tired, irritable, and confused before becoming weak and, in the extreme, passing out. If an individual eats large amounts of sugar, the blood sugar can rise and fall abruptly, causing reactive or rebound hypoglycemia. However, there is little evidence that low blood sugar can become a significant source of difficulty in a significant number of children suffering from ADHD-like symptoms.

A study by Timothy W. Jones (1995) and a team from the Yale University School of Medicine has tested one possible mechanism by which eating sugar might impair the functioning of healthy children. After the ingestion of the equivalent of the sugar content of two cans of Coca-Cola, children developed a drop in blood sugar 3–5 hours later with accompanying symptoms of hypoglycemia: "pounding heart, feeling shaky, feeling weak, having difficulty concentrating, headaches, feeling anxious, slowed thinking, and feeling sweaty." There was a corresponding rise in epinephrine (adrenaline) levels in the blood. Auditory evoked potentials measured in the brain indicated a dulling effect on the brain's responsiveness. Young adults in the same study did not develop these marked reactions.

This study does not confirm that children who suffer from ADHD-symptoms on a regular basis are suffering from *chronic* problems with sugar. It does show that hypoglycemia with associated *acute* behavioral and mental effects can be caused when normal children eat a large amount of sugar without other food to slow down its absorption and to provide more lasting sources of energy. Children should be discouraged from gobbling down large amounts of unadulterated sugar, especially if they have hypoglycemic rebound symptoms. Obviously, it's also a good nutritional principle to stay away from "empty calories"—foods that satisfy the palate but not the whole body.

Block (1996) takes a different position, claiming that "low blood sugar, or hypoglycemia, is the most significant underlying problem I find in children who exhibit behavioral problems," but she doesn't seem to check her theory or her diagnosis of individual children by administering glucose tolerance tests. Instead, she bases it on commonplace symptoms such as being "shaky and irritable when hungry."[9] Block herself recognizes that the hundreds of studies on the relationship between sugar and behavior have been largely negative, but she is critical of them. Her views are discussed further in Chapter 10.

Why So Many Different Approaches Work

Why would children seem to be helped by changes in their diet, in particular, limiting their sugar intake, providing sugar free snacks, making snacks readily available, and encouraging frequent small meals? A parent who employs this strategy is likely to be less punitive and more encouraging to her child whom she now sees as suffering from a medical problem. The parent is also required to pay special attention to the child. The child is likely to see the parent as more caring and more willing to respond to his or her desires for snacks. By providing extra attention to the child, the implementation of any rigorous diet is likely to be helpful. It requires cooperation between the parents and child toward a common goal. It becomes a family therapy project. More realistic educational or recreational projects would probably be even more helpful.

Acupuncture, Biofeedback, Meditation, and Other Alternative Therapies

Advocates of the ADHD/Alternative movement often expect me to support their efforts but I believe there are several problems with all of these approaches.

First, whether they advocate acupuncture or herbs, these alternative approaches are likely to reinforce the myth that the problem lies in the child's individual body or mind. The promotion of this metaphorical medical disorder, ADHD, as well as alternative physical treatments, blames the child and exonerates adults and adult institutions, such as the schools, of any responsibility.

Second, alternative practitioners, if they become focused on a fad of their own, are likely to overlook the broad range of known medical disorders that can cause ADHD-like symptoms.

Third, by focusing on the body, they risk rejecting the reality that the behavior of children is far more influenced by their psychological and social environments, and that most ADHD-like symptoms signal a conflict between children and the adults in their lives.

On the other hand, as psychiatrist and alternative healer James Gordon describes in *Manifesto for a New Medicine*, I'm sure many children could be helped by non-judgmental, non-medical approaches that improve their sense of empowerment, self-control, and concentration. Gordon gives the example of helping a child find his power animal. Meditation, relaxation exercises, acupuncture, and many other interventions that bring a measure of accomplishment, self-determination, and peace to a child will be helpful. If they involve a responsible, caring relationship with an adult, they will be all the more successful.

In short, anything that improves the self-esteem and competence of children, from martial arts to dance, from football to camping, is going to be helpful—as long it does not pin "the problem" on the children or imply that they have something wrong in their brains or minds. The quality of the relationships with the adults will be key to how helpful the program can become for the children.

Even People with Physical Diseases

When genuine physical disorders are diagnosed in children, such as diabetes or phenylketonuria, specialists are likely to treat children with much more compassion and understanding, and with much more emphasis on gaining the child's cooperation, than do psychiatrists and pediatricians who diagnose ADHD and prescribe Ritalin. The modern treatment of diabetes, for example, involves teaching children to take control over their own treatment. It encourages these children to view themselves as "normal" as much as possible. It motivates them to improve their overall physical and mental health. Good medical care in general, unlike the way many doctors treat children for "behavior disorders," requires enlisting the child and parent in a mutually cooperative treatment program that enhances the child's self-discipline and autonomy.

PART THREE

THE POLITICS OF THE ADHD/RITALIN LOBBY

Chapter 14

WHO'S BEHIND ALL THIS?

Part I: The Pharmaceutical Company and Its Allies

I do not suggest that either they [the drug companies] or we [the American Psychiatric Association] are evil folks. But I continue to believe that accepting such money is, in the long run, inimical to our independent functioning. We have evolved a somewhat casual and quite cordial relationship with the drug houses, taking their money readily... We seem to discount available data that drug advertising promotes irrational prescribing practices. We seem to think that we as psychiatrists are immune from the kinds of unconscious emotional bias in favor of those who are overtly friendly toward us.... We persist in ignoring an inherent conflict of interest.

—Fred Gottlieb,
APA Speaker of the House (1985)

In fact, the field of psychiatry has become an economically driven profession.
—George Pollock, APA Treasurer (1986)

By now many readers must be asking, "How is it possible that critical information on Ritalin and other drugs is being withheld from the public and even from doctors? Why isn't any research being done on long-term harmful effects from these drugs, even though they are given to children for years at a time? Why do doctors encourage the use of drugs that have so little good effect and do so much harm? Why do professionals continue to believe in something as unscientific and farfetched as ADHD?"

The answers to these questions lie in the politics of psychiatry and what I call the Psychopharmaceutical Complex.[1] This chapter focuses on politics and economics because these are the forces that drive the ADHD/Ritalin movement. We begin with the self-avowed "partnership" between the American Psychiatric Association (APA) and the drug companies, and look at two parent groups that might as well be working for the drug companies. In a sense, they are.

In the next chapter we will look at the role of federal agencies in supporting ADHD/Ritalin.

Psychiatrists Face a Shrinking Market

In the 1970s, the APA was going broke. Many psychiatrists were having difficulty filling their practices. Always near the bottom of the medical income scale, psychiatrists were floundering economically. Competition from non-medical professionals was cutting heavily into private practices. Psychologists, social workers, counselors, family therapists, and other non-psychiatrists were taking over the mental health field. They charged smaller fees and yet often provided better service as "talking therapists." With a larger proportion of women among the new breed of therapists, they drew increasing numbers of women patients to them for therapy.

Psychiatry discussed its economic crisis in its newspapers and journals, as well as within its conferences and board meetings. Psychiatry had to convince the American public that psychological suffering should remain under the ultimate control of physicians, including psychiatrists. To do this, psychiatry had to convince the public that emotional or spiritual suffering is rooted in genetics and biology, requiring drugs, electroshock and other "medical" interventions.

A major step was to revise the *Diagnostic and Statistical Manual of Mental Disorders*, the ultimate source of "official" diagnoses, in order to make the diagnoses sound more medical.[2] This resulted in the evolution of the concept of ADHD into its present form. By elaborating on ADHD as a "disorder," psychiatric interventions with drugs became more justified.

However, rewriting and publicizing the diagnostic manual requires money. Deep in financial trouble, the APA did not have the resources to mount a national PR campaign on behalf of psychiatry.

Drug Companies to the Rescue

In the early 1980s, APA made a decision that changed its history and that of our society. It decided to create an economic and political partnership with the drug companies. The partnership would enable psychiatry to use drug company funds to promote the medical model, psychopharmacology, and the authority and influence of psychiatry. Backed by the multi-billion dollar drug industry, psychiatry hoped to defeat the threat from non-medical professionals, such as psychologists and social workers. Within a scant few years, APA transformed itself from a failing institution into one of the most powerful political forces in the nation. It developed lobbying groups in state capitals and in Washington, DC; gained a stronger influence in the media and the courts; and distributed increasing numbers of drugs to escalating numbers of people.

An Openly Discussed Survival Plan

This is not the story of a covert "conspiracy." Psychiatry's decision to save itself by going into partnership with the drug companies was an openly discussed survival plan whose historical details I have documented in *Toxic Psychiatry* (1991). As illustrated by the quote from APA official Fred Gottlieb at the head of the chapter, ethical issues were raised within the APA about becoming so dependent on drug company financing. But these occasional ethical voices were easily drowned out by a pragmatic political leadership whose eyes were glued on expanding psychiatry's economic base and influence.

Psychiatric News (1997b) the official newspaper of the American Psychiatric Association now brags about revenues from drug company ads in APA's newspaper and journals: "pharmaceutical advertising alone could hit $4 million for 1997." Drug companies also pour money into the APA through grants, by funding special projects, by paying for "fellows" at the APA, and by massive support for local and national professional meetings. Beyond that, drug companies support everything from professorships, lecture series, and labs at medical schools to Continuing Medication Credits (CMEs) for physicians and most of the drug research conducted in the world.

By funding the largest chunk of research, the drug companies build relationships of dependency and cooperation with researchers and research centers. This prevents important, critical research from taking place—such as follow up studies on Ritalin-induced shrinkage of brain tissue or on the irreversibility of stimulant-induced biochemical changes in brain cells.[3]

Becoming "Partners"

Is it an exaggeration to speak of a "partnership" in describing the relationship between the American Psychiatric Association and the drug companies? To the contrary, the APA itself openly boasts of its "partnership" with the drug companies. The boast came in response to my criticism. A report in the *New York Times* questioned how the sleep medication Halcion, banned in England, could be prescribed for then President George Bush in the United States. The newspaper published my response explaining that APA received a "gift" of $1.5 million cash from Upjohn, the manufacturer of Halcion, at the time that Halcion was coming under international fire.[4] APA's deep financial dependency on Upjohn makes it impossible for the organization to take any actions that would seriously threaten the company.

In rebuttal of my published letter, the medical director of the APA, Melvin Sabshin (1992), defended his organization by praising its "partnership" with the drug companies. According to Sabshin, "Dr. Breggin attacks a responsible, ethical partnership that uses the no-strings resources of one partner and the expertise of the other...."

Upjohn uses the same language in defense of itself against criticism from neurologist Fred Baughman, Jr. (1992). The company admits to a "partnership" with the APA.[5] Apparently the APA and the drug company are also cooperating in developing the language of their responses to criticism. Even after the exchange of letters, the APA continued to flaunt the theme of "our partners in industry" in a mass mailing to its membership.[6]

Can any reasonable person doubt the inherent conflict of interest in a financial partnership between drug companies and organized psychiatry? Could huge cash giveaways from Upjohn to APA have no impact on APA's attitudes toward the drug company and its products? In fact, Upjohn contributes a great deal more than this one donation of $1.5 million to the psychiatric coffers. I was focusing on one particularly egregious, identifiable example.

Is There "Collusion" between Drug Companies and Organized Psychiatry?

Partnership may not be a strong enough word to describe the relationships between APA and the drug companies. In an opinion column for *Psychiatric News* entitled "APA and Drug Companies: Too Close for Comfort," psychiatrist Lester E. Shapiro (1991) identifies the closely shared interests of APA and the drug companies:

> I am aware that the interrelationship of APA and the pharmaceutical industry is a complex one. We share research needs, appropriate product evaluation, planning for long-range goals, and the overarching considerations inherent in biopsychosocial patient care.

Using the emphatic word "collusion" to describe APA-drug company relations, Shapiro concludes:

> It is far better that we engage in a serious examination and dialogue of the issues I have raised than to act in collusion with an industry whose goal is to increase drug usage by broadening indications for their drugs, advocating long-term administration, minimizing adverse side effects, overstating effectiveness, de-emphasizing adjunctive treatments, or denigrating generic drugs.[7]

This is a stunning indictment from within the psychiatric establishment itself. Shapiro's detailed observations are equally remarkable: The APA colludes with drug companies whose interests lie in broadening marketings, encouraging long-term use, minimizing the dangers of drugs, and belittling alternatives to drugs.

In its introduction to Shapiro's column, *Psychiatric News*, the official newspaper of the American Psychiatric Association, admits the truth of it: "Many of APA's scientific and educational programs depend on support from pharmaceutical companies. Some psychiatrists have questioned whether taking money from these companies compromises APA's integrity and professional mission."

David Brody (1997) is another rare psychiatrist who raises issues about drug company funding of psychiatry. He laments the huge outpouring of pharmaceutical company support for APA's 1997 annual meeting, repeating one psychiatrist's comment that it "made it seem as though APA was a subsidiary of Janssen or Lilly."

Brody suggests that "APA prohibit industry-supported symposia and/or exhibits at the annual meeting." The cost of the meetings for individual members would be "significantly greater" without drug company sponsorship, he observes, but it would help to preserve the "quality of our scientific meetings" against the dangers of "profit-driven" medicine.

From Partnership to Dependence

Marc Czarka, director of pharmaceutical affairs for Eli Lilly Benelux, also describes Eli Lilly's relationship with the APA as something more than a "partnership." In defending his company against charges of suppressing criticism of Prozac by doctors and consumers in Europe, Czarka made a remarkable concession to a European journal. According to the *Bulletin*:[8]

> Czarka concedes that Lilly funds the American Psychiatric Association and that, with other pharmaceutical companies, it sponsors and helped create the Belgian League of Depression in 1995. "It's useful for us because, unlike American law, European law does not allow us to talk directly to potential patients," says Czarka. "The league does that for us."

The drug company executive seems to view APA as a kind of front group for his company's interests.

Here in the United States, Gary Tollefson, a psychiatrist and Lilly executive, has bragged about Lilly's "partnership with the academic community" and "peer review medical journals." According to conservative political columnist Arianna Huffington (1997b), who witnessed these remarks, Lilly is also in partnership with Congress: "The company went from zero soft-money contributions in the 1992 election cycle to $746,675 in 1996." The company also gave to politicians, including Newt Gingrich. When Huffington called a Congressional staffer to request information about Lilly and the FDA, she was told bluntly that he would do no such thing because Lilly had made campaign contributions to his boss.

When the pharmaceutical industry *funds*, *colludes* with, or has a *partnership* with organized psychiatry—truth is the loser, along with the public and patients. The combined interests of drug companies and organized psychiatry have much too much control over research, as well as the flow of information and the practice of diagnosing and medicating psychiatric patients. Meanwhile, a Congress well-fed by the drug companies is not likely to investigate their collusion with organized psychiatry.

The Psychopharmaceutical Complex

The Psychopharmaceutical Complex is a close association, a "partnership" in Melvin Sabshin's adoring words, a "collusion" in Lester Shapiro's more skeptical view. It brings together the drug companies, their researchers and doctors, government agencies, various medical organizations including the American Psychiatric Association, medical schools, and insurance providers. All of the groups benefit enormously from the wide spread use of psychiatric drugs in America, including the insurers who believe it's much less expensive for them to fund drugs than psychotherapy.

Many private philanthropic organizations are also closely aligned with the Psychopharmaceutical Complex. The National Mental Health Association, for example, accepts large sums of money from Eli Lilly and Company, the manufacturer of Prozac, and in turn puts out "educational" advertising that promotes the concept of depression as a "disease" and the use of medication to treat it.[9] The advertisements, disguised as educational commentaries, have been heard on the radio throughout the country.

To start with, we will focus on six major players in the Psychopharmaceutical Complex:

1. The American Psychiatric Association, the largest and most powerful group representing the interests of American psychiatrists;

2. CibaGeneva Pharmaceuticals (the manufacturer of Ritalin), now a subdivision of the giant pharmaceutical company, Novartis;

3. CHADD (Children and Adults with Attention Deficit Disorder), an influential parents organization that receives money from Ciba/Novartis and other drug companies;

4. The U.S. Department of Education (DOE);

5. The National Institute of Mental Health (NIMH);

6. The Food and Drug Administration (FDA).

All bear responsibility for society's current epidemic of drugging children.

Who Is Novartis?

At the top of the Psychopharmaceutical Complex stands the multi-billion dollar drug industry. As one of the richest and most powerful industries in the world, it exerts enormous influence throughout government and society. The focus is on Novartis, whose division, CibaGeneva or Ciba-Geigy, makes Ritalin; but the observations could apply equally to many other drug companies.

Novartis: a Big-Bucks Merger

The company that manufactures Ritalin is a giant among giants. When Ciba combined with Sandoz to create Novartis in 1996, it was advertised as "the largest corporate merger... New company Novartis captures number one world-wide position in life sciences... number two global rank in pharmaceuticals."[10] The press release boasted that "Ciba has recorded double-digit annual earnings growth over the past five years." The combining of Ciba and Sandoz created a $27 *billion* giant and it has been thriving with sales of $18.5 *billion* in 1996 and an "operating profit" of $3.2 *billion*.[11]

To justify their high prices for health products, drug companies claim to spend relatively huge sums of money on research and development. Novartis (1996) spent almost twice as much on marketing and distribution as on research and development. Much of what gets called research and development is in reality devoted to marketing—for example, reinterpreting research or developing research to meet public criticism or other promotional needs.

The Ciba financial report does not break down sales for Ritalin. However, IMS America, which provides marketing facts for industry, estimates an increase in consumer purchases of Ritalin from $95.3 million in 1991 to $349.3 million in 1995.

Novartis also announced its creation through media advertisements, including a giant full page ad in *USA Today* on February 20, 1997. The ad asks rhetorically, "Who's harnessing the world's most advanced scientific thinking to develop new medicines in the 21st century? Novartis. The world's leading Life Sciences company. Formed by the merger of Ciba and Sandoz." Lavish spending on advertisements encourages the media industry to be sympathetic to and protect the drug companies when controversies whirl up around them. However, *USA Today*, unlike many other newspapers, has continued to publish columns and reports critical of the over-medication of children, including my February 2000 Op-Ed column about parents retaking repsonsibility from the medical doctors.

Selling an Industrial Product

It is important to remember that medical and psychiatric drugs are industrial products in the same way that cars, clothing, or toys are industrial products. Drug companies are among the most profitable industries in the world.

They are subject to the same market pressures for sales and for profits as any other giant industry. They will take the same extreme measures when their profits are threatened. While some of their products are evaluated for safety by the government, the same can be said of cars, clothing, and toys as well. The government cannot possibly guarantee the overall quality of scientific research, drug promotion, and drug prescription practices. Instead, the government too often becomes part of the problem by responding to political pressure to be lenient on the drug companies.

Ciba Acts Like... a Profit-Making Corporation

The magazine, *Mother Jones* (1993), named Ciba to its "Toxic Ten." They chose Ciba, "a Swiss-based agrochemical and drug multinational" to "represent" the problem of companies using a double standard, using lower foreign standards to withhold information on environmental impact statements required in the United States. Without providing background information or evidence, *Mother Jones* declared, "In behavior shocking by any standard, Ciba-Geigy tested herbicides on human subjects in the 1970s in Egypt and India."

Recent research findings show that Ritalin can cause cancer in some animals.[12] Now there's another possible cancer threat—this one from Ciba's industrial practices. In an ironic tragedy for a company purporting to devote science to the interest of America's children, Ciba has been suspected of causing increased cancer rates in children in the surrounding community in the Toms River region of New Jersey.[13] Local citizens' committees "long suspected that waste from the pharmaceutical giant has fouled soil and water in the region." But Ciba denied the allegations and claims to have "spent millions to clean up the waste-disposal site."

While these various acts don't involve Ritalin, they reflect on Ciba's central motivation—making a profit, sometimes regardless of the human cost. In this regard, Ciba probably differs little from other giant industries seeking to satisfy their investors in a highly competitive market place. But the public too often forgets this fact, that drug companies make industrial products, and then try desperately to sell them.

The Physician Sales Force

Physicians are the ultimate distributors and salespersons for pharmaceutical products. The companies of course have their own distribution and sales teams; but they must rely upon physicians to get the product to the patient. Drug companies spend a great deal of money appealing to medical organizations and to physicians to win their overall sympathy and loyalty as well as their support for particular products. Novartis, the parent company of Ciba, has a sales force of 2,300 in the United States alone.[14] Most doctors seem to get their basic drug information from drug company sales reps.

In psychiatry the dependence on the drug companies is even greater than in medicine in general. People who suffer from medical illnesses—pneumonia, Parkinson's disease, or heart disease—don't usually have to be convinced that they have real physical diseases that require treatment by medical doctors. They may not always want to go to the doctor but they will usually concede that they suffer from physical illnesses that lie within the province of physicians.

Psychiatry, by contrast, must convince unhappy or troubled people to become "patients." To do this, psychiatry must first convince the public that anxiety, depression, or ADHD are genuine diseases that require a medical intervention in the form of drugs. Drug companies—by supporting "educational" campaigns with their partners—have become the financial engine for advertising and promoting psychiatric interests.

Like most drug companies, Ciba/Novartis spends a great deal of money to influence psychiatric opinion in favor of its drugs. It sponsors seminars, pumps dollars into psychiatric conventions, and helps support journals with its advertising. Unfortunately, the dollar amounts are concealed. Except for newspaper and journal advertising, the American Psychiatric Association will not release figures on how much it receives from drug companies. The drug companies will not say how much they contribute to psychiatry.

Is Ciba/Novartis Cheating on the Internet and in Its Publications?

There are federal laws that limit the advertising claims companies can make about their drugs.[15] Drug companies are limited to presenting material that the FDA has allowed in the approved label for the medication, and they must do it in a fair, balanced manner. It must not be *misleading, deceptive* or *false*.[16]

Novartis Pharma (1997) is the corporate division that deals with pharmacology. On its web site, the company spouts the ADHD/Ritalin ideology:

Attention Deficit Hyperactivity Disorder (ADHD) is a neurobiological disability... Although the exact cause of ADHD is unknown, researchers believe it to be the result of an imbalance or deficiency of specific chemicals in the brain... Novartis has developed a drug that appears to correct a deficiency of certain chemicals in the brain.

Ciba's promotional remarks illustrate several important aspects of its PR campaign. The company makes an unfounded speculation that ADHD is a physical disorder and ties this to the need for children to take drugs. Toward this end, the company lists the ADHD discussion under central nervous system disorders, even though ADHD has never been proven to be a disease of the brain. The company also claims that it has developed a drug that may correct the presumed biochemical deficiencies in ADHD. Even Paul Leber (1994), the doctor then in charge of the approval of psychiatric drugs at the FDA, has said there's no evidence that ADHD is a disease.[17]

Ciba uses a similar strategy in its ADHD booklet for classroom teachers.[18] It describes multiple presumed mental and neurological disabilities associated with learning disabilities and with ADHD. It then tells teachers the false speculation that ADHD "is caused by neurological differences in the child's brain." Miraculously, according to Ciba, the drugs used to treat ADHD have no negative effect on the brain at all:

[T]hey appear to work by correcting for a lack of certain necessary brain chemicals in the nervous system. Parents should be aware that these medicines do not "drug" or "alter" the brain of the child. They make the child "normal" by correcting for a neurochemical imbalance.

Ciba's claim that Ritalin makes the brain normal is also utterly false. Instead, the drug drastically alters the brains of animals and children alike, regardless of the presence or absence of an ADHD diagnosis. The closing sentence of the booklet reminds the teacher, "Work closely with the student's physician." This almost inevitably means obtaining a prescription for Ritalin.

Ciba is not allowed to make these misleading statements in its official FDA-approved label or advertising. For example, the label states unequivocally, "Specific etiology of this syndrome is unknown." The approved label also declares, "There is neither specific evidence which clearly establishes the mechanism whereby Ritalin produces its mental and behavior effects in children, nor conclusive evidence regarding how these effects relate to the condition of the central nervous system." There are no claims in the label about correcting biochemical imbalances or making the brain normal. Instead, the label provides evidence that Ritalin does in fact "deter" the brain with the production of adverse effects.

How does Ciba get away with seemingly false advertising on its web site and in its booklet? In both cases, the drug company does not actually mention the *name* of its drug. The written material is clearly aimed at promoting a biological viewpoint leading to the prescription of medication, but without naming the company product.

The booklet and the web site are so clearly talking about Ritalin that the FDA could probably insist that Ciba adhere to ethical advertising standards even though the company never actually prints the word "Ritalin." But the FDA is relatively inactive in monitoring advertising.[19] Ciba can rest easy.

Aggressive from the Beginning

In *The Myth of the Hyperactive Child*, Peter Schrag and Diane Divoky (1975) describe the aggressive advertising techniques through which Ciba primed the drug pump by helping to create the concept of drugging children to control their behavior:

At the heart of that success lies an aggressive promotion and sales campaign pushing not only the drug but the ailments it is supposed to mitigate, if not to cure, a brilliant blend of social mythology about bright happy classrooms with bright happy children and carefully selected citations from the medical literature which, on closer inspection, totally fail to support the conclusions that the advertising suggests.[20]

Schrag and Divoky document how Ciba pushed its advertising claims and promotional materials too far time and again, and how occasionally the FDA would rein them in. Schrag and Divoky describe in detail the drug company's aggressive promotional tactics including presentations to PTA meetings and other parent groups by teams made up of a physician and a Ciba salesperson. Eventually the FDA cracked down on these direct-to-consumer promotions. Ciba, early on, also funded many of the researchers who went on to dominate the field, such as C. Keith Conners and Leon Eisenberg.

Misinformation for Doctors in Ciba's Journal Ads

Ciba has always spent heavily on advertising Ritalin in journals read by doctors. Because the FDA regulations on balance and fairness in advertising are not usually enforced, many drug company ads gloss over adverse effects and exaggerate therapeutic effects.[21] Ciba's ads for Ritalin have been no exception over the years.

Ciba ads for Ritalin have often involved two carefully designed multi-color art pages followed by a third page with the required FDA-approved label details in fine print. Over the years, the Ritalin ads have been very misleading. In a February 1974 issue of the *American Journal of Psychiatry*,[22] the first two pages of a Ritalin advertisement display photos of a young boy happily attentive in school. The ad copy quotes a journal article, "an effective agent in the alleviation of the hyperkinetic disorder." There is no mention whatsoever that the "alleviation" is very short-lived and wholly confined to the control of behavior. Placing the boy in a classroom lends the impression Ritalin must improve academic performance, and the ad copy says nothing to dispel that false impression. Ritalin's more serious adverse effects, including addiction and psychosis, are unmentioned except in the fine print on the third page, and so the claims made in bold letters are not balanced by a description of adverse effects.

Similarly, a two-page Ciba ad for the long-acting form of Ritalin in the 1986 *American Journal of Psychiatry* lists no adverse reactions at all on its main page, while also failing to mention the short-lived nature of the behavioral effects or the lack of improvement in academic achievement. Instead the ad displays a picture of a child happily sitting still and raising his hand in class. Only the fine print on the back page mentions any of Ritalin's adverse effects or limitations.

In recent years, Ciba seems to have cut back on its advertising in journals, perhaps finding it far cheaper and more effective to advertise directly to the public through its own website, through booklets aimed at parents and teachers, and especially through the parents' group, CHADD

The Politics of Defining a Drug's Uses and Adverse Effects

The public does not tend to think of psychiatric drugs as industrial products that will be marketed and promoted as vigorously as the companies can get away with. Although it should, the public does not bring the same skepticism to claims about "medical" drugs as it would, for example, to claims about tobacco and alcohol products, colas, cosmetics, and the like.

Instead, most people believe that modern psychiatric medications are fine-tuned to brain chemistry and hence to specific psychiatric disorders. As I document extensively in *Toxic Psychiatry* (1991), *Brain-Disabling Treatments in Psychiatry* (1997a), and *Your Drug May Be Your Problem* (1999, with David Cohen) these are false claims. Public belief in them is driven by the concerted campaigning carried on by the Psychopharmaceutical Complex.

Drug companies tend to try to get the FDA to approve their drugs for a variety of purposes, usually as loosely and broadly defined as possible. They want the potential market to be as large as possible. After a period of bargaining and concessions on both sides before the drug is marketed, the drug gains FDA approval for one or more disorders. Over the years, the number of FDA approved indications for the drug may increase or decrease in number in a process that continues to involve political pressures, bargaining, and accommodations. In recent years, the FDA has loosened rules governing media advertising, unleashing a deluge of magazine and TV advertising for psychiatric drugs for special uses such as "social anxiety disorder."

The same process takes place in regard to listing adverse drug effects in the label. The drug company wants as few as possible to be listed and it wants to minimize the danger from those that do get listed. Again there is a period of haggling and give and take with the FDA out of which grows the final label with its list of adverse effects. The list often grows as the drug is used over the years and reports of new adverse effects stream into the FDA. Often, however, it becomes a political process in which the FDA is pressured not to give the drug a bad name that will harm its marketing. I have described these fundamentally political processes in some detail in discussing both Prozac and the FDA in general.[23]

Ciba Pushes Its Claims for Ritalin beyond the Limits

Ritalin was first approved under relatively lenient FDA standards in late 1955. Despite widespread Ritalin addiction and abuse through the world, up until 1969 Ciba did not indicate these problems in its label. On January 24, 1969 the U.S. Bureau of Narcotics and Dangerous Drugs gave notice of its intention to place Ritalin under drug abuse controls.[24] The FDA also required the drug company to place a prominent warning in its label about addiction and abuse. It took the government many years before it forced Ciba to do the right thing.

In 1969 Ciba was still promoting Ritalin as an antidepressant "which brightens mood and improves performance." Claiming "wide clinical applications" in its label, Ciba even advocated Ritalin for "increasing response to psychotherapy." Based on a National Academy of Sciences review (circa 1970), the FDA rejected the company's 1970 label claims for depression, chronic fatigue, and psychoneurosis.[25]

Ciba's Magic Ritalin Elixir

One astonishing Ciba (1970) product, Ritonic, claimed to "improve mood and maintain vitality." In addition to Ritalin, it contained male and female hormonal replacements,[26] calcium supplement, and B vitamins! The cocktail tonic was intended "for patients who are losing their drive, alertness, vitality and zest for living because of the natural degenerative changes of advancing age." Who could resist?

After years on the market, when the FDA tightened its scrutiny of Ciba labeling, Ritonic went to the deserved final resting place of all magic elixirs—oblivion. As the *Medical News Letter* (1969) declared, "There is no evidence justifying the use of such a heterogeneous drug combination for these symptoms." In fact, there is added danger in mixing several drugs at once and even more danger in recommending the combination for elders who are much more susceptible to adverse reactions. None of this led to Ciba pulling Ritonic off the market in the years before the FDA cracked down.

The FDA Re-Evaluates Ritalin

In a re-evaluation of Ritalin by the FDA, Scoville (1970) noted that "the longest study" submitted for efficacy and adverse effects in children was 6 weeks in duration. Only "short-term efficacy" was supported by the data. At that time, Ritalin's label was also found to be inadequate in regard to various adverse reactions. The FDA's medical reviewer wrote, "Adverse effects have been described in published articles which have not been included in the labeling—some effects apparently quite common. These include abdominal pains and weight loss, which deserve study and follow up. Paradoxical increase in symptoms, and statistically significant tachycardia [increased heart rate] are not adequately described in the present labeling..."[27] The label had described tachycardia as "rare."

History indicates that Ciba is as honest in its claims as the FDA forces it to be. Even if the FDA had the requisite political courage, the agency does not have the resources to keep on top of the drug companies to ensure their honesty in promoting their products.

Ciba's 3 R's of Ritalin

When addiction and abuse problems with Ritalin could no longer be so fully hidden from the public in 1996, Ciba developed a multi-color pamphlet "For the Parent" that it mailed to 110,000 doctors and 100,000 pharmacists, "hoping they will pass them on to parents and school nurses."[28] The package contained a glossy letter to the doctor, sample brochures, and information sheets for the parents. It was another brilliant PR stroke, truly making lemonade out of lemons.

The striking cover of the Ciba promotional has three large R's scrawled across it in a child's hand, while the title declares, "The 3 R's of Ritalin— Read, Respect, Responsibility." The pamphlet purports to warn against the diversion and abuse of Ritalin, but children are asked to "respect Ritalin" much as they would a person: "Respect yourself. Respect others. Respect Ritalin." As we have seen, children sometimes tend to treat Ritalin more like a person than they treat themselves—attributing to Ritalin their good and bad behavior. CHADD is listed as a suggested resource.

Ciba also put out glossy booklets on ADHD for the parent and for the teacher written by Larry B. Silver (1989, 1990), clinical professor of psychiatry at Georgetown Medical School. Child-like lettering and drawings again lend charm to these clever advertisements.

Like other aggressive drug companies, Ciba also sponsors symposia, gaining favor with leading figures in the field. On May 11, 1993, for example, the company sponsored The Fourth Annual Decade of the Brain Symposium at the prestigious National Press Club in Washington, DC. The brochure from a mass mailing declared, "The symposium will highlight the importance of developmental neuroscience in providing an understanding of the management and prevention of childhood mental and neurological disorders." Of course, there is no neuroscience behind the diagnosis or treatment of ADHD. But pseudo-scientific rallies like these lend an air of science to the process of drugging children.

Drug Company Researchers— How Many Masters Can a Doctor Serve?

The drug companies themselves finance, design, and carry out all of the research that goes into the approval process for their drugs.[29] At dozens of steps along the way, the drug company can influence the outcome of the research, but probably no step is as important as selecting and sponsoring favorably-inclined researchers.

Some well-known psychiatrists require a page or more just to list the drug companies they work for. Here's an example picked at random from a recent disclosure statement in small print from a drug company sponsored symposium.[30] Sheldon Preskorn is Professor and Vice Chairman of Psychiatry at the University of Kansas School of Medicine and Director of Psychiatric

Research Center. He is or has been a *principal investigator* (the doctor in charge) on drug studies funded by *thirty-five drug companies* including Ciba. Preskorn has also been on the *speakers bureau* of Ciba and *more than a dozen* other companies. On top of all this, Preskorn has been a consultant to *sixteen* drug companies.

Obviously Preskorn is deeply trusted and well paid by the world's drug companies while he simultaneously plays a leading role in American psychiatry. When a doctor like Preskorn teaches young psychiatrists, directs a psychiatry department, or conducts research, can he remain independent and objective? Or are his economic and professional interests too intermingled with those of the drug companies? Regardless of how Preskorn himself responds to these potential conflicts of interest, the widespread dependency of psychiatric leaders on the drug companies will tend to push the profession toward promoting drugs.

Massive Fraud by Two Drug Company Researchers

As I'm writing this section, the *Wall Street Journal* reports a case of massive research fraud—skewed in favor of the drug companies—by doctors used by multiple corporations. Novartis (Ciba) is among them.[31] Richard L. Borison and Bruce I. Diamond, "distinguished clinical researchers," and professors at the Medical College of Georgia, are going on trial for committing fraud in conducting research for drug companies. The research includes studies for the FDA approval of numerous drugs that are now on the market. What's so interesting is not the accusations of fraud committed by investigators in the hire of drug companies. That's happened before. The FDA keeps a list of researchers who can no longer be used. What's critical is the degree to which many drug companies went along with these doctors—and continued to make use of their research results. Some drug companies used these doctors despite their obvious skewing of research, even complying with their seemingly blatant attempts to skim off research money for themselves.

According to the *Wall Street Journal*:

> Some drug companies acknowledge they complied with Dr. Borison's requests to send payments to companies he controlled or even to his house, instead of the medical college. The companies also didn't question the researchers' practice of obtaining approval from outside human-test review boards, including one 2,500 miles away, instead of the one across the street that the college says they were supposed to use.

The *Wall Street Journal* report makes clear that drug companies raised no concerns in the face of obviously suspicious behavior:

Prosecutors and medical-college officials are incredulous that none of the drug companies appeared to notice anything wrong. The companies, which are required to monitor clinical trials to ensure integrity of the data and patient safety, overlooked or ignored obvious signs that the two professors at the Medical College of Georgia here didn't follow proper procedures, investigators say.

Companies lavished bonuses on the doctors for recruiting so many patients so quickly—patients who sometimes didn't exist and didn't fit the criteria for the studies.

Indeed, the researchers were "showered" with research money from companies, including Novartis (Ciba), Eli Lilly, Glaxo Wellcome, Bristol-Myers Squibb, Zeneca, Sandoz, Smith-Kline Beecham, Johnson & Johnson, Abbott Laboratories, Hoechst, Warner-Lambert, and even Japan's Otsuka Pharmaceutical Company. Much of the money ended up in the personal accounts of the doctors who reported income of over $1 million a year.

Dr. Borison's behavior was so pro-drug company that he was criticized by the FDA for a study in which he claimed Thorazine was more effective than its generic equivalent, chlorpromazine. It turned out that the V.A. hospital in which he supposedly conducted the research did not have the generic equivalent in stock for the alleged experiment when the research was supposedly conducted. How could the study have been carried out without the drug being available? Furthermore, some of the supposed patients were not in the hospital at the time.

The chairman of the medical college institutional review board called about two dozen drug companies to tell them that the doctors had been charged with fraud and endangering patients. He was disturbed at how little the drug companies were concerned, especially about the welfare of the patients. From the perspective of the profit motive—getting the drugs approved—these doctors were in many ways ideal drug company researchers.

A January 9, 1998, brief report in the *Chronicle of Higher Education* states that Diamond has *pled* guilty and has promised to testify against Borison who has pleaded not guilty.

How Novartis Reacted to the Disclosures of Fraud

Some drug companies became suspicious of Borison and Diamond's research long before the two were indicted. The U.S. division of Solvay told the *Wall Street Journal* that the company stopped using the researchers' data in the early 1990s after realizing that the doctors weren't supervising the projects properly.[32] A Solvay spokeswoman said it was "incredulous" that some companies continued to work with the doctors and are still planning to use their data.

Novartis—the parent company of Ciba—has taken a different approach. According to the *Wall Street Journal*, Novartis continued to use Borison and Diamond until April—shortly before their indictments. Novartis states that it is auditing the research results but claims, "As far as we know, the protocols were carried out properly." Is that a reasonable assumption when the two men are under indictment for 172 criminal charges relating to their research? Shouldn't the drug company, at the least, show concern for the welfare of the patients who were involved in those studies? Shouldn't the company be concerned about the actual safety and efficacy of any drugs that came through their research with flying colors?

Meanwhile, the FDA is taking a different approach than Novartis. It has declared that it will eliminate all the data from the Borison-Diamond research.[33]

Rumblings within the Establishment

Leaders within the medical establishment have begun to raise serious issues about drug company control over scientific efforts in the field of pharmacology. Writing in May 2000 in the nation's most esteemed medical journal, *The New England Journal of Medicine*, Thomas Bodenheimer, M.D., questioned the "alliance" he found between the pharmaceutical industry and the clinical investigators who conduct drug trials. Dr. Bodenheimer described the growing trend for drug companies to hire commercial research outfits to produce research favorable toward their products. He documented how drug companies control the design of clinical trials, the gathering and analysis of the data from the trials, and the final spin that is placed on the research.

Dr. Bodenheimer found that drug companies attempt to control whether or not research results get published, and squelch papers that do not serve their economic interests. Ultimately, some drug companies provide secret authorship for papers that end up being published under the names of respected researchers. He warned that the pharmaceutical industry runs the risk of "potential public and physician skepticism about the results of clinical drug trials."

The "alliance" between the drug companies and clinical investigators, like the "partnership" between the drug companies and the American Psychiatric Association, corrupts research and results in the fraudulent development and marketing of drugs.

Ciba Targets the Child Market

Since Ciba admits that it doesn't know the long-term adverse effects of Ritalin on children, by condoning and encouraging the long-term administration of Ritalin, the company is participating in medical experimentation on millions of unwitting children and parents in America in the 1990s. Ciba, in fact, has been ahead of other drug companies in focusing on the child market. On the extremely meager basis of 46 children and adolescents in one controlled study lasting "up to 8 weeks," they managed to get FDA approval in 1991 to give the powerful antidepressant, Anafranil (clomipramine), for the treatment of obsessive compulsive disorder, to children age ten and older. As they point out, "It is unknown what, if any, effects long-term treatment with Anafranil may have on the growth and development of children."[34] Once again, Ciba experiments on America's children.

What the company itself admits to knowing in its label for Anafranil is frightening enough. It causes a variety of mental abnormalities, sometimes more easily detected in the larger adult studies, including somnolence (excessive sleeping) or insomnia, other sleep disorders, nervousness, memory impairment, anxiety, impaired concentration, depression, confusion, abnormal dreaming, agitation, depersonalization, and emotional lability. In children, it also can cause panic reactions and aggressive reactions. It can produce psychosis and mania. A variety of other symptoms were also caused, including tremor, dizziness, sweating, various gastrointestinal problems, fatigue, and weight gain. It's easy to see how a child on Anafranel could develop one ADHD-like adverse drug reaction, leading an unwitting physician to add Ritalin to the treatment regimen.

Some of Anafranil's adverse effects occurred in nearly one-quarter or more of their small sample of children, including somnolence (46%), tremor (33%), dizziness (41%), dry mouth (63%), constipation (22%), anorexia (22%), and fatigue (35%).

Ciba (1991) announced Anafranil to America's physicians with a glossy 28-page "guide to obsessive-compulsive disorder" entitled "OCD: When a habit isn't just a habit." Calling OCD "The Hidden Epidemic," it dismissed psychological causes and treatments, and speculated on biochemical causes as if they were scientifically based. One of their vignettes is about a 14-year-old girl. The back of the booklet provided a "'screening' quiz that you may want to give selected patients in your practice." A prepaid postcard enabled anyone to get additional free copies of the lengthy brochure.

CHADD—Parents United with Ciba

Nowadays Ciba has an ally that does extraordinarily effective, if devious, advertising and campaigning on its behalf. This partnership has led the International Narcotics Control Board and the Drug Enforcement Administration (DEA) to raise the possibility that the relationship might constitute the illegal promotion of an addictive drug. The ally—Ciba's best partner—is CHADD, an organization of parents whose leadership supports biological explanations and drugs for the problems that they have with their children.

Parents Who Pack a Drug Company Wallop

CHADD—Children and Adults with Attention Deficit Disorder—was formed in 1987 as a parent-based organization and quickly became a major player in mental health politics. Its leaders are parents who have strongly embraced ADHD diagnoses for their children and treat them with Ritalin or other drugs. CHADD now claims 30,000 members in 600 chapters nationwide. Revenues in 1995 and 1996 were approximately $2 million.

A substantial portion of CHADD's support comes from CibaGeneva Pharmaceuticals. The 1996 annual report also lists financial grants from four other major drug companies, Abbott, Glaxo Wellcome, Pfizer, and SmithKline Beecham.[35] The amounts are not specified.

The partnership between CHADD and the manufacturer of Ritalin is both ideological and financial. Many CHADD projects are underwritten by Ciba, including its national conventions. "Spreading the Message... Annual Highlights" on its website in June 1997 describes the organization's new Public Service Announcement (PSA) campaign "which was made possible through a grant from Ciba Pharmaceuticals." By June of 1995, they boast, their ad campaign reached 400 television stations, and resulted in 80,000 calls on their toll-free phone line. It would be impossible to exaggerate the value to a nonprofit organization in having a profit-making partner who is willing to commit money to publicize the organization. Ciba's support is undoubtedly the most important factor in CHADD's rapid growth in membership and power.

The information release also declares "CHADD Goes Bilingual" with its Fact Sheet series, and again gives "Thanks to a generous grant from Ciba Pharmaceuticals." In November 1995, CHADD held its first international conference which drew 2,300 attendees. It too was supported by Ciba.

Donations from Ciba to CHADD apparently began in 1989 with $170,000. According to CHADD's report to the IRS on Form 990 for tax exempt organizations, Ciba contributions peaked at $448,000 for the fiscal year ending June 30, 1995. In that year, additional contributions came from Abbott Laboratories ($79,500) and Burroughs Wellcome ($18,000) for a total of more than half a million dollars from drug companies in one year.

Probably as a result of the controversy, Ciba's contributions declined to $137,000 in 1996 and to $65,000 in 1997. Also, CHADD was already becoming well-established in good part due to Ciba's previous help. In addition, other drug companies began to contribute. For the year ending June 30, 1997, Richwood Pharmaceutical, the maker of the amphetamine Adderall, gave $118,000. Abbott Laboratories (Cylert) gave $27,000, SmithKline Beecham (Dexedrine) gave $2,500, Glaxo Wellcome (Wellbutrin) gave $3,500, Wyeth Ayerst (Effexor) gave $9,150, Pfizer (Zoloft) gave $5,000, and Alza (maker of a testosterone skin patch) gave $10,000. The sources of money reflect industry interest in marketing stimulants and antidepressants to the child market, and perhaps the hope for using skin patch technology.[36]

CHADD's Biological Ideology

A CHADD *Educators Manual* was written by Mary Fowler (1992) in collaboration with ADHD/Ritalin advocates such as Russell Barkley. The document is remarkable for its blatant description of how "ADD is not very hard to spot." In Fowler's view, the *complaining voice of an irritated adult* is apparently sufficient to suggest a diagnosis of ADHD for the offending child:

> Attention Deficit Disorder is a hidden disability. No physical marker exists to identify its presence, yet ADD is not very hard to spot. Just look with your eyes and listen with your ears when you walk through places where children are—particularly those places where children expected to behave in a quiet, orderly, and productive fashion. In such places, children with ADD will identify themselves quite readily. They will be doing or not doing something which frequently results in their receiving a barrage of comments and criticisms such as "Why don't you ever listen?" "Think before you act." "Pay attention."

CHADD takes the view that "ADD children" have a neurologically based disorder. They have promoted the term "neurobiological" that increasingly crops up in the media and the professional literature. They insist that ADHD exists independently of any environmental stressors or any difficulties that teachers or parents may have. Harvey Parker, a founder of CHADD, states that ADHD is one of "a number of disorders which we now consider neurobiological, and which were heretofore considered emotional or behavioral difficulties, and which we used to attribute to family or personal issues rather than having an organic basis."[37]

A CHADD (undated) brochure proclaims the blamelessness of parents in headlines: "Dealing with parental guilt. No, it's not all your fault." After claiming that ADHD is biological, the brochure argues:

> Frustrated, upset, and anxious parents do not cause their children to have ADD. On the contrary, ADD children usually cause their parents to be frustrated, upset, and anxious.

The child is always to blame for everything, while parents and teachers remain blameless.

CHADD (1993a) is fond of citing Zametkin's badly distorted PET scan study of ADHD adults that claims to show a biological component. CHADD incorrectly maintains that brain scan studies and other research "have convinced researchers that ADD is a neurobiological disorder and not caused by a chaotic home environment."[38]

CHADD commands enormous media attention on both a national and local level. As I went through newspaper after newspaper in writing this book, CHADD dominated the information flow about ADHD and Ritalin. Recently my wife, Ginger, and I stopped for lunch on a ride in the country-side and browsed through the local county newspaper. There was a lengthy letter from a local CHADD spokesperson saying that Ritalin should not be considered controversial and that the local school board should not waste its time investigating how many children are being medicated.[39] The CHADD chapter coordinator took a position that the FDA specifically rejects: "No prescription drugs are allowed in the market before they have passed scrutiny on the basic criteria of safety and effectiveness." Similar pro-Ritalin propaganda is churned out on a regular basis all over the country by national, state, and local CHADD representatives. The FDA, however, acknowledges that the brief, relatively small 4–6 week controlled trials cannot detect many potentially serious adverse effects.[40]

CHADD produces publications, lobbies in Washington with a loud voice, and holds large annual conventions. It works closely with leaders in biological psychiatry and in 1995 gave awards to Russell Barkley and Alan Zametkin. Barkley and Zametkin are both on the Professional Advisory Board of CHADD, along with many other leaders of the ADHD/Ritalin movement, including C. Keith Conners, Barbara D. Ingersoll, Judith Rapoport, and James Swanson. CHADD also has an ADHD "Hall of Fame" into which it has inducted several lifelong biological idealogues, including C. Keith Conners and Paul Wender in 1995 and James Swanson and Judith Rapoport in 1996.[41] Peter Jensen, the NIMH stiumlant advocate, is also a member.

CHADD has become a promotional and lobbying arm for biological child psychiatry and behavioral pediatrics. Honoring its leaders dovetails perfectly with its policies. As we shall demonstrate, it also became a covert political partner for Ciba.

Most dismaying, as we shall also document, the special education services of the U.S. Department of Education are heavily influenced by CHADD or by CHADD's ideological sympathizers.

No Kidding

One of CHADD's "Fact Sheets" (1993b) sports a cartoon strip by syndicated cartoonist Scott Stantis. In the first box, a doctor is telling two parents that their child's ADD is caused by a "chemical imbalance in the brain." In the second box the doctor explains that ADD is not caused by parents or teachers. In the third box, the parents say goodbye as they leave with their child. In the fourth and last box, as their tiny child looks up blankly at them, the parents raise their hands above their heads and shout in unison, "Yahoo! It's not our fault!!!."

When I first saw the cartoon, I thought it was an ironic criticism of simple-minded "biochemical imbalance" theories and a criticism of parents too eager to reject responsibility for their children. I was puzzled that CHADD wanted to print it.

I was wrong. The CHADD "Fact Sheet" explains that cartoonist Scott Stantis is "the parent of a child with ADD." CHADD's entire thrust is, in effect, "Don't blame us as parents and don't blame the teachers, either." Any existing conflict or stress in the school or family is seen as caused by the child's "disorder." Against all common sense, they take the position that in nearly all cases children make adults upset, not vice versa.

As "Suggested Reading For Children," CHADD recommends Quinn and Stern's book, *Putting On The Brakes*, which compares children to broken cars and shows them PET scans that supposedly show that they have abnormal brains.[42]

Not Guilt but Responsibility

It is not useful for parents to feel guilty. Guilt is a painful, self-defeating emotion that can paralyze us. It can overwhelm us, rendering us unable to change the behavior that contributes to our feelings of guilt. As a psychiatrist and therapist, I have seen compulsive guilt feelings drive parents to deny any responsibility for their children. In trying to ward off their anguished guilt, they make believe they have no responsibility at all.

Taking responsibility is very different from feeling guilty. When we take responsibility, we open our minds to every possibility—including our own contribution to our child's problems. We don't blindly or hatefully accuse ourselves. But as parents, we look closely at our own contribution to our child's well-being. We also critically examine the role of other people in our children's lives, including our spouse, extended family, siblings, neighborhood children and parents, babysitters, teachers, coaches, and anyone else who can have an impact on them.

If we begin instead with a conviction that our child has a biological disorder, we may temporarily stave off guilt—but we also give up responsibility. We sacrifice our perceptions of reality—and potentially our child's well-being—to feeling good about ourselves. Underneath, our guilt is likely to smolder. What's needed instead is a sense of how important we are to our children's well-being and a determination to work continually to improve ourselves as parents.

False Facts from CHADD about Ritalin

CHADD views Ritalin in such a positive light that its claims for the drug, if made by the manufacturer, would constitute unethical, illegal advertising. In a sheet entitled "Stimulant Medications,"[43] CHADD makes many points as if they are factual, including "Ritalin use is not followed by withdrawal when it is discontinued," "Ritalin does not lead to drug addiction," "Ritalin does not make a person a 'zombie'," "Ritalin does not appear to interfere with growth," and "Ritalin does not cause personality changes or psychosis." As documented in the first several chapters of this book, every one of these claims is false.

Why would a parent group tell falsehoods that make a drug look safer for children than it is? Why would these parents put the image of the drug above the welfare of their children? The motives must be complex, involving profound psychological issues about the attitudes of these parents toward their children. But CHADD also has political motivations for making claims for the drug that even Ciba itself couldn't legally claim. CHADD is supported by Ciba. The inflow of money apparently began around the same time, 1989, as these false facts were put together.

Pushing the DEA to Get Soft on Ritalin

In 1994, CHADD made a most extraordinary political move: It petitioned the DEA to drop Ritalin from Schedule II to Schedule III.[44] As described earlier in the book, in 1971 the federal government classified Ritalin in Schedule II where it joined drugs such as cocaine, opium and morphine.[45] Drugs in this category must have a "high potential for abuse" that can lead to "severe psychological or physical dependence." They may be used medically with severe restrictions, including stricter prescription requirements and pre-approved production quotas.

On October 11, 1994, attorneys for CHADD petitioned the Drug Enforcement Administration (DEA) to reclassify Ritalin from Schedule II to the less stringent Schedule III.[46] CHADD argued that Ritalin was safe and effective, and largely free of abuse and addiction. It declared, "Because MPH [Ritalin] is rapidly converted in the blood stream to an inactive agent, the effectiveness of MPH is restricted to the time in which the child is medicated. Thus, even with long-term usage, MPH does not have continuing effects which could lead to addiction."

This is an entirely false observation. Cocaine is probably more addictive than Ritalin or amphetamine precisely because it is even shorter acting. The more short-acting the stimulant, the more "punch" it has in creating euphoria and the more suffering it causes during abrupt withdrawal. Both the punch and the added anguish during withdrawal contribute to continued abuse.

It was very much in the interest of Ciba to lobby the DEA to lower Ritalin into Schedule III. It would remove the stigma of Ritalin as a highly controlled substance similar to cocaine and morphine. It would stop the requirement for physicians to write new prescription instead of refills. The drug company would escape from government supervision and control of its production quotas. Ciba would be able to manufacture as much of the drug as it wanted, regardless of the dangers of massive amounts being diverted for illegal use. Despite the benefits the petition would accrue to Ciba, CHADD never mentions that it has financial ties to the manufacturer in its carefully documented 22-page analysis.

Defying Science

As a highly addictive Schedule II drug, Ritalin's production quotas are determined by the Drug Enforcement Administration (DEA) of the U.S. Department of Justice. CHADD argued that production quotas were unnecessary because of Ritalin's safety. In defiance of scientific knowledge, CHADD (1994) wrote to the DEA:

> Strict control over dangerous and addictive substances is important and must be maintained. However, MPH [Ritalin] is not a dangerous and addictive substance, and in fact is a beneficial and relatively benign medication which assists millions of children daily.

This, of course, conflicts with three decades of widespread Ritalin abuse and addiction. It contrasts with the DEA's (1993) conclusions:

> Methylphenidate [Ritalin] is a central nervous system stimulant with a high potential for abuse and diversion for illegal purposes. DEA must determine the amount needed for legitimate medical and scientific needs while ensuring that an oversupply does not occur. These limits or quotas are set up to prevent the diversion of the drug for illegal purposes.

Success in forcing the DEA to change Ritalin from Schedule II to Schedule III would contradict the efforts and viewpoint of the International Narcotics Control Board which observes "Methylphenidate, due to its high abuse potential, was one of the first substances to be placed under international control in Schedule II of the 1971 Convention on Psychotropic Substances."[47]

"Attention: Ritalin Shortage"—Engineering a Crisis

On October 1, 1993, Arthur J. Emmett, Senior Vice President for Medical & Public Affairs of Ciba sent a "dear doctor" letter to America's physicians. The outside of the envelope sports a huge black banner in capital letters: "ATTENTION: RITALIN SHORTAGE." The opening line of the letter warns of impending disaster: "We regret to inform you that we anticipate that pharmacies will soon be experiencing shortages of Ritalin (methylphenidate USP)."

Ciba's letter blames the situation on a delay at the DEA in approving the production quota for the year. The company declares, "We recognize that this could be a difficult situation and regret any inconvenience to you and your patients." It gives an 800 number.[48]

It was a brilliant PR stroke by Ciba. The headline in the *New York Times* announced, "Blunder Limits Supply of Crucial Drug."[49] Coming out in the widely read Sunday edition, the article blossomed into a public relations dream for the manufacturer of Ritalin, CibaGeneva, as it portrays the desperation of parents who couldn't find the "crucial drug." It even describes ADHD as "a neurobiological problem that affects up to 3.5 million children in this country...."

According to the article, a clerical mistake at the DEA resulted in delayed approval for a production quota, resulting in "shortages." In fact, few if any parents couldn't obtain the drug; and the massive diversion of Ritalin into the black market rolled on.[50]

The *New York Times* article was also a media coup for Wade F. Horn, executive director of CHADD, who argued for relaxing controls on Ritalin and ridiculed the danger of Ritalin addiction. Claiming there was little or no evidence that Ritalin was being diverted into illegal markets and abused, he quipped: "I've heard of crack houses, but I haven't heard about any Ritalin houses." In fact, Ritalin is sold illegally throughout the country in the same black markets as cocaine.

CHADD also brought up the drug-company concocted shortage panic of 1993. It argued that the medication would become less expensive if it were not classified in Schedule II. In reality, the price of the drug is probably determined much more by what the market will bear than by any drug company costs which have long ago been outstripped by profits.

CHADD's petition, produced with considerable input of time and energy by a Washington D.C. law firm, is a most remarkable lobbying effort by a non-profit foundation. But was it really a non-profit effort? No, not when it takes money from Ciba.

Controversy Hits the Media

On October 20, 1995, The Merrow Report aired on PBS with a story "ADD: A Dubious Diagnosis?" The show, on which I appeared as one of the experts, raises many issues about CHADD and Ciba. Although I pointed out the issue in earlier publications, including *Toxic Psychiatry* (1991), this was the first time that CHADD's drug company funding became a media scandal. John Merrow, the creator of the program, criticized CHADD for not telling the DEA that it is funded by Ciba, even while it's taking actions consistent with being a Ciba lobby group. The show questioned why CHADD's publications, paid for by Ciba, don't mention the drug's addictiveness.[51]

The DEA was not the only agency that felt deceived by CHADD The American Academy of Neurology, which cosigned CHADD's petition to the DEA, withdrew its support after learning of the drug company ties. The Department of Education also found out through the Merrow Report that CHADD was funded by the drug company. As a result, the department pulled a $100,000 ADHD/Ritalin video that CHADD produced for it. Unfortunately, the video was already being distributed to educators.[52]

CHADD (1995a) defended taking funds from Ciba:

CH.A.D.D would not be able to conduct important educational activities without such support. CH.A.D.D used these grants for educational projects such as creating and distributing a television and radio public service announcement (PSA); translating our fact sheet series into Spanish; and operating a toll-free information line.

In psychiatry, advertising campaigns are always called "educational activities." That's why it's so important to remember that drugs are products that are marketed by drug companies and by organized psychiatry.

CHADD further denied that funding by Ciba influences any of its policies or pronouncements concerning medication, or that Ciba encourages CHADD to pursue policies advantageous to the company. Yet nothing could have been more advantageous to Ciba than to have a parent-based "consumer" group minimize Ritalin's addictiveness while petitioning the DEA to loosen its controls over the drug.

Are CHADD And Ciba Breaking International Law?

The International Narcotics Control Board, an affiliate of the United Nations World Health Organization, has shown concern about CHADD's promotion of Ritalin, its attempt to pressure the DEA into easing up controls over the drug, and its association with CibaGeneva. In its 1995 report, the board wrote:

The competent authorities of the United States have informed the board of their concern at the sharp increase in the use of methylphenidate, especially the preparation sold under the trade name Ritalin. Treatment of ADD with Ritalin is being actively promoted by an influential "parent association" that has received significant financial contributions from the leading manufacturer of the preparation in the United States.

In its 1996 report, the board repeated its concern about "questionable promotional activities for methylphenidate."[53]

On June 27, 1995, the international board wrote to the United States government about its concern over America's mounting production and use of Ritalin.[54] The board also voiced concern about drug promotion efforts of parent organizations, especially the danger of encouraging "an indiscriminate use of methylphenidate." The International Narcotics Control Board then raised an ominous question about the funding of parent groups by drug companies, suggesting that this might be in violation of international law:

Finally, the board is concerned about reports, not yet confirmed, that some kind of financial transfer has taken place between pharmaceutical companies and one/some of the non-governmental organizations/parent associations active in the field of promoting methylphenidate use for ADD.... [A]ny financial transfer from a pharmaceutical company with the purpose to promote sales of an internationally controlled substance could be identified as a hidden advertisement for the substance. As such activities are in contradiction with the provisions of the 1971 Convention (Article 10, para 2), I would be very grateful if you could investigate this matter and inform the board about the outcome of this inquiry as soon as possible.

The Drug Enforcement Administration (1995c) stated, "it came to the attention of DEA that Ciba-Geigy, the manufacturer of Ritalin products, has contributed $748,000 to CHADD" as of 1994. The DEA acknowledged the INCB's concerns that CHADD's financial connections to Ciba "may be contrary to international treaty obligations." But the DEA said it would not take this accusation into account when evaluating CHADD's petition about Ritalin. However, the DEA warned CHADD "it is possible that this information may, at a later date, be evaluated to determine if such contributions have unduly influenced or compromised the petitioner's data."[55]

It seems unlikely to me in the present pro-drug and pro-drug company political climate that the DEA will carry out its threat and investigate CHADD.

CHADD Defends Itself

On February 28, 1996, CHADD responded to the International Narcotics Control Board with a letter from its national president, Mary McDonald Richard. It denies that CHADD "promotes the use of methylphenidate," stating that it advocates a broad approach including "medication only when indicated and prescribed by a physician." It rejects the idea that Ritalin is over-used or dangerous: "When used under the supervision and direction of a physician, methylphenidate is a safe and effective medication."

Apparently retreating before adverse publicity, in March 1996 CHADD withdrew its petition to the DEA to transfer Ritalin from Schedule II to Schedule III. The International Narcotics Review Board of the United Nations (1996b) applauded: "Attempts to ease control of methylphenidate and to proliferate its uncritical use have been successfully thwarted."[56]

NAMI: More Parents United to Control Their Children

CHADD has followed the model of its adult counterpart, called NAMI. This politically powerful organization boasts a national membership of

140,000. NAMI, the National Alliance for the Mentally Ill, is a parent group that was formed in 1979. Local chapters use the acronym AMI, as in CAMI, the California Alliance for the Mentally Ill.

Another Partnership with the Drug Companies

NAMI, like CHADD, is supported by drug company money.[57] Eli Lilly, the maker of Prozac, recently pointed out that "With a network of 71 local affiliates, 14,000 members and 150 legislative key contacts, CAMI is a presence in California legislative activity."[58] Eager to participate in this legislative process, Lilly gave CAMI a grant to purchase 160 fax machines: "The machines will ensure rapid dissemination of vital patient information in addition to federal and state legislative alerts." Once again, a major drug company finds that a parent group can act as its publicist. Like CAMI, Lilly benefits from the concept of "mental illness" as a "brain disorder" treatable with drugs. Lilly praises CAMI's success in getting articles placed in newspapers, "placing experts on talk shows," and "a barrage of posters and brochures [that] was aimed directly at supermarkets, pharmacies and other public facilities."

Who Are the NAMI Leaders?

NAMI parents usually have adult offspring who are severely emotionally disabled. Their leadership tends to promote biochemical and genetic explanations, drugs, electroshock, psychosurgery, and involuntary treatment. NAMI also tries to suppress dissenting views by harassing professionals who disagree with them.[59] Now NAMI has developed an affiliate, NAMI-CAN—the National Alliance for the Mentally Ill; Child and Adolescent Network.[60]

Your Child Has BBBD

NAMI-CAN, like CHADD and the drug companies, believes in BBBD—biologically based brain diseases. According to Carol Howe, a founder of NAMI-CAN, her motivation began when her son was diagnosed at the age of seven with schizophrenia. Her stated goal as a founder was to prove that her child, and children like him, have brain diseases. This would absolve her of any personal responsibility for his condition. NAMI-CAN organized to become "hard hitting advocates" to fight against "the denial by professionals, and therefore the general public, that biological brain disorders could afflict children."

In other words, the purpose of the organization was to promote a specific biopsychiatric viewpoint that exonerates parents for any role in causing the suffering of their children. The agenda was not aimed exclusively at children with severe diagnoses, such as schizophrenia. It quickly came to include all children with psychiatric diagnoses, including depression, anxiety, and ADHD.[61] Any child with one of these diagnoses, according to Howe and to NAMI-CAN, has a "brain disorder" or a "neurobiological disorder" with "demonstrable brain malfunctions." Howe is quite specific:

> NAMI and NAMI-CAN focus their advocacy specifically on children with brain disorders that are long lasting, and, unless successfully treated, are disabling.

Remember, they are not talking about high blood pressure, diabetes, cerebral palsy, leukemia or some other known medical disorder with known medical consequences. They are talking about upset children and children in conflict with their parents and schools—children diagnosed with "depression," "anxiety disorders," and "attention-deficit hyperactivity disorder."

A local southern California AMI, in collaboration with a local government mental health agency, published a booklet that illustrates the NAMI theme of "we are not responsible."[62] The first page of their booklet quotes biopsychiatrist Nancy Andreasen's book, *The Broken Brain*: "People who suffer from mental illness suffer from a sick or broken brain, not from weak will, laziness, bad character or bad upbringing." The back cover contains the clever motto, "*no fault* brain illnesses."

Whose fault is the California AMI group talking about? Clearly, the parents, teachers, and other adults in the child's life are enabled to feel that they play no role in the development of the child's difficulties. The child may also feel exonerated of personal responsibility but at what cost? The cost to the child is a diagnosis that says "brain disease."

NAMI's ideology seems to come down to this: The existence of a psychiatric label is proof the child suffers from a chronic, potentially disabling brain disease for which parents and other adults have no responsibility. It is a claim biopsychiatry has often hinted at making, but seldom dared to fully embrace in public. The claim vastly empowers both psychiatrists and parents, while relegating the child to the status of a broken machine—but it still has no scientific basis whatsoever.

In her insightful analysis of NAMI-CAN, Louise Armstrong (1993) points out that the average member may have little idea about or identification with the authoritarian ideology of its leadership:

> Those mothers I met in my travels who were NAMI-CAN members did not appear to have much in the way of information in the broader poli-

tics or alliances of the leadership, or in NAMI's role as participant in what Peter Breggin has called the "psychopharmaceutical combine."[63]

Controversy over NAMI's Stance

The going wasn't initially trouble-free for NAMI-CAN. According to founder Carol Howe (1994), they met opposition from state and local governments, including the head of the federal government's Child and Adolescent Service System Program. He wrote to the head of NAMI to warn that "never have children's issues fared well in adult-centered organizations, and nothing that has been said or printed has convinced me that an experience with NAMI will be any different."

Despite this kind of opposition, by 1994 NAMI-CAN had developed over 100 groups. Parent groups like NAMI-CAN and CHADD have now learned power politics to the degree that they dominate the field of child mental health.

Forcing Grown Children to Take Drugs:
Parent Groups and Drug Companies United

Parent groups, drug companies, and biological psychiatry commonly work together toward their common ends. All are served, for example, if patients can be forced to take drugs against their will. The drug companies, of course, are given an involuntary consumer. Psychiatrists find their jobs made easier when they can make their patients take toxic agents to subdue their behavior. NAMI-CAN leaders also favor involuntary medication; it gives them more control over their offspring.

In recent years, some civil rights inroads have been made on behalf of patient rights, but they are being eroded by this combination of drug companies, organized psychiatry, and the parent groups. In California a court decision has expanded the right to refuse treatment with psychiatric drugs. According to journalist Vince Bielski (1990):

> A year after the informed-consent law took effect in California hospitals, the combined might of the California Psychiatric Association, an organization called the California Alliance for the Mentally Ill and a few Sacramento legislators—with the financial backing of the nation's major pharmaceutical companies—has come very close to overturning the landmark patient's rights decision in the Legislature.

Bielski describes contributions made by several drug companies, including Ciba, to legislators leading the campaign to overturn the patient rights law. The most powerful lobbyist, according to Bielski, was the California Alliance for the Mentally Ill (CAMI) which was itself being funded by pharmaceutical companies.

Future Disclosures

The material in this chapter was developed without the opportunity to examine in-house, secret pharmaceutical company data concerning the development and marketing of stimulant drugs. As a result of the burgeoning class action suits, these secret documents may soon be made available to attorneys and to medical experts, and someday to the public. As a medical expert in product liability suits against the manufacturers of other classes of drugs, such as tranquilizers, antipsychotic drugs, and antidepressants, I have had the opportunity to look in detail at otherwise secret documents contained within the walls of pharmaceutical companies. I routinely discover an enormous amount of deception and manipulation. I have written about these findings in the greatest detail in regard to Eli Lilly & Co., the maker of Prozac. In books such as *Talking Back to Prozac* (1994), *Brain-Disabling Treatments in Psychiatry* (1997), and the forthcoming *Antidepressant Fact Book*, I have documented the egregious but usually successful efforts by Eli Lilly & Co. to hide the dangers of Prozac from the profession and the public.

The new product liability lawsuits against Novartis are described in chapter 1. The civil suits charge the company with fraud and conspiracy in the development and marketing of Ritalin and the over-promotion of ADHD as a disorder. CHADD and the American Psychiatric Association are named as co-conspirators. When given the go-ahead by the courts, the suits should provide attorneys and medical experts with the opportunity to delve into the internal workings of Novartis. The results should be enlightening.

We turn now to the role of several federal agencies, closely tied with NAMI and CHADD, who join the drug companies in pushing Ritalin and other drugs on America's children.

Chapter 15

WHO'S BEHIND ALL THIS?

Part II: The Taxpayers' Money

School personnel need to recognize that hyperactive behaviors in the classroom can be dealt with by using educational strategies rather than medical intervention.... Teachers and parents who neglect available educational approaches and suggest or readily agree to drug therapy may be abrogating their professional or personal responsibility to the child.

—Saul Axelrod and Sandra L. Bailey,
Exceptional Children (1979)

Scientific research tells us ADD is a biologically-based disorder that includes distractibility, impulsiveness, and sometimes hyperactivity. While the causes of ADD are not fully understood, recent research suggests that ADD can be inherited and may be due to an imbalance of neurotransmitters—chemicals used by the brain to control behavior—or abnormal glucose metabolism in the central nervous system.

—U. S. Department of Education,
Attention Deficit Disorder: Beyond The Myths (undated)

Parents in Pittsburgh have filed suit against a school district and a psychiatric facility for subjecting their elementary school children to ADHD research without informing the parents or asking their permission. The study, called the Pittsburgh School Wide Intervention Model or P-SWIM, involved 1,500 children over a decade.

The lawsuit alleges that a research questionnaire asked 5–10 year old children if they tortured animals or forced sex on anyone. The parents report that the research upset their young children so much that it caused bedwetting and nightmares. The attorney for the parents said that research data on the children was gathered from several sources, including the questionnaires, interviews with the children, and observations in the classroom and at recess.

Associated Press reporter Jeffrey Blair (1997) quoted an outraged parent, "These children were being labeled. It is disheartening to find out that a child can be subjected to a [test] without a parent's consent."

The research was overseen by William Pelham, Jr., a psychologist who was associated with the University of Pittsburgh's Western Psychiatric Institute and Clinic. Pelham now works at the State University of New York at Buffalo. Among ADHD researchers, Pelham leads the pack in getting federal funding. As we describe in *The War Against Children of Color*, Pelham is the recipient of at least three drug-related NIMH grants totalling more than $700,000 per year.

In hearings about the controversial Pittsburgh program, Pelham testified that he had given workshops in nearly 100 school districts in three states. What did he say to the teachers and school officials about managing behavior? In an editorial in the *School Psychology Review*, Pelham (1993) makes a stirring call for training school psychologists in how to identify young pupils who may need psychiatric medication. In his workshops in the nearly 100 school districts, he almost certainly was pushing the ADHD/Ritalin viewpoint that he espouses in his publications.

What has happened that our schools can be used for psychiatric research on children seemingly without the permission of parents? How can an extreme advocate of psychiatric drugs be invited into so many school districts to give workshops on the management of behavioral problems in children? How long has the government been committed to funding Ritalin advocates like Pelham? Which federal agencies are involved?

The previous chapter described how the American Psychiatric Association, CibaGeneva Pharmaceuticals, and CHADD go about selling ADHD and Ritalin. We now examine the role of three federal agencies: the U.S. Department of Education (DOE), the National Institute of Mental Health (NIMH), and the Food and Drug Administration (FDA).

Schools Push the Fourth "R"

Teachers, much like parents, are under enormous pressure to find shortcuts for handling their more difficult children. A recent critical analysis of American education found that many teachers feel "overworked, underpaid, under appreciated—and poorly prepared."[1] Too often they are left hanging on an educational limb as they try to teach rebellious students with outdated curriculums in over-crowded classrooms.

Meanwhile, the educational establishment propagandizes teachers to turn to Ritalin as a solution to management problems with difficult students. Teachers, again like parents, need support in their efforts to teach America's children without resorting to drugs. They cannot on their own reverse the tide of the entire society toward the quick cures that are being sold by the Psychopharmaceutical Complex.

Writing more than two decades ago, Edward Levin and his colleagues (1977) seem to be describing contemporary schools when they cite data that 96% of teachers think they can "recognize" a hyperactive child, and that 70–80% would inform parents, the school principal, or specialists about the problem. Many teachers already felt confident about referring parents for Ritalin. Levin's group commented:

> It is very likely that there are teachers who set standards of comportment that are too rigid for their students... It is seldom, if ever, the case that a teacher complains of a child being hypoactive.

Nowadays, schools not only recommend medication to parents, school nurses or office personnel then dispense the drug at noon to make sure that the children get their dose before the start of the afternoon classes. The Drug Enforcement Administration has warned that "Many schools have more methylphenidate stored on a routine basis than most pharmacies have in stock."[2] The International Narcotics Control Board (1996b) reports that 20% or more of children are taking stimulants in some American schools.

It is no exaggeration to say that teachers are being heavily propagandized to believe in ADHD. In a sample of 147 elementary and middle school teachers from a suburban district, "over 85% of the teachers indicated they had attended at least one workshop regarding ADHD."[3] Almost without exception, such workshops will be presented by professional advocates of ADHD/Ritalin. They will convince the teachers that medication is far more effective and appropriate than improved teaching strategies in dealing with children who seem inattentive, restless, bored, distractible, or fidgety in class.

School guidance counselors are also instructed in how to identify possible ADHD children. Their goal is to "direct and advise the parents" toward further evaluation, and to resources such as CHADD and its biologically oriented network of professionals. Despite their psychological and social traditions, counselors are now being instructed to inform parents "that ADHD is a physiological problem."[4]

When teaching in a masters level counseling program in the education department at Johns Hopkins University, I saw firsthand that young students and professionals are eager to understand the needs of their children and to meet them. They believe in the basic principles of counseling—to empower the child's natural abilities rather than to focus on the child's problems or limitations. But what are they being taught in most classrooms and in the standard journals?

Writing in *Elementary School Guidance & Counseling*,[5] three educational psychologists declare that *almost* anything can cause ADHD-like symptoms—including brain damage, malnutrition, and food additives. They don't mention boring, overcrowded classrooms and inadequate teaching. What do they recommend? Medications and behavior modification techniques. What don't they recommend? Improved teaching.

The "R" They Left Behind

While pushing Ritalin, our schools have fallen behind with the most important "R" of all. A recent expose in the *Baltimore Sun* declared, "Millions of children aren't learning to read properly during the crucial early grades of school—not because they can't but because their schools aren't teaching them how."[6] According to an NIH study, 40% of all school children are poor readers and half of these have severe problems. In Baltimore, 89% of students rated below satisfactory. The key to rectifying the disaster, NIH reports, is "intensive training in sounds of the language and sound-letter relations, while exposing students to stories that engage their interest." In other words, good teaching. Poor teacher training was identified as the root of the problem.

America's educational establishment, including the U.S. Department of Education, has fallen down on the job, virtually abandoning its responsibility to our children. In poorly taught classrooms, frustrated children have trouble "behaving" and "concentrating." Fertile ground for the "4th R."

The U.S. Department of Education: Teaching Teachers to Diagnose

How have the schools—teachers and counselors alike—become so involved in pushing drugs instead of improved education? Part of the answer lies in the U.S. Department of Education (DOE).[7] A recent news feature aptly declares:[8]

> The U.S. Department of Education promotes the [ADHD/Ritalin] trend by distributing brochures about attention disorders and how to treat them. It publishes a directory of support groups, doctors who specialize in the field, and where to get information on treating it with drugs.

The DOE funds a series of ADD Centers at major universities aimed at proving the usefulness of the ADHD diagnosis and Ritalin. The series of Executive Summaries[9] written by these centers fails to consider the single most important issue of all—potential adverse drug effects from the long-term treatment of millions of children.

Despite the many warnings about the dangers of using the medical model in educational settings,[10] a recent DOE publication, *Attention Deficit Disorder: Beyond The Myths*, calls it a "fact" that ADHD is biologically based, genetic, and probably caused by a biochemical imbalance. The government pamphlet also states that "scientists" "have ruled out most of the factors controlled by parents."

The DOE also publishes *Attention Deficit Disorder: What Teachers Should Know*[11] which urges teachers to become the frontline for psychiatric diagnosing. It begins with a direct instruction: "The child who repeatedly disrupts your class and who seldom completes assignments may not be deliberately troublesome, but could be showing signs of Attention Deficit Disorder (ADD)." The pamphlet then informs teachers about "Identifying ADD in Your Students."

The DOE document even encourages teachers to make the provisional diagnosis: "While teachers are not required to make the final diagnosis of ADD, you can help these children by recommending that a child who frequently demonstrates these behaviors be checked for ADD or other learning problems." After noting that 60–90 percent of children with ADD are treated with medication, the DOE seems to suggest that legality is all that stands in the way of teachers recommending medication: "Due to legal issues, a teacher should not recommend medication; however, you may suggest the parent take the child to a doctor for examination." Given such encouragement from the federal agency, it is no wonder that many teachers readily recommend that parents take their children for evaluations for ADHD and Ritalin.

The DOE also describes the "team" that so many parents have found themselves confronting: "the administration will call a conference with a team of parents, teachers, administrators, health care professionals, school psychologists, and other specialists."

The U. S. Department of Education also promotes the ADHD/Ritalin viewpoint by funding organizations like the National Information Center for Children and Youth with Disabilities (NICHCY).[12] Using language developed by CHADD and Ciba, NICHCY's 1997 Fact Sheet on ADHD calls it a "neurobiologically based disorder." It states that "Scientific evidence suggests that AD/HD is genetically transmitted and in many cases results from a chemical imbalance or deficiency in certain neurotransmitters, which are chemicals that help the brain regulate behavior." The few resources cited include CHADD and its publications.

NICHCY's 1997 web site publishes a lengthy "NICHCY Brief Paper" by Mary Fowler (1994), former Vice-President of Government Affairs for CHADD, and a lobbyist for ADHD/Ritalin. The author thanks her DOE project officer "for her time in reading and reviewing this document...."

Teaching Classroom Techniques 101

In *Attention Deficit Disorder: Beyond the Myths* (undated) the U. S. Department of Education makes a variety of common sense suggestions for how to teach children diagnosed with ADHD. The suggestions include such simple concepts as "maintaining eye contact with students; using gestures to emphasize points; and providing a work area away from distractions." Our final chapters will review many of these basic principles for parents and teachers to implement. Meanwhile, we should ask, "Why should these suggestions be limited to children identified as having problems? Why shouldn't they be a part of any normal classroom? Aren't these suggestions part of the ABC's of adequate teaching for any child in any class?"

Many teachers and educators are appalled that the DOE feels it necessary to approach teachers with such a low level of expectations concerning their teaching and classroom management skills.[13] Only a deeply flawed educational system would need the DOE to provide these simple instructions to the nation's teachers.

Children labeled ADHD do not differ from other children in what they need. If a child doesn't focus in class, it means that the child doesn't have a relationship to the teacher that fulfills the child's educational needs. Think about that: If the teacher were empowered to grab this child's imagination, the child would pay attention. Thus, even overcoming inattention and impulsivity in the classroom is a matter of creating a relationship—in this case, an educational relationship.

Creating positive educational relationships is of course much harder to do with some children than with others. That's the challenge of teaching, not an excuse for diagnosing and drugging a child. But even the best teachers can find it difficult to perform adequately in many of today's schools.

Even the PTA

Even the national PTA has joined the propaganda campaign. In 1996 its journal published an article on ADHD jointly authored by Ellen Schiller of the U.S. Department of Education,[14] Peter Jensen from NIMH, and James Swanson who runs the federally-funded ADHD center at the University of California, Irvine. They repeat the ADHD/Ritalin message:

> Once parents and teachers ... recognize that children with ADD are not lazy or "bad," but have a biological disorder, they can stop blaming themselves or their children and take appropriate steps to prevent a pattern of failure.

Sneaking in ADHD As an Official Disability

During the debate over federal legislation for the handicapped,[15] Congress was heavily lobbied to include ADHD as a disability that would entitle these children to special educational services provided through the schools. The ADHD/Ritalin advocacy bloc seemingly lost this round when the bill was passed without the inclusion of ADHD. However, on September 16, 1991 the Department of Education signed a special memorandum setting guidelines for how children diagnosed ADHD could be made eligible for services under "other health impaired."[16] As a result, school districts can get approximately $420 per child per year for ADHD children under the health impaired category. The children may get little more than the services of a nurse or clerk handing out a dose of Ritalin while the money goes into a general fund for special education.[17] This adds additional pressure to label children ADHD in order to bring in general purpose funds.

In addition, the Office of Special Education Programs (OSEP) began to fund special centers for the study of ADHD and for disseminating information to educators, researchers, and parents concerned with "the needs of children with ADD."[18]

Thus, the ADHD/Ritalin lobby, as a result of concerted political efforts, has embedded itself in the federal educational bureaucracy.

Portrait of a School District—and One Lone Reformer

Chappell Dew (1997) was an elected member of the Horry County Board of Education, District One, in the Myrtle Beach area of South Carolina with almost 19,000 students enrolled in kindergarten through 8th grade. He became very concerned about the amount of medicating with Ritalin that was taking place through the schools. He began to demand facts and figures[19] and to go to the press with his data.[20] Based on the figures provided by the school district to the board, Dew made some additional calculations from which the following data are drawn. In the 1996–1997 school year, almost 3% of the boys were already receiving Ritalin in kindergarten. The percentage peaked in the 4th grade with 10.2% of the boys and 2.5% of the girls getting Ritalin handed to them in school.

This data did not include children who received Ritalin-SR, a sustained release Ritalin tablet that can be given at home to last throughout the school day. It also did not include another 50 students who were recorded as receiving medication but who were not identified by grade level in the raw data. It also excluded children taking other stimulants, as well as a presumably small number of children who receive only a single dose before or after school.

The figures show a slight decline in usage in 1996–1997 which may have been brought about in part by Dew's efforts to publicize the problem. He believes it may also have been caused by increased prescription of Ritalin-SR tablets that are given once in the morning before school.

In the Horry County School District, 28% of the children are identified as African-American. Only 24% of the children receiving Ritalin at school are black, a figure that conforms to other research and to my general impression that comparatively fewer black children take Ritalin.[21] However, Dew came up with a disturbing observation which he communicated to me and to my wife, Ginger, who is Executive Director of the Center for the Study of Psychiatry and Psychology. Dew wrote to us: "I am somewhat frightened by the fact that in Horry County, 24% of the students prescribed Ritalin are Black yet 54% of students receiving Ritalin two times per day [in school] are Black. Perhaps we are trying to subdue their 'violence' as you postulated in *The War Against Children*."[22]

With increased reliance on long-acting stimulant preparations such as Concerta increasing numbers of children will recieve their medication at home and remain uncounted in school surveys.

Teachers Chastised

As a result of Chappell Dew's work, the school district sent a memo to all elementary school principals about an addition to the Teacher Handbook:[23]

> Under no circumstances should a teacher EVER recommend or suggest Ritalin or any other form of medication.

In a follow up administrative directive to all elementary school principals, superintendent of schools Gerrita Postlewait (1997) ordered teachers to stop recommending or referring students for Ritalin. She sternly warned:

> According to some parents, we still have teachers who are suggesting to individual parents that they take their children to a physician to see if they can "get him on Ritalin...." As I'm sure you are aware, use of the drug Ritalin is an extremely controversial topic, both nationally and locally. Elementary principals, especially, need to strongly remind school personnel that we never suggest to parents that they obtain medication for a child.

One Against the Many

Chappell Dew's efforts illustrate the healthy impact that one individual can have in his own community in terms of publicizing the Ritalin epidemic. He is neither a professional educator nor a health worker but owns a large hardware store in North Myrtle Beach where he is a community leader.

Unfortunately, CHADD and NAMI have cultivated or placed untold numbers of individuals strategically in most communities of any size in the country. They are situated on the boards of schools and mental health clinics, as well as in the media. They include many individual health professionals.

Dew's own county has a local psychiatrist who estimates that 5–10% of children have ADHD. Several pediatricians also promote Ritalin in his county and an active local CHADD group meets in several of the elementary schools. In addition, the state Department of Education gives free seminars in support of the ADHD/Ritalin viewpoint. Even though Chappell Dew was responsible for alerting the media, nearly all the coverage went to the ADHD/Ritalin community.[24]

It is a sad commentary on contemporary social values that leaders like Chappell Dew are in the distinct minority and that they face overwhelmingly powerful lobbying groups with unlimited access to the media.

Economic and Academic Advantages to the Diagnosis

While Ritalin cannot improve a child's academic achievements, the diagnosis of ADHD can lead to improved test results. How? Journalist Trish Ready (1997) from Washington State remarks:

> If a student is diagnosed with ADD, they can take standard entrance exam tests untimed; that would include GEDs, SATs, LSATs, MCATs…you name it. Some claim that wealthy white parents are trying to buy their kids a better chance for the college of their choice.

Ready also zeroes in on how schools take advantage of the diagnosis:

> Schools also benefit from kids being diagnosed with ADD as a learning disability. The federal government gives schools approximately $420 per ADD kid; state funds are also available for learning-disabled students. At a time when school budgets are being slashed to the bone, disabilities are valuable for school funding.

The amount of $420 is not a lot per child per year but it does go into a common pool where it can be used in a discretionary fashion for children with handicaps.

Yet another advantage accrues to individual teachers. Ready quotes psychology professor Keith Hoeller:

> Teachers and parents have been given tools for social control. They have set up a system whereby, when teachers have problems with kids, kids have a learning disability. The teachers send kids to counselors and then psychologists.

Psychologist Gerald Coles, author of *The Learning Mystique: A Critical Look at Learning Disabilities*, observed that the diagnosis reached "epic proportions" because it is consistent "with an explanation of school failure that finds fault with the child and protects the institution."[25]

Teachers and parents are likely to mistake obedience for academic improvement when children are subdued and "behave better" in school and at home. Children who "sit down and shut up" may mistakenly seem to do better in their studies even though their learning ability has been impaired.[26] Compliance should not be mistaken for academic improvement.

ADHD Fraud and Social Security

Social Security has recently begun to include ADHD as a disability.[27] One result has been the increased diagnosing and drugging of children from poor families who desperately need the $400–$600 per month to live on.[28] Philadelphia officials are investigating unscrupulous mental health clinics and professionals who encourage the process in order to collect fees for services such as diagnosing and medicating children.

Eileen DeFranco, a middle school nurse in Philadelphia, calls this diagnosing children for profit "pure unadulterated child abuse." "It's sad," she said, "that we have to be advocates for kids against their parents and doctors." An Ohio school counselor recently told me about parents who coach their children on how to "fail" ADHD testing in order to qualify for Social Security disability payments.

With one in four children living in poverty,[29] many parents can easily fall prey to doctors who encourage them to increase the family income through disability checks for their "ADHD child." No one will be too surprised that small "store front" clinics might rip off Social Security even at the cost of abusing children. But this is minor stuff compared to the big rip off—the ADHD/Ritalin lobby and its institutionalized abuse of children.

The inclusion of ADHD as a disability under Social Security has helped to motivate successful lobbying efforts by parent groups, such as CHADD, to make ADHD into a respectable diagnosis. Parents or guardians are not required to use the money for therapeutic or medical purposes. They can spend it in any way as long as it benefits the child. The rules have been interpreted to allow the purchase of a TV, video game, or automobile.[30]

These observations should not be used to undermine the already weakened safety net for children in this country. We don't do enough for children in regard to such basic needs as health care and educational opportunities. Instead, I favor making disability determinations based on legitimate illnesses, not diagnoses with no merit such as ADHD.

What's Happening to Our Teachers and Our Schools?

Most parents reading this book will have immediate concerns about what to do when their children are diagnosed ADHD as a result of difficulties in school. I will address these problems in the series of chapters on empowering oneself as a parent and dealing with teachers and schools. But there is a broader problem that all of us should face. We need to know, "What in the world has gone wrong in our schools that so many of our teachers cannot adequately teach so many of their students without drugging them?" Teachers may also want to look more deeply at these issues, perhaps to be inspired to take some action.

The Department of Education pamphlet, *Attention Deficit Disorder: What Teachers Should Know*, concludes its recommendations by stating, "Recent research suggests that providing more stimulation and variety can improve the performance and behavior of students with ADD." Do students have to be labeled ADD before they can be provided with stimulation and variety in their education? Right now the answer is often "Yes."

Numbing the Minds of Teachers

A recent *Time* story by Steve Wulf confirms the size of the problem in the educational system:

> Six hundred experienced teachers surveyed in 1995 were brutal about the education they had received, describing it as "mind numbing," the "shabbiest psycho-babble," and "an abject waste of time." They complained that fragmented, superficial course work had little relevance to classroom realities. And judging by the weak skills of student teachers entering their schools, they observed, the preparation was still woefully inadequate.

Wulf points out that behavior and classroom management is not taught on a hands-on classroom basis in most teacher's colleges. Instead it's presented in large lectures in the first or second year. This leaves little likelihood that students will be able to recall or to make practical use of the information at a later date amid the stresses of everyday teaching.

Teacher remediation, rather than student medication, would go a long way to solving the problem of ADHD. The motto should be, "Educate, don't medicate." As Wulf confirms, there is widespread recognition of the need for reform in teacher education. But it is likely to be held back by the ready availability of drugs as an alternative solution to problems in the classroom.

Cookie-Cutter Schools

Ken Livingston (1997) raises the question of why so many teachers have become so enthusiastic about ADHD and Ritalin. With the end of corporal punishment in most school systems, one explanation is "Drugs have replaced the reprimand." Livingston then goes on to suggest that the problem lies more deeply in the failure of schools to meet the individualized needs of children:

> But it seems to me that the real problem may be that the concept of compulsory, cookie-cutter education needs rethinking. In spite of the rhetoric in schools of education about the importance of taking into account the individual needs of children in a classroom, the current system of public education is designed to make that nearly impossible.

Commenting on current-day America, Livingston reminds us that "when it is difficult or inconvenient to change the environment, we don't think twice about changing the brain of the person who has to live in it."

Overcoming the Real Attention Deficit

Even before the ADHD/Ritalin movement, there were repeated calls for the reform of the nation's schools. When I was a full-time consultant in mental health and education at the National Institute of Mental Health in 1967–8, a "crisis in education" was widely recognized and discussed.

Instead of reform, the schools became more bureaucratic and unwieldy. Meanwhile, educators and commissions continued to confirm the escalating failure. In 1990, for example, the Carnegie Council on Adolescent Development produced a report, *Turning Points: Preparing American Youth for the 21st Century*. The Council, consisting of business leaders, governors, presidents and deans of universities, school superintendents, and professors, focused on middle schools where students entering their adolescence are educated. Its report underscored dramatic changes and new pressures confronting young people, including sexual promiscuity, drugs, the breakdown of social relationships in the community, and a lack of adult guidance. It found that schools too often contribute to the problem:

> A volatile mismatch exists between the organization and curriculum of middle grade schools and the intellectual and emotional needs of young adolescents. Caught in a vortex of changing demands, the engagement of many youth in learning diminishes, and their rates of alienation, substance abuse, absenteeism, and dropping out of school begin to rise.

Instead of diagnosing and blaming the children for these problems, the report holds adult institutions responsible:

> Many large middle grade schools function as mills that contain and process endless streams of students. Within them are masses of anonymous youth…. Such settings virtually guarantee that the intellectual and emotional needs of youth will go unmet.

Among the Carnegie Council's recommendations are:

- The creation of small communities of learning within the larger schools
- A better core curriculum
- Greater attention to the students' actual educational needs
- The availability of at least one concerned adult to take a special interest in each child
- The involvement of families and communities in education

These steps would go a long way to reversing adult inattention to children and, in the process, so called Attention Deficit-Hyperactivity Disorder.

While they won't come in time to help individual parents and their children who find themselves faced with difficult choices right now, these observations can empower parents to organize and to demand changes in their schools. It can also empower parents to realize that the problem often does not lie in their children but in the schools. Strengthened by this perspective, parents can reassure their children and become more demanding of the teachers and the school. In the extreme, parents who can afford to may want to pull their children out of public school in favor of a selected private school or home schooling.[31]

Fake Science at NIMH

The National Institute of Mental Health (NIMH) is the federal agency most responsible for supporting establishment psychiatry through funding research, through research carried on at the institute, and through "educational" efforts. In the past two years, NIMH has lent its considerable weight to promoting psychiatric drugs for children. It co-sponsored a 1995 conference with the FDA[32] and followed up with a 1997 journal article by Benedetto Vitiello and Peter Jensen from the Child and Adolescent Disorders Research Branch. In a section of the article entitled "Marketing and Financial Aspects," Vitiello and Jensen heap praise on "the vision and efforts of a few key industry leaders" in marketing drugs to children. They conclude by quoting a "pledge" from a drug company representative to be "strong advocates for the development of safe and effective pediatric psychopharmacological agents."

Assuming the role of drug company advocacy and promotion, the NIMH officials seem wholly innocent in regard to any awareness of potential conflicts of interest between drug companies and researchers, parents, or children. The many warnings about the dangers of psychiatric drugs for children that were voiced in the unpublished proceedings of the conference itself are hardly mentioned in the published article.[33] The future of the nation's children is darkened by NIMH's testimonials to drug industry marketing practices that target children.

Brains Not People

NIMH for several decades after its creation was devoted to a spectrum of human activities from the psychological and social through the biological. In keeping with the new politics of psychiatry, NIMH has remade itself into a brain research center. *U.S. News & World Report* confirms "NIMH now focuses its studies almost exclusively on brain research and on the genetic underpinnings of emotional illness... The decision to reorder the federal research portfolio was both scientific and political."[34]

When I was on the staff at NIMH in 1966–1968, the institute had a strong psychologically and socially oriented wing that was concerned with the effect of family, schools, and society on the mental health of children. I worked in an area concerned with innovations in education aimed at improving the well-being of children. By the early 1970s, all that was changing.

In taking the "being" out of human being, NIMH has literally become a biological research center with little or no focus on psychology, family life, schools, or any personal or environmental factors that influence the feelings, thoughts, and actions of human beings.[35] The institute's policies are an extreme expression of "scientism"—the simple-minded application of physical principles to the study of human life.

In a 1993 booklet, *Learning Disabilities: Decade of the Brain*, NIMH describes its mission:

> Scientists supported by NIMH are dedicated to understanding the workings and interrelationships of the various regions of the brain, and to finding preventions and treatments to overcome brain dysfunctions that handicap people in school, work, and play.

Such heavy and exclusive focus on brain dysfunction is absurd in the field of psychological health. If it were possible to translate human emotional suffering into brain malfunctions, psychiatry would become identical to neurology which in fact does treat brain abnormalities. Instead, ADHD has no known roots in physical disease or brain dysfunction.

A Congressionally-mandated PR campaign for biopsychiatry, called "The Decade of the Brain," was partly NIMH inspired. This government-funded advertising benefits the entire Psychopharmaceutical Complex, including the drug companies and organized psychiatry.

With an increasingly biological climate in psychiatry, NIMH has fully committed itself to financing research that promotes the use of medication for the behavioral control of children.[36] It has also provided a federal pulpit for ADHD/Ritalin extremists such as Paul Wender, Alan Zametkin, and Judith Rapoport.

NIMH Attacks the DEA

The Drug Enforcement Administration (DEA) of the Justice Department is the only federal agency to show genuine concern about the dangers of the stimulant prescription epidemic. NIMH is so drug oriented that it has attacked the DEA. Peter Jensen, when he was the chief of the child and adolescent disorders branch at NIMH, declared:[37]

> They have an agenda here, unfortunately. They have to worry about the potential for abuse. I think the DEA, unfortunately, has been beating this drum when it [Ritalin] is not a major drug of abuse. The DEA concern has

been really irresponsible [sic] claims based on emergency room reports. They are not epidemiologists.

In fact, DEA concerns spring from many sources, including the escalating use of Ritalin, the wide-scale theft of the drug, black market distribution rings, and surveys on abuse among high school students. I found a report in one of our local newspapers that 95 Ritalin pills were stolen from an elementary school clinic.[38]

Jensen should know better. Ritalin has a long history as a drug of abuse going back to the 1960s.[39] NIMH, not the DEA, is being irresponsible toward America's children. The DEA should be commended for its honest stand based on scientific evidence.

I have been told by a DEA official that the agency has no plan to pursue Ciba for marketing Ritalin directly to the public through its funding of CHADD The official did feel that the agency's efforts had forced CHADD and Ciba to be more public about their relationship.[40]

NIMH Supports the ADHD/Ritalin Lobby

Even before NIMH became one-dimensional in its devotion to biology, it was supporting research into hyperactivity and ADHD. The grants began as early as 1961 in the amount of $32,000 and escalated each year to $862,048 per year by 1970.[41]

The deluge of NIMH money in support of ADHD/Ritalin not only continues to this day, it has recently swelled. NIMH gives millions in research funds to many of the most high profile members of the ADHD/Ritalin movement, including Rachel Klein, Magda Campbell, Paul Wender, Russell Barkley, Howard Abikoff, James Swanson, C. Keith Conners, William Pelham, Joseph Biederman, Lawrence Greenhill, Stephen Hinshaw, and a host of others. Many of these individuals have been receiving NIMH funds for decades in their endless efforts to promote the drugging of children. Nearly all the money goes to lifelong ADHD/Ritalin advocates. None goes to critics.

In a major escalation of its effort to justify the widespread use of stimulants, NIMH is now funding a series of multi-million dollar studies around North America to demonstrate their effectiveness culminating the new clinical trials on preschoolers.[42]

None of NIMH's funding is aimed at discovering or elaborating on the dangers of the long-term use of Ritalin, Adderall, and other stimulants. This neglect of the health of America's children is scandalous and can only be explained by subservience to the political power of the drug companies. If NIMH wished, it could easily reach out to fund much-needed critical examinations of the ADHD/Ritalin concept, including studies of long-term adverse drug effects. Unfortunately, as a faction in the Psychopharmaceutical Complex,

NIMH will never do anything so threatening to the interests of the drug companies and organized psychiatry.

Current NIMH Publications Promote the ADHD/Ritalin Lobby

A 1994 NIMH publication, *Attention Deficit Hyperactivity Disorder: Decade of the Brain*, states that ADHD is not usually caused by "poor home life" or "poor schools." It presents speculations on brain function as if they were scientific observations. It twists the truth by presenting graphics of Zametkin's brain scans as if they really can distinguish between the brains of adults with and without ADHD.[43]

The NIMH pamphlet estimates that 2 million children have ADHD while it pushes drugs in a most astonishing fashion. It claims that "Nine out of ten children improve on one of the three stimulants" when, in fact, most children end up not taking them for any length of time. Speaking as if with the voice of science, NIMH claims that 80% of children diagnosed ADHD will need a stimulant as teenagers and that 50% will need it as adults. The NIMH booklet claims that the drug "rarely stops working"—an unfounded claim for a drug that cannot be shown to have any beneficial effect after 4–18 weeks. It recommends CHADD to parents without disclosing the parent group's drug-company connections.

The booklet has one saving grace. It ends up contradicting its own earlier assertions by stating, "problems with home or school environment can make children seem overactive, impulsive, or inattentive."

NIMH is not embarrassed about its connections to the drug companies. NIMH researchers such as Judith Rapoport have taken direct funds from drug companies.[44] The funds, until our recent disclosures, were funneled to them through an intermediary foundation. Ciba, the manufacturer of Ritalin, is among the companies to funnel money into NIMH. In its 1993 pamphlet which provides a very rosy picture of stimulants, NIMH cites a Ciba publication[45] as one of its recommended sources for "teachers and specialists." It also lists the two drug-company financed parent groups, CHADD and NAMI, as resources.

Scientifically speaking, the billions of dollars spent on trying to connect brain dysfunction to psychiatric or psychological problems have been an utter waste. No solid connection has been found between any common psychiatric label and a physical disorder of the brain.[46] The flood of money, however, has been a boon to government agencies, psychiatric organizations, drug companies, and mental health professionals.

NIMH is not the only federal agency to join ranks with the ADHD/Ritalin community. A publication of the federal Alcohol, Drug Abuse, and Mental Health Administration (ADAMHA) (1984) entitled "Cocaine and Stimulants" discusses the abuse of a wide range of stimulants including various forms of amphetamine, caffeine, and even over-the-counter cold medications with stimulant properties. Somehow, it fails to mention one of the worst offenders, Ritalin.

The Food and Drug Administration

To rely on the FDA is in many ways to rely on the drug companies themselves. Not only does the FDA tend to avoid confrontations with politically powerful drug companies, all of the research used for FDA approval of a drug is under the control of the corporations.[47] During the FDA approval process, the drug company designs the research, selects and pays the researchers, and then collects and interprets the data. After that, it presents the data to the FDA and begins a lengthy process of haggling over the implications. Occasionally, the FDA will catch especially notorious examples of researchers who fudge for the drug companies, such as Drs. Borison and Diamond,[48] but more often the drug companies get away with being cozy with their paid researchers.

Deteriorating Circumstances at the FDA

While the FDA has been criticized over the years, the situation has been further deteriorating during the recent period of deregulation. A *Washington Post*[49] headline accurately describes the situation: "Slowing the Flow of Federal Rules: New Conservative Climate Chills Agencies' Activism." The article cites new rules to speed up FDA approval of drugs, while the agency itself loosens its drug approval standards. Another headline says it even more vividly:[50] "Medical Firms Take a Scalpel to the FDA."

Recently the FDA has made two drastic changes that enormously favor big business. It is planning to implement regulations that would allow the drug companies to use much more judgment concerning the adverse drug reaction reports that they send on to the FDA.[51] This would not only blind the FDA to the actual reports being sent in to the companies, it would blind the public as well. The adverse drug reaction data would remain under the control of the companies where it is not subject to the Freedom of Information Act. This should not be allowed to happen.

In discussing Ciba's advertising policies, the FDA's ineffectiveness in monitoring ads was described.[52] It's getting worse. Recently the FDA has loosened its requirements on how much the drug company must communicate when advertising directly to the public. As a result, there's been an outbreak of drug company advertising on television.[53]

What Can You Tell about a Drug in Two Weeks

Ritalin was first approved in the 1950s. In response to a Freedom of Information request, the FDA told me that it was unable to produce the original documents from that long ago. However, the FDA had a more recent chance to evaluate Ritalin when Ciba applied for approval of Ritalin-SR, a sustained release tablet. The long-acting pill is intended to enable parents to give their children a dose before school that will last throughout the school day.

After Ciba finished collecting its data and submitted the Ritalin-SR application on April 22, 1977, it was five years before the FDA finally approved it with a March 30, 1982 letter.[54] Does this long period of time indicate that the FDA required elaborate, lengthy studies? No, it means that the FDA used to be as slow as molasses. The Ritalin-SR drug trials used for approving Ritalin-SR lasted exactly *two weeks in duration* and involved a total of 90 children.[55] Studies of such short duration and small size could not possibly determine the safety or efficacy of a drug.

Despite the short duration and small size of the trials, 10 patients on Ritalin-SR and 8 on Ritalin showed "Treatment Emergent Symptoms"—adverse effects that weren't there before they started taking the drug. For the Ritalin-SR group that's an adverse reaction rate of 22%. The FDA Summary Basis of Approval states "none of these [adverse drug reactions] were considered serious."

Were they serious? A separate FDA document entitled "Clinical Review"[56] lists a series of reactions to the Ritalin and the Ritalin-SR. For Ritalin-SR, here are four of the ten reports:

> **Patient # 5**: Increasingly poor behavior. Minor anxiety.
>
> **Patient # 11**: Behavior worse at Visit 2 and Visit 3 [total of 3 visits in study].
>
> **Patient # 30**: Behavior vacillated; overly quiet or excessive crying. Poor appetite.
>
> **Patient # 31**: Laughs at everything. Restless sleep. Fidgety.

Despite the FDA's contrary opinion, these reactions would seem potentially serious both in terms of intensity and frequency. Nor is this a complete list, since there were apparently six more cases of treatment emergent symptoms for the Ritalin-SR patients. The list was not made with an eye toward reporting adverse reactions but rather to determining if Ritalin-SR is effective throughout the desired period of time.

In fact, Ciba and the FDA apparently did not consider these clinical vignettes to reflect adverse drug reactions. In the summary of adverse drug reactions "which may in any way be related to the pharmacological action of the drug," only three reactions are mentioned: a "mild decrease" in concentration, "mildly moody" during treatment, and an episode of vomiting.[57] This would indicate that the company somehow managed not to report the cases cited in the FDA's "Clinical Review" as adverse reactions!

In my experience evaluating FDA and drug company documents, it is not uncommon for the FDA to accept corporate interpretations of adverse drug effects, even when they leave out or minimize important dangers. In the hundreds of pages sent to me by the FDA concerning the approval process for Ritalin-SR, the subject of adverse reactions gets only a few sentences—a paragraph or two—amid hundreds of pages devoted to evaluating the physical composition of the pill.

While the company and the FDA found it necessary to test the drug's effect on children for only two weeks, they studied the physical stability of the pill for 24 months.[58] The priority isn't the safety of the child but the stability of the product!

The reader may pause at this moment and suggest, "But this happened a while ago and we have new studies which don't show such a high rate of adverse reactions." Remember, this study was monitored by both the drug company and the FDA, and it failed to take seriously seemingly obvious drug reactions. This is what goes on all the time, study after study, including countless ones that get published in the literature. It continues to go on in the contemporary FDA approval process as well.[59]

No placebo control group was required in the FDA's approval process for Ritalin-SR, so the studies showed nothing about the real effectiveness of the long-acting preparation. Instead, the FDA allowed Ciba to compare the SR preparation to the company's regular Ritalin tablet in patients who were already receiving Ritalin. It turned out that Ritalin-SR was about as effective as Ritalin. But was either Ritalin tablet doing any good at all? The FDA didn't bother to ask. It acted as if the effectiveness of Ritalin were a proven fact—even though the original studies for FDA approval were so old (and outdated) that they could not be found.[60]

As an interesting aside, Ciba wanted to advertise Ritalin-SR on the basis that children would not have to suffer from "ridicule over pill taking" from their peers if they could avoid having to take the pill during the school day.[61] The FDA would not allow the company to make this claim.

The FDA: a Watchdog with No Bite?

Too often the FDA allows the manufacturers to exert their will over the drug approval process.[62] The FDA has approved psychiatric drugs of questionable efficacy, even when effectiveness is measured from the drug company's perspective. The agency allows drug companies to go for years—sometimes indefinitely—without listing severe adverse drug reactions in their labels. The FDA has supported the continued use of drugs such as the sleeping medication Halcion that have been banned in England and elsewhere.

Pressure from the drug companies and from members of Congress who receive money from them makes the FDA overly concerned about the interests of the drug companies.[63] Paul Leber, until recently the physician in charge of the FDA's psychiatric drug approval process, once reassured industry that he wouldn't let FDA-enforced label changes "cause injury to industry."[64] At the time, pressure from my own media campaign and the publication of my book, *Psychiatric Drugs: Hazards to the Brain*, made the FDA take seriously the need for compelling the drug companies to put more honest information into their labels concerning the high risk of neurological damage from the neuroleptic or antipsychotic drugs, such as Haldol and Thorazine. The drug companies, out of self-interest, had resisted doing this. How could the FDA accomplish anything if it was unwilling to harm the economic interests of the drug companies? Not surprisingly, the labels' final changes failed to make clear the seriousness or frequency of the hazards of the drugs.

When the FDA was originally formed, there was enormous resistance from the drug companies and from organized medicine in the shape of the American Medical Association. Every attempt was made to dilute the agency's proposed powers. Naturally the drug companies and organized medicine wanted the watchdog to be as toothless as possible.

How toothless has the watchdog become? Now the drug companies and the AMA go to Congress to support funding for the FDA so they can get their drugs approved faster and more easily. An advertisement was recently placed in the *Washington Post* at budget-cutting time, asking Congress to "Restore FDA funding." The ad was sponsored by the FDA's former enemies—organized medicine and the drug companies, represented by the American Medical Association, the Association of American Medical Colleges, the National Medical Association, the National Health Counsel, and PhARMA.[65] The National Health Counsel is a consortium of powers in the health industry. PhARMA is the trade organ of the Pharmaceutical Research and Manufacturers of America, including companies like Eli Lilly (Prozac) and Novartis (Ritalin).

How come *these* folks are now supporting funding for the FDA?

Buying a Pet

The consumer group Public Citizen has also used the pet metaphor to describe the potential results of upcoming federal legislation aimed at weakening the FDA:[66]

> By attaching dangerous provisions to legislation that would speed up the FDA drug approval process, industry hopes that their $33.5 million in political contributions to Congress over the past six years will buy the right Washington mix of access, influence, and outcome to transform the FDA from a sharp consumer watchdog into a toothless industry pet.

The FDA's transformation to industry pet has already taken place. Now it's just a matter of obedience training.

A Cover Up at the FDA?

An earlier chapter looked at the risk of irreversible brain damage from methylphonidate (Ritalin, Concerta), from amphetamine (Dexdrine, Adderall), and from methamphetamine (Desoxyn or Gradumet).[67] Neither the FDA nor the respective drug companies have chosen to take the risk seriously. The danger is unmentioned in the labels for these drugs as found in the current *Physicians' Desk Reference* and approved by the FDA.

The FDA often requires mention of much less serious dangers with much less scientific substantiation. For example, based on large doses in animal studies, the possibility of fetal damage is mentioned in regard to methamphetamine. Similarly, as we have seen, a supposed "weak signal" danger of Ritalin-induced liver tumors in animals led the FDA to require a label change and a Dear Doctor letter to the nation's physicians.[68]

The FDA, seemingly in concert with the psychiatric and psychopharmacologic community, almost always tries to avoid disclosing that psychiatric drugs can permanently impair brain structure and function. For example, the FDA does not require studies of adverse effects on brain function in the form of neuropsychological testing of human subjects during drug approval trials. When a psychiatric drug is approved for marketing, patients have not been given testing to see if their mental functions have been impaired during the drug trials. Nor does the FDA require that drugs be studied to see if the brain recovers from the biochemical imbalances that they inevitably create. Even when it is known that a drug causes the loss or disappearance of receptors in the brain—as all the stimulants can do—the FDA does not require any studies to determine if the brain recovers from this drastic malfunction.[69] In regard to Ritalin and amphetamine, there are indications that the changes may be irreversible but there has been no attempt to thoroughly study the problem.

If the FDA or the drug companies were conscientious in protecting America's children, the evidence for irreversible brain damage caused by stimulants would be trumpeted to the profession and the amphetamines would be withdrawn from the market. At the same time, there would be a deluge of studies to determine if Ritalin can cause similar permanent brain damage in animals and humans, especially growing children. Instead, the dangers have been engulfed within a "code of silence."

Diet Drug Disasters and the FDA

Earlier chapters looked at recently disclosed dangers associated with the diet drugs fenfluramine (Pondimin) and dexfenfluramine (Redux) in regard to brain damage and heart valve abnormalities. Before the withdrawal of the two diet drugs because of the heart defects, Una McCann (1997) and others at NIH had already confirmed that both Pondimin and Redux can also cause an incurable, potentially fatal disorder called primary pulmonary hypertension. The FDA (1997b), in reporting the pulmonary hypertension as a Public Health Advisory, noted that Pondimin, first marketed in 1973, had been approved for *more than twenty years!* Dexfenfluramine was approved in 1996. These various disclosures have important implications for the FDA's lack of responsiveness to major health threats. They also confirm that drugs can continue to pose a potentially serious but unrecognized public health risk even after they have been used for decades. This speaks directly to the current national experiment with the widespread use of stimulants.

Twenty-three patients have had heart surgery after taking fenfluramine. Three died post-operatively. The heart valve defect may appear in 30% of patients.[70] Yet it took decades for doctors to begin to realize the dangers of the fenfluramines, including the apparently common heart valve abnormalities.

In response to the shock of this sudden withdrawal of Redux and Pondimin from the market, Laura Johannes and Steve Stecklow asked questions in a *Wall Street Journal* front page story: "How could the U.S. Food and Drug Administration have approved a drug that a year later proved so dangerous it had to be withdrawn from the market?" The *Wall Street Journal*, as an organ of industry, was not likely to point to the answers which are embedded in the Psychopharmaceutical Complex.

Chapter 3 noted that the FDA and the drug companies continued to fail to respond to research showing that the two diet drugs cause brain cell death.[71] The similarity of these drugs to amphetamines, as well as their Prozac-like serotonergic effects, should raise additional grave concerns about the use of both the stimulants and the Prozac-like drugs called SSRIs (selective serotonin reuptake inhibitors).

Concern about the harmful effects of over-stimulating serotonin in the brain finally led the FDA to approve a two-year study of potential brain toxicity from Prozac and dexfenfluramine.[72] The principal researchers include Harold Sackeim of Columbia's College of Physicians and Surgeons. Sackeim is a leading electroshock treatment advocate who recommends extra-large doses of electricity, claiming that they cause no harm to the brain or mind.[73] The study will be conducted by Wyeth-Ayerst, the maker of dexfenfluramine (Redux) who is already minimizing the dangers in their press release. All this makes me skeptical about the potential objectivity of the study and in fact nothing has been reported despite the passage of several years. Members of the Psychopharmaceutical Complex, including drug companies and their handpicked researchers, are not likely to come up with findings that impugn the safety of drugs.[74] Furthermore, now that fenfluramine and dexfenfluramine have been removed from the market due to the production of heart valve abnormalities, the studies may be jeopardized.

It is always imperative to remember that psychiatric drugs are industrial products subject to all the hype, misinformation, and media spin techniques that characterize the marketing of any other multi-billion dollar product. Caveat emptor—buyer beware—applies to psychiatric drugs as much as it does to new cars, cosmetics, or any other mass market product that competes through advertising and promotion. The growing realization that psychiatric drugs are in fact products that can be fraudulently developed and promoted helped to pave the way for the Ritalin class action suits described in chapter 1.

The next chapter looks at the increasing focus on selling this product—psychiatric drugs—in the children's market.

Chapter 16

BRAVE NEW WORLD OF CHILDHOOD

Growing Up on Psychiatric Drugs

[T]he application of Ritalin to hyperactive children is leading to a situation in which social problems are increasingly defined as medical ones.... There is a tendency to look for the solutions to complex social problems in the behavior of individuals, not in the surrounding environment. Thus the unruly child at school and at home is perceived as in need of medical attention. Peer groups, parents, teachers, and administrators thereby avoid responsibility for aberrant behavior and its ultimate correction.

—T. Alexander Smith and Robert F. Kronick,
International Journal of Addictions (1979)

Even "good" psychopharmacology decreases the need to scrutinize the child's social environment and may permit a poor situation to continue or grow worse. Should dysfunctional family patterns and overcrowded classrooms be tolerated just because Ritalin improves the child's behavior?... Should society use a biological fix to address problems that have roots in social and environmental factors? If it consistently does, how might society be affected?... The rise in the use of stimulants is alarming and signals an urgent need for American society to reevaluate its priorities.

—Lawrence H. Diller,
pediatrician who prescribes Ritalin (1996)

A recent report in *Science* by Eliot Marshal confirms the escalating use of stimulants. A study from Duke University surveyed eleven counties between 1992 and 1996, and found that more than 7% of the children were receiving stimulant drugs. Given that boys are far more frequently medicated, the data suggests that more than 10% of the boys were being given the drugs. The researchers found that many of the children had few if any signs of ADHD, and did not meet the formal criteria for the diagnosis.

The Duke report followed a study of elementary school children in Virginia that found that 8–10% of elementary school children were receiving stimulants in school. This figure was undoubtedly an underestimate, since many children are given long-acting Ritalin in the morning without having to take any later on at school. While the *Science* report raised questions about medicating so many children, it quoted child psychiatrist Peter Jensen as defending these medication rates as appropriate.

It's going to get worse before it gets better. The drug companies are competing with one another to develop more efficient methods of medicating children with stimulants. Two new long-acting preparations of methylphenidate (Ritalin) have entered the market, Concerta from ALZA Corp. and Metadate ER from Medeva. Meanwhile, Novartis is also working on another long-acting form of Ritalin.

An August 22, 2000 column in the *Washington Post Health* magazine by Jennifer Huget praises Concerta because it will enable parents to give a child a morning dose that lasts throughout the entire school day. The child and the parents therefore won't need the school to hand out the drug. Of course, it is positive to keep the schools out of the medication process, and it's good for children to avoid public embarrassment. But the newspaper report, which reads like a drug company press release, fails to mention the downside. First and foremost, longer-acting drugs are more dangerous. When the child develops an adverse effect, such as a potentially fatal cardiac arrhythmia or a painful stomachache, the adverse drug reaction is likely to persist for a longer time due to the continuing presence of the drug in the bloodstream. Second, by making it more efficient and more secret from the rest of the world, parents will feel more comfortable about drugging their children.

A Fun-Filled ADD Evaluation Package

Consider what inducements parents are offered nowadays. For those who are tired of the same old boring medical consultations for their children, physician Corydon G. Clark (1997) offers families an "EVALUATION/ TREATMENT FUN PACKAGE" to Las Vegas, complete with "2 nights FREE room accommodations in one of Las Vegas' premier Strip casinos, Monday through Thursday only; Coupons worth $900 for discounts for meals, shows, and many other Las Vegas attractions!" There's a note that "normally it is possible to play golf, tennis, etc. year-round." Oh, yes, you can also get your child evaluated at Clark's "A.D.D. Clinic." He offers a toll free number.

What sort of political and social climate would allow a doctor to post such an advertisement? The climate of America today. Meanwhile, less flamboyant professionals are nonetheless climbing on the Ritalin money train. Child psychiatrist Daniel Amen (1997), for example, offers day-long workshops around the country that conclude with the theme, "Building a Thriving ADD Practice (step by step)."

Camp Ritalin

Canada is in second place in the rate of prescribing Ritalin with an astonishing 32% rise in Ritalin use from 1995 to 1996.[1] Murray Campbell (1997) describes what she calls "Camp Ritalin" outside of Toronto for children "who have really struggled in school or in other settings where they don't fit." IMS Canada, which provides its data to industry, calls Ritalin a "godsend." The US and Canada leave all other countries far behind. Australia and Germany, followed to a lesser extent by France and Mexico, have also been reporting increased use, and there are indications of a world-wide trend.[2] I can plot the world-wide marketing of Ritalin from the calls I get from foreign media asking me to comment on efforts to promote the drug. Two years ago I was already debating Ritalin on Australian television. Now I'm hearing from Germany and England.

A Ritalin Patch Instead of a Boy Scout Patch?

When I was a child, the only patch I knew about was the one I wore on my Boy Scout uniform. In the age of technology, we now have another evolving possibility—the Ritalin "transdermal patch" that delivers the drug trouble-free to parents and teachers who no longer have to keep track of doses and cajole the children into taking them. The skin patch methodology, well along in development by Sano Corporation, has already been tried experimentally for giving psychiatric drugs to children labeled with ADHD.[3]

C. Keith Conners, venerable ADHD/Ritalin advocate, heralded the new approach as relieving children and their caregivers of the daily responsibility and stigma of pill-taking. The news was announced at an NIMH conference—which demonstrates where the government stands. In a remarkable example of the Psychopharmaceutical Complex at work, the research is being financed by both the government and Solvay Pharmaceuticals, which is contributing $100,000 per year. Thus the FDA, NIMH and industry are cooperating in an effort that is guaranteed to speed up the approval of drug patches for children. These patches will almost surely escalate the sale of stimulants and other drugs in the children's market.

While a great advance for ADHD/Ritalin advocates, it's a step toward Brave New World for our children. Now parents won't even have to fuss over the responsibility of handing pills to their children once or twice a day. They can have the doctor stick on a patch and then forget about it.

An August 13, 1997 advertisement in the *Seattle Times* seeks children diagnosed with ADHD, ages 6 to 12, for clinical trials with a skin patch that delivers a "well tolerated, non-stimulant drug."[4] Notice the break in scientific research design. Potential patients are already being told not to anticipate serious adverse effects. Unless this is a miracle drug without any serious adverse effects, it's also a breach in informed consent. That safety pitch is aimed at convincing parents to sign up their kids. But any drug that is toxic enough to modify behavior will have serious hazards.

Saturation in the Adult Market

Why the growing focus on the children's market for psychiatric drugs? It's simple enough: The psychiatric drug market for adults is becoming saturated. Mary Leonard described the motivation behind pharmaceutical company efforts to find a pediatric market for psychiatric drugs:

The search has intensified because drug manufacturers see a potentially lucrative market among 8- to 15-year-olds now that growth in the saturated adult market—28 million Americans took antidepressants last year—has slowed. According to Dr. Gary Tollefson, a Lilly vice-president and psychiatrist who oversees Prozac research, the company "feels very good" about fresh results from the largest controlled pediatric study on Prozac...

Elyse Tanouye confirmed this new marketing thrust in an April 1997 story in the *Wall Street Journal*: "Antidepressant makers also need a new market as growth slows in the adult segment." According to the marketing research company, IMS America, 28 million Americans took antidepressants last year, many more than APA's official estimate of 16 million adults suffering from depression. The market is flattening, and the pressure to find new consumers drives the companies toward the relatively untapped market of America's children.

Berkeley professor of psychology S. Mark Breedlove (1997) writes: "More chilling is the possibility that a billion-dollar-a-year Prozac market may need an infusion of new, young customers whether or not they benefit from the product."

Already Bombarding Children

The manufacturers of the new serotonergic antidepressants, like Prozac, Zoloft, Paxil, Celexa, and Luvox have already taken a big bite into the children's market. By 1997, an estimated 580,000 prescriptions per year for these drugs were written for children age five and older.[5] That's on top of the several million children getting stimulants and the hundreds of thousands more being prescribed other psychiatric drugs.

None of these 580,000 prescriptions for antidepressants were written on the basis of scientific evidence. None was FDA approved. There have been no studies confirming their usefulness in children and many indicating they are useless and dangerous.

We can expect that growing economic pressure will enable the drug companies to begin generating research to support their marketing aims, because where there's a will, there's a way. In fact, as we have seen, NIMH has been conducting controversial stimulant drug clinical trials on little children on behalf of industry.

A Winner Keeps on Winning

Psychiatric drugs are the second most profitable pharmaceuticals, close behind cardiovascular drugs in sales. Psychotherapeutic drug sales in the United States exceeded 7 billion in 1996.[6] Prozac and Zoloft were ranked number three and five respectively among all drugs. That reflected slippage for Prozac which used to be number one—but the drug is making a comeback down the throats of children. Prozac took second place in the period of January–June 1997 with US sales of $917 million during those six months.[7] Zoloft remained in 5th place with $588 million and Paxil entered the top ten at number 8 with $449 million. Their combined sales for the first half of 1997 was $1.95 *billion*.[8] An even more recent financial report indicates a 17% jump in sales for Eli Lilly's Prozac for the quarter ending September 1997 with a three-month total of $705 million.[9] Prozac accounted for nearly one-third of its company's total revenues.

Children: The Expanding Drug Market

The escalating profitability of SSRI antidepressants—Prozac, Zoloft, Celexa, Luvox, and Paxil—in part reflects their strong showing in the children's market. While this book focuses on the stimulant drugs, there is a massive new threat from the increasing promotion of antidepressants for children.[10] An especially disturbing report appeared in the October 20, 1997 *Newsweek* which presents the SSRI antidepressants as lifesaving for children.[11] Depression in children is treated as a disease that has nothing to do with trauma or loss in the child's life. NAMI, the biologically oriented parents group, is given extensive coverage, including its 800 number. *Newsweek* indicated that Prozac prescriptions for children have increased 80% in two years.[12]

Drug companies are in the process of seeking FDA approval for the use of the latest antidepressants in children. At the head of the pack in vying for FDA approval are Eli Lilly (Prozac), Pfizer Inc. (Zoloft), Bristol-Myers Squibb Co. (Serzone), American Home Products (Effexor), and SmithKline Beecham PLC (Paxil).

Remember, it's all about marketing—drugs are an industrial product. But when the National Institute of Mental Health declares that "mental diseases affect 15–20 percent of the American public annually,"[13] it's not considered an advertising campaign, it's considered an educational campaign. In reality, selling "mental illness" to the American public is one of the most vigorous and successful advertising campaigns in history.[14] This new marketing strategy entails marketing the "disorder" as well as the drug. It is now being directed at the drugging of America's children.

While doctors can give these drugs to children without FDA approval, the official imprimatur of the government will enormously liberate them to overcome their own concerns, to respond to parental pressure for drugs, and to begin prescribing them more freely.

A Warning from the Old Guard Itself

The drugging of children has gotten so out of hand that psychiatrist Leon Eisenberg sounded an alarm to the *Boston Globe*:[15]

> "This whole trend toward giving pills to children as a solution to everything, particularly in the absence of evidence that they work, is fundamentally unethical," says Leon Eisenberg, a professor of psychiatry and social medicine at Harvard Medical School. "It's driven by the convenience of the doctor, the profitability of the drug company, and the notion that there is nothing more meaningful to life than biochemistry."

Eisenberg should know well of what he speaks. With financial support from NIMH and the drug companies, he and C. Keith Conners became "the country's most influential proponents of the use of stimulants for hyperactive children" more than two decades ago.[16]

NIMH sponsored a two-day symposium on Alternative Pharmacology of Attention Deficit-Hyperactivity Disorder. Proposed ideas ranged from caffeine to a nicotine patch, from decongestants to a variety of adult medications. Reporting on the NIMH conference, Susman (1996) describes drug company interest in finding new medications to compete with Ritalin:

> The symposium also heard from pharmaceutical industry representatives who, like John Heiligenstein, MD, senior clinical research physician at Eli Lilly in Indianapolis, and Albert Derivan, MD, of Wyeth-Ayerst Laboratories in Philadelphia, say their companies are seeking to develop medications for ADD. Heiligenstein said, "There is a lot more interest at Lilly to look at this condition. We see an opportunity to develop a first-line treatment or at least a co-equal treatment."

The use of Prozac-like drugs in children is especially threatening since Prozac remains one of the most frequently mentioned drugs for adverse reactions in the FDA system of spontaneous reporting.[17] For many years Prozac was first. It still leads the pack in total adverse reaction reports over the years. Last year, it was third in the number of reports of adverse reactions. Since reports for individual drugs decline over years of use, this is a very high rank for a drug that has been around for a decade.

Drugs that affect the brain are by far the most commonly reported for adverse effects.[18] Central nervous system agents were first among ten categories in 1995, with more than three times as many reports as the next category, and more than one-quarter of all mentions. This is important to keep in mind in terms of the willingness of doctors to give these kinds of drugs to an ever-increasing number of children.

Prozac for Children

Although not approved for children by the FDA, Prozac is increasingly prescribed as an alternative to stimulants for ADHD. Prozac has a stimulant profile very similar to Ritalin and Dexedrine. In *Talking Back to Prozac* (1994) we pointed out that all of the major clinical effects of Prozac and related drugs, such as Zoloft and Paxil, are similar to the stimulants. Prozac can cause euphoria, agitation, irritability, aggression, insomnia, weight loss, and, in the extreme, psychotic mania. It can lead to "crashing" with depression and suicidal feelings. It can also narrow attention and cause obsessive focusing. It sometimes produces robotic behavior.

While the chemical effects on the brain differ from those of the stimulants, Prozac-like drugs have sufficiently similar clinical effects to encourage doctors to use them as substitutes for Ritalin or Dexedrine. There is no evidence for their usefulness in children and they are at least as dangerous as stimulants.

The rush to drug America's children with antidepressants is taking place amid increasing evidence that they are of no benefit whatsoever for children or youth.[19]John and Rita Sommers-Flanagan reviewed studies of antidepressants in children for *Professional Psychology* and concluded that neither the older ones nor the newer Prozac-like antidepressants "have demonstrated greater efficacy than placebo in alleviating depressive symptoms in children and adolescents." Researchers have begun to question the ethics of prescribing any antidepressants to children and youth.[20] The situation is summed up in a headline in *Clinical Psychiatry News*: "Though data lacking, antidepressants used widely in children."[21]

Probably, the newer antidepressant drugs are more dangerous for children than adults. Both the brains and minds of children are less developed and less able to resist the toxic effects.[22] Prozac, for example, tends to cause mania in approximately 1% of depressed adults, but initial results from controlled clinical trials involving depressed children age 7-17 suggested a menacing rate of 6%.[23] The final report by Graham Emlsey (1997) and his colleagues from the University of Texas confirmed this high rate of Prozac-induced mania in children but buried the data almost out of sight in a section concerning study drop outs (p. 1033).

A retrospective study of hospital charts from the University Pittsburgh by Jain and his colleagues found that nearly one-quarter of young people age 9-19 developed manic-like or manic symptoms on Prozac, and that many more suffered irritability and insomnia. A study by Mark Riddle (1990/1991) and other researchers from Yale University found that 50% of children age 8-16 developed two or more mental or behavioral disturbances on Prozac, including sleep disorders, loss of inhibition or self-control, agitation, and manic-like symptoms. Also from Yale, a group led by Robert King (1991) documented the emergence or intensification of suicidal and violent tendencies in six of forty-two children age 10–17 who were treated with Prozac. Although the King study was conducted before the highly publicized school shootings, one twelve-year-old boy on Prozac developed nightmares about shooting his classmates and had difficulty distinguishing his nightmares from reality. I have reviewed these studies in more detail in *Reclaiming Our Children* (2000), where I have related the prescription of psychiatric drugs to some of the school shootings.

In 1995 at a conference on psychiatric drugs for children sponsored by NIMH and the FDA, it was reconfirmed that drug advocates have been unable to prove that any of the antidepressants are beneficial to children. NIMH's Benedetto Vitiello referred to "the fact that the antidepressant effect in children is still unproven." The FDA's Thomas Laughren confirmed Vitiello's remarks.

Xavier Castellanos of the Child Psychiatry Branch of NIMH recently confirmed that there are no well-controlled studies involving the use of the new Prozac-like drugs (SSRIs) for children.[24] Yet hundreds of thousands of children are getting them.

Tragically, the fact that antidepressants for children have repeatedly failed to prove effective seems to mean very little to drug companies or to organized psychiatry and pediatrics. Worse yet, there is a large body of evidence that Prozac-like drugs cause very high rates of psychosis and behavioral abnormalities in children.

Putting on a Happy Face with Prozac

Meanwhile, Eli Lilly is conducting an enormously costly PR campaign for Prozac with three-page advertisements in many of America's major magazines, such as *Time*, *Newsweek*, and *Cosmopolitan*. A laudatory report in *Psychiatric Times* describes the campaign as an educational breakthrough for informing the nation about the biological basis of depression.[25] Lilly anticipates that the ad will be seen by "tens of millions of consumers who read the more than 20 U.S. magazines in which the ad is scheduled to run." Is this a multi-million dollar blockbuster PR campaign to sell drugs? Heavens, no. According to Lilly, the purpose is to "promote depression awareness and education." The recent 17% growth in Prozac sales is attributed to this ad campaign.[26]

The lavish Prozac ads begin on the left side of the magazine page with a black, white, and gray picture of a little cloud that is crying big tears. Beneath the weeping cloud are the words, "Depression hurts." On the right hand page is a bright yellow sun, much like a smiley face without the smile, set on a blue background. Beneath it are the words "Prozac can help." The third page contains the FDA-required small print about toxic effects. The art work has a child-like quality, an advertising technique that subtly associates the drug with helping children.

After calling the Lilly ads "morally indefensible," syndicated columnist Arianna Huffington (1997a) focuses on the message of the child art work:

> More troubling is the fact that the childish drawings are clearly aimed at stressed-out parents too busy to deal with children who are acting up, having trouble at school or simply being moody. The solution is simple: Drug them up to your expectations.

In a follow up column, Huffington (1997b) disclosed that the FDA has told her that Lilly has filed preliminary papers for beginning the approval process for Prozac for children. The company had denied this to her.

The Prozac and Ritalin professional lobbying groups are closely related. Child psychologist Barbara Ingersoll, one of the most vociferous advocates of Ritalin/ADHD, has now thrown her hat into the Prozac ring as well. Huffington quotes Ingersoll:

> Children on Prozac tell us they are not as angry and not as temperamental, behave better and feel better. It is a tremendous development. We can see a future where mood disorders will be treated not as exotic, uncommon conditions in children but more like dental cavities or poor vision. [In the future] there won't be a stigma for kids on Prozac—the stigma will be on not taking Prozac.

Huffington concludes that Eli Lilly is "just a big-time drug pusher."

Ordering the Drug Companies To Conduct Studies on Children

President Bill Clinton ordered changes in the testing of prescription drugs to make manufacturers include data on children in their studies for drug approval if the drug seems likely to be used on children.[27] Some effort will also be made by the FDA to demand that drug companies produce studies of the effects on children if their drugs are already being widely used in the pediatric market.

On the surface, this seems like a positive step—but in a society dominated by business interests, it's a good idea to look beneath the surface. Up to now the manufacturers of psychiatric drugs haven't needed to get FDA approval for children because doctors are willing to prescribe the drugs for kids without the FDA imprimatur. The companies therefore resisted pressure to begin testing on children.[28]

It costs money to do a whole new battery of drug tests and it raises the specter of discovering new adverse effects in children. If one company were to make the investment of money or risk the new studies, it would put the company at a competitive disadvantage in a market where the drugs are being prescribed for children anyway. That changes if *all* the companies are required by the government to test their products on children. The government regulations do away with the competition. With *all* the companies required to test their drugs on children, they will be eager to do so, because that will open up the children's market even further for all of them at once, adding the FDA's imprimatur on child drugging. Meanwhile, the National Institute of Mental Health has taken the drug companies further off the hook by takng it on itself to conduct the most controversial sttimulant drug testing on preschoolers (chapter 1).

Isn't there a chance that testing on children will disclose that drugs like Prozac, Zoloft, Paxil aren't effective on children? No, not much chance, because the FDA, working *with* the drug companies, will make sure that everything comes out right, much as they originally did with Prozac.[29] The FDA is in no mood to offend these enormously powerful corporations. Besides, with *billions* of dollars at stake, the drug companies will find research strategies and researchers that are largely FDA-proof, much as they have in the past.[30] Nonetheless, the continued failure of any antidepressants to be approved for children has kindled a small flame of hope the FDA will adhere to an ethical line on this issue.

Treating "Shadow ADHD"

Leading psychiatrists waxed enthusiastic for journalist Jane Brody (1997) of the *New York Times* as they advocated medication for patients with "shadow syndrome"— "a mild form of well-recognized neuropsychiatric disorder like depression, attention-deficit disorder, obsessive-compulsive disorder, mania or autism." Notice the inclusion of ADHD.

The new term, "shadow syndrome," has the same old persistent psychiatric intention—to medicate more and more people. Soon we shall be hearing of "shadow ADHD" as a justification for prescribing even more Ritalin. Other terms for shadow syndrome are "subthreshold," "subclinical," and "subsyndromal."

Significant names in biopsychiatry lent their authority in Brody's article to extending psychiatric diagnosis beyond the customary limits. Frederick Goodwin, who resigned as Director of NIMH after Ginger and I campaigned against his racist federal programs aimed at children,[31] told the *New York Times* that some of these "milder states" could be more disruptive than more well-defined syndromes. Lewis Judd, another former head of NIMH, repeated his well-known advocacy of using Prozac for "subclinical" depression.

Psychiatric Drugs: The New "In Thing" for Youngsters?

We are entering a unique time. The tobacco industry has been severely criticized for appealing to children with Joe Camel ads and other tactics. While adult smoking has been reduced, minors are smoking more than ever.[32] A series of lawsuits, combined with pending FDA controls, may to some extent, at least, put a crimp in tobacco industry interests.

On January 15, 1998, John Mintz and Saundra Torry of the *Washington Post* broke the story, "Internal R.J. Reynolds Documents Detail Cigarette Marketing Aimed at Children." According to the newspaper report, internal memoranda show that the nation's second largest cigarette company "sought for decades to reverse the declining sales of its brands by developing aggressive marketing proposals to reach adolescents as young as age 14 years old..." The Joe Camel ad campaign was a key element in this marketing strategy. The disclosure of these documents aroused expressions of outrage from members of Congress and the former commissioner of the FDA, David A. Kessler. Yet this marketing strategy is being pursued right now by the manufacturers of psychiatric drugs who are pushing various forms of "speed" for children. Desperate for ever-increasing profits and to compete successfully with each other, the drug companies as a group are now trying to saturate the children's market...and not just children as young as age 14 but also preschool children. Yet, as we have seen in this chapter and in chapters 13 and 14, this promotional campaign directed at the children's market is being openly applauded and abetted by officials from the FDA, NIMH, and the Department of Education.

As the FDA cracks down on tobacco, and approves increased numbers of psychiatric drugs for children, the results seem inevitable. The ADHD/Ritalin movement seems to have an insatiable appetite for drugging America's children. Unlike the tobacco industry, the cloak of science and medicine gives them total respectability—even though the product they are pushing is a stimulant and commonly abused street drug. More and more young people will turn to handling their emotional struggles with psychiatric drugs instead of tobacco. More and more, they will do so through illegally obtained stimulants, if not directly through a physician's prescription. Prozac-like antidepressants that can also have stimulant effects will also be used both legally and illegally. All this is already taking place. As Arianna Huffington headlined her syndicated column, "Exit Joe Camel, but here comes Joe Prozac."

Which is worse, cancer-causing, addictive tobacco or brain-disabling, addictive psychiatric drugs like Ritalin? There's recent animal research suggesting that Ritalin can cause cancer.[33] We have evidence that Ritalin can cause the same kind of down-regulation of receptors in the brain that led to the death of brain cells from Redux and Pondimin. I cannot begin to choose between the two evils—cigarettes and speed. Children and youth should be protected from both tobacco and stimulant drugs. Since originally writing the above paragraphs in the first edition of this book, it is encouraging and gratifying to have helped to motivate the former anti-tobacco attorneys to turn their attention to Ritalin.

The Vulnerability of Affluent Children

Economist Lester C. Thurow (1997) makes the following point:

Values follow economic realities. Individual fulfillment now ranks higher than family in public opinion polls. "Competitive individualism" grows at the expense of "family solidarity." The ideal is "choice," not "bonds." In the language of capitalism, children have ceased to be "profit centers" and have become "cost centers."

He is talking about relatively affluent families. Even for them, children have too often become an economic and emotional burden. It seems easier to confine the children within their own heads with toxic drugs than to deal with them as human beings. Ironically, the wealthiest families are giving their children the worst psychiatric care. This is because they tend to trust and even to revere psychiatry and to pursue the latest drug fads. When psychoanalysis was in vogue, everyone was in therapy. Now it's Prozac and Ritalin.

The Vulnerability of the Poor and the Inner-City Community

As described in chapter 1, Harvard Medical School psychiatrist Joseph T. Coyle warned in the February 2000 *Journal of the American Medical Association* about an escalation in the drugging of two–four year old toddlers. Since many of the children were on Medicaid, he was especially concerned about a growing trend to medicate children who live in poverty.

A disproportionate number of poor children land in foster care. In an extraordinary 1997 four-part series on the drugging of children in Washington state, journalist Steve Goldsmith documented that 19 percent of children who enter the foster care system end up on psychiatric drugs. The most frequently prescribed drug was not Ritalin, which took second place (3.6% of children). In first was the old antidepressant, imipramine (Tofranil) (4.4%). It is not approved for treating psychiatric problems in children. Behind Ritalin came other antidepressants, desipramine (Norpramin) (1.4%), and fluoxetine (Prozac) (1.1%), followed by lithium, Dexedrine, Cylert, and the antipsychotic agent, Mellaril.

Every class of adult psychiatric drug was given to these children, sometimes with disastrous results, including death. Goldsmith (1997a) quotes

NIMH's Peter Jensen, "We know very little about the safety and efficacy of a number of these medications."

Drug companies, as well as government agencies and researchers, often view the African-American poor as an underdeveloped market. Of course, they don't call it "an underdeveloped market;" they call it "under-served." Drug advocates lament that the "African-American community believes that children are being overmedicated."[34]

In the mid-1990s, as Ginger Breggin and I describe in *The War Against Children of Color* (1998), reform efforts through the Center for the Study of Psychiatry and Psychology took me into many of America's inner cities from Harlem to Watts. It was part of a largely successful effort to stop the federal government from developing a massive program to perform intrusive biological research on inner city children in the hope of finding genetic and biochemical causes for violence.[35] In my travels and workshops, I found that inner-city African-Americans as a group seem far more concerned about the dangers of medicating their children than are suburban parents. Perhaps because they feel such threats to their children on a daily basis, they seem to view their children as more precious. The long and tragic history of racist medical experiments in America also makes them more cautious.[36]

Urban African-Americans in general tend to understand the dangers of medical social control better than more affluent whites and to offer a more organized and spirited opposition to the drugging of their children.[37] Protests over ADHD/Ritalin in Philadelphia were described as a "furor" with the holding of hearings by the City Council:[38]

> Parents are accusing Philadelphia school teachers of administering drugs to their children without parental consent. School district officials maintain that they are in the middle of an agreement made only by the child's doctor and the child's parent. Members of the African-American community are accusing the district of using Ritalin to target African-American children as a way of mind control. Council members are trying to clarify what policies, if any, the school district has broken regarding the distribution of drugs in the public schools.

Some parents accused teachers of harassing them until they agreed to go along with drugging their children.

Similar controversy also erupted in Baltimore, Washington, D.C., and around the nation, partly inspired by our campaign against the violence initiative. Journalist Diane Granat (1995) observed:

> Minority parents also have complained that Ritalin and other medications are being pressed on their children as a way of forcing them to social norms.

"We call it the racism pill," Dixie Jordan, a Native American parent, said at a recent NIMH conference on psychopharmacology and children. "This is a pervasive feeling in many minority communities because schools have not created an environment that is hospitable to our children."

There is a grave danger in the reality that lower socioeconomic families are likely to have more children suffering from ADHD-like symptoms. In Michael Valentine's (1997) words, "There is a big risk that this labeling and medicating of children will eventually become a social control issue for lower SES [socioeconomic status] and minority students." The danger is increased by the reality that a disproportionate number of African-American students are diagnosed in the schools with Serious Emotional Disturbance (SED), a diagnosis which often overlaps with ADHD as well.[39] It is also increased by the poverty in the inner city which leads some parents to want to have their children diagnosed with ADHD so that the family can benefit from Social Security disability payments. With their susceptibility to hypertension, there is also a special danger for black youngsters in being exposed to a drug that routinely elevates the blood pressure.

At the moment, America's more affluent white suburbs are embracing ADHD/Ritalin more than any other group but it is only a matter of time before resistance in the black community is overcome by the propaganda barrage and by economic pressures.

Whatever our origins—African-American, Latino, Native American, Asian, European—we should fear for the future of all of America's children.

What If a Better Drug Comes Along?

Ritalin and the other stimulants work by subduing the mind and behavior of the child, reducing spontaneity and autonomy, and producing apathy, compliance, and robotic submission to boring activities. Since psychiatric drugs in general work by disabling the brain and mind, there seems little chance of the development of a "better" drug that is not a more disabling drug.[40]

From a somewhat different perspective, Schrag and Divoky warned in 1975 that a *better* drug for controlling children would be an even more dangerous drug. The dangers of Ritalin, they already knew, included such dramatic problems as growth suppression, psychosis, and addiction. They also already knew that it had no long-term efficacy. It was almost too easy to criticize Ritalin:

In the final analysis, all the controversies about efficacy, safety and side effects, though highly significant, tend to be misleading. They turn attention from social and political considerations to individual medical questions and therefore conceal the most fundamental issue.

The more fundamental issue, according to Schrag and Divoky, is the blind faith in both the benevolence of the institutions pushing the drugs, and society's willing acceptance of the need to take pills to accommodate to these institutions.

The real danger lies in someday finding a "magic pill" that will make children happy to do whatever their families, schools, and government want them to do. At present, it is still possible to appeal to the fact that stimulant drugs are highly dangerous; but new drugs may some day at least seem to render this argument less effective. Then society will have to face the more essential question—what Schrag and Divoky describe as the base impulse to make our children conform at the cost of their physical, mental, and spiritual individuality.

Warnings about America's Future

The Drug Enforcement Administration (DEA) (1995c) has observed:

> Most European physicians are extremely reluctant to prescribe methylphenidate or any other stimulant for what they believe to be a conduct or behavior problem in children.... Quite clearly, the United States is the only country in the world that has so thoroughly embraced the notion that a large number of our children are suffering from a "neurobiological" disorder that needs to be treated with a potent psychostimulant as a first-line treatment for behavioral control.[41]

America has yet to heed repeated warnings from the International Narcotics Control Board (1996):

> The board reiterates its request to all Governments to exercise the utmost vigilance in order to prevent the overdiagnosing of ADD in children and medically unjustified treatment with methylphenidate and other stimulants.

Gene Haislip, a recently retired DEA official, warns "We have become the only country in the world where children are prescribed such a vast quantity of stimulants that share virtually the same properties as cocaine."[42]

Millions of children are being made to take stimulants and millions more are being given other psychiatric drugs. The number of child victims of the Psychopharmaceutical Complex is escalating every day. This leaves nothing to be encouraged about.

Persisting in Senseless Treatments

Many people are surprised and even shocked that psychiatry persists in promoting antiquated treatments such as electroshock and even psychosurgery.[43] Similarly, many are aghast at the widespread prescription of psychiatric medications to children when there is so little evidence to support it.

Psychiatry's persistence in using obviously senseless and harmful treatments contradicts the idea that psychiatry is a science that makes inevitable progress in a similar fashion to engineering, chemistry, or physics. It's not so. Psychiatry as a whole is not a scientific enterprise. Psychiatry is more like a two-party political system with the biological and environmental parties constantly vying for power.

Biological psychiatry is now the party in power. Its fate rises and falls not with science but with politics. Politics, as always, is driven by money. This is nowhere more obvious than in the current successful promotion of stimulants like Ritalin and Adderall. Over three decades, ADHD/Ritalin advocates have failed to develop a sound scientific basis for their approach. Yet this has not prevented them from collaborating with the drug companies and other interest groups to dominate child mental health in recent years.

What does America's future hold in regard to the increased drugging of its children? It holds as much as Americans will tolerate. Organized psychiatry is always looking for voids to fill. The drug companies are always looking for new markets. Only an outraged citizenry can stop this massive psychiatric drug abuse of our children.

PART FOUR

HOW WE CAN HELP OUR CHILDREN

Chapter 17

EMPOWERING YOURSELF AS A PARENT

Love your children, care about them, respect them, do as much as possible to have them grow and develop, teach them social skills, and teach them how to identify and express their feelings and to become uniquely human; but, at the same time, care about them enough and love them enough to give them guidance, structure, limits, and control as they need it.

—Michael R. Valentine, educator,
How to Deal with Difficult Discipline Problems (1988)

Parents are blamed, but not trained. Millions of new mothers and fathers take on a job each year that ranks among the most difficult anyone can have, taking an infant, a little person who is almost totally helpless, assuming full responsibility for his physical and psychological health and raising him so he will become a productive, cooperative, and contributing citizen. What more difficult and demanding job is there? Yet, how many parents are trained for it?

—Thomas Gordon, *P.E.T.: Parent Effectiveness Training* (1970)

While advocates of the ADHD diagnosis and drugs often speak of empowering parents by releasing them from feelings of guilt, more often they are disempowering parents by stripping them of responsibility for their children. The disempowerment of parents is one of the most destructive aspects of the ADHD/Ritalin movement.

While parenting is the hardest job of all, there's no hope for our children unless parents retake responsibility from the "experts" and determine for themselves to take the most sensible, effective, and loving approach to their children. We may seek professional guidance but we must never relinquish parental intuition, common sense, or love.

Seven Parenting Principles to Remember

The following principles are worth returning to whenever we feel unsure about ourselves as parents. Most of us have to remind ourselves about these principles on a regular basis.

First, don't worry about who's to blame.

Blaming is not a good approach to solving problems. Blaming is driven by feelings of helplessness on our part which we then turn into angry and hateful feelings toward ourselves or other people. When you feel yourself "blaming," you need to take a deep breath and stop. Focus instead on your ability to remain rational and loving, and then on your ability to focus on your child's needs from a rational and loving perspective.

If you decide that you have contributed to your child's problem, blaming yourself will only paralyze and confuse you with guilt. Instead, be *glad* that you've identified yourself as part of the problem; that makes it easier for you to become part of the solution. We have more power over ourselves than over other people, so if we're a source of the problem, we can much more easily and directly fix the problem. It's always most effective to look to ourselves first as the source of any problem in our family.

Even if we find that someone else is responsible for our child's problem, such as the school or a teacher, we need to let go of our anger in order to be helpful in encouraging the school or teacher to change.

If we feel our children are to blame for "their own problems," we are not likely to be helpful. Children do not respond well to being blamed. Even if we don't scream at them, "You're to blame!," they will sense the negative message coming from us.

Second, without blaming yourself, assume parental responsibility for your child's well-being.

Once you've set aside blaming and guilt, remind yourself, "I'm the parent." Look to yourself for the ultimate answers, not to the teacher, the psychiatrist, or some other expert. You are responsible for your child and have the right, and the duty, to decide when and if your child needs help.

Third, look to yourself as a possible contributing factor.

Before modern biological psychiatry began to destroy genuine family values of parental responsibility for children, it was assumed that parents had a great deal to do with how their children behave. If we saw a child who was out of control, we felt like chiding the parents to provide more rational discipline. If we saw a child who was hungry for attention, we wondered if the youngster was getting enough love at home. Conversely, if a child seemed especially mature or confident, we assumed he or she was getting something good from mom and dad.

The changes we need to make in ourselves as parents are never-ending as we get to know new aspects of our children's needs. You may have to spend your next weekend and maybe your next vacation rebuilding a relationship with your child—or perhaps building one for the first time. If your son is out of control, dad may have to do something radical—like finding an hour every day to do something with him that will build a relationship of caring, empathy, and mutual concern.

Fourth, remember that no one knows your child as well as you do.

A teacher who has your child in class or a doctor who sees your child in an office has only a limited view. Don't be bamboozled by diagnostic terminology. Remember, Attention Deficit-Hyperactivity Disorder, as fancy as it sounds, is largely a checklist of behaviors that reflect conflict between children and adults surrounding school and family life. If your child isn't focused on school work or doesn't listen very well at home, that's not a disease to be diagnosed by a doctor. How to view your children's behavior and what, if anything, to do about it must remain ultimately up to you.

Fifth, accept that each child needs something different from us as parents.

It's easy to justify ourselves as parents by saying, "I didn't have any trouble with Janie and Jimmy, so what's the matter with Joanie?" On the surface it seems to make sense: If you've raised five children without a serious problem, then there must be "something wrong" with the sixth who seems to have a lot of problems.

In reality, no two children are born into the same family. It has never happened. Except for twins, each child enters at a different time in the family's life. And even individual twins tend to react and to be treated differently. The family structure, including grandparents and siblings, is likely to be markedly different for each child. Parents themselves change with time and with new childrearing experiences.

Here's a key to parenting: Every child asks something different from us as parents. Who knows where all these differences in our children come from? Explanations vary from karma to genetics. I simply don't know the answer to how and why people are born and then grow up to be so different. I've puzzled over it and I just don't know. But I do know this: We cannot sit back smugly as parents thinking that the way we are is ready made for the way our kids are. It isn't so. We have to learn to adapt to our children, even to accommodate them at times.

Sixth, remember that having children is a sacred trust requiring a grateful, loving acceptance.

Especially in modern times we have begun to view our children as burdens. They cost too much and, worse, they take too much time. We want parenting to be more convenient. Like fast food or drive-thru tellers.

Being a parent is not convenient. It is very inconvenient. In fact, it is almost always far more inconvenient than the parents ever could have anticipated.

Sometimes we may regret how very inconvenient children can become. That's understandable. But we must not be driven by our desire to make parenting easier. Nurturing and guiding a human life should be accepted as one of the most deeply meaningful life experiences—something we cannot escape but can only embrace.

Seventh, rethink how you spend your private time with your child.

Above all things in life, your child needs a good relationship with you. Nothing is more important than frequent, regular, private, uninterrupted time between a parent and child. A child never outgrows the need for parental love and approval. I have seen parents in their seventies improve their grown children's lives by finally managing to build a good relationship with them. In large and busy families, it can be difficult to give each child periods of undivided attention but these times are central to every young person's development.

Your child needs times when he or she is the absolute center of your interest and attention. That doesn't mean taking your child shopping with you—unless perhaps it's what your child has chosen to do. It doesn't mean doing chores with your child. Making your child the center of your attention involves activities that the child desires and that encourage some degree of intimacy, like walking and hiking, talking and eating together, reading aloud together, playing together—just the two of you for the sake of your relationship.

The single most common denominator of children in trouble is the lack of a meaningful personal relationship with one or both parents. As you firm up your relationship with your child, you may also be able to communicate about the source of your children's problems.

If You Are Told That Your Child Has a Problem

It is often a shock when someone tells us that one of our children has a problem. With the escalating diagnosis of ADHD, many parents are confronting this for the first time. The following six principles are aimed at fortifying and further empowering you as a parent when someone says, "Your child has a problem."

First, carefully assess the situation to determine if you believe that your child has a problem or if instead your child is being held to an unrealistic or inappropriate standard.

As parents or teachers, it's easy to hold children to a standard that is too narrow or restrictive. When they don't meet our standards, we become impatient and frustrated. Meanwhile, children vary enormously in regard to their activity level, their impulsivity, their talkativeness, their self-centeredness, and their attention span. The children with the roughest edges may become the adults with the most to contribute. The children with the smoothest edges may suffer through life in quiet despair.

Second, children are almost always diagnosed ADHD and put on stimulants because they are in conflict with adults at school or at home. Beneath the conflict, the child may have important unmet needs.

Understanding the importance of conflict between children and adults is so central to helping children that I will devote an entire chapter to it. Conflicts can be overt and even physical, or they can be very subtle, waged beneath the surface over failures to meet the expectations of parents or teachers.

If we decide that our child does have a problem—that our child is inattentive, impulsive, and hyperactive—then our child needs *special attention* rather than drugs. Our task as a teacher, parent, or other caring adult is to identify the child's unmet needs and then to find ways to meet them.

Third, even if your child fits into the diagnosis ADHD, it does not mean that there is anything wrong with the youngster.

Children often meet the formal diagnostic criteria for ADHD without having anything at all wrong with them. When children find themselves in conflict with adults, they always display "symptoms." But when the conflicts are resolved, the child will usually respond. Sometimes the improvement in the child's outlook and conduct may occur almost overnight, sometimes it may take longer. It depends upon the depth of the psychological injury caused by the conflicts and the capacity of the parents and other adults to transform themselves to transcend the conflict.

In my experience, children who become psychiatrically labeled are often more energetic and more spirited than most. To fulfill their special promise, they need a more disciplined, interesting, and loving child-oriented environment. They may require more attention from us than other kids but they will also provide us more satisfaction. They are likely to become our most creative, outstanding and responsible members of society—providing we don't label, drug, and demoralize them before they grow up.

Fourth, if your child is already on Ritalin or any other psychiatric drug, as a parent you've lost control of the situation. It's time to retake your child from the experts and the drug companies.

You probably did not make the decision lightly to start your child on a psychiatric drug. You probably went along with medication because you were pressured to do so. You may have felt you were out of alternatives. You may have been frightened into believing that your child would fail in school and even in life without drugs. You were almost certainly misled into believing that the medications are more safe and effective than they are. It's time to regroup, to regain your moral commitment to yourself as your child's parent and advocate, and to determine that there must be other ways than drugging your child.

Giving drugs to children too often amounts to giving up on them. The teacher gives up figuring out better ways to teach and the parent gives up figuring out better ways to parent. This is because a stimulant, when it works, makes children less demanding. Remember, children on Ritalin are children who have gotten into conflict with adults. Don't "win the conflict" or give up on your child by going along with drugs.

Fifth, be cautious about abruptly removing your child from stimulant drugs, since withdrawal can produce dangerous reactions.

Remember that it can be dangerous to stop a child's stimulant medication too abruptly and without proper clinical and parental supervision. Children can become very emotionally disturbed, depressed, fatigued, and even suicidal when stopping Ritalin or other stimulants. They may also go through a temporary period of worsening behavior with increased hyperactivity, impulsivity, and inattentiveness. Some may even turn to illegal drugs to ease their discomfort. The longer the treatment and the higher doses, the greater the potential danger during withdrawal. While many children do well when these drugs are stopped, others will experience serious difficulties. Most important, parents should stay in close touch with how their child feels.

Withdrawal from psychiatric drugs, including stimulants for children, is described in my 1999 book co-authored with David Cohen, *Your Drug May Be Your Problem: How and Why to Stop Taking Psychiatric Medications.*

Sixth, seek help for yourself as a parent before sending your child for individual help.

If you've concluded that your child is having serious problems that could be helped by a professional intervention, start by seeking that intervention for yourself and for any other significant adults in the child's life. If you learn how you can help your child, it will be much more beneficial than having someone else try to do it. As a therapist, I'd rather see mom, dad, grandma, and grandpa, without the child, before bringing the child into family sessions. The point is to re-establish the basic truth—parents are responsible for children. When adults come up with a good plan for how to help a child, the child will respond.

In my clinical practice I never give guarantees, except in regard to preadolescent children. I can almost always guarantee parents that if they improve their capacity for unconditional love and for implementing a limited number of rational rules in their child's life, the child's sense of well-being will vastly improve. As the child feels better and learns from the parents about unconditional love and rational rules, the child will become more loving and rational.

One alternative is to join a parent effectiveness training group. As chapter 12 documented, a number of studies have shown that parent training can help parents improve their methods of dealing with their children and that this improves the child's "ADHD."

I favor family sessions with everyone who's actively involved with the child, including parents, older siblings, and significant relatives in the child's life. Don't label your child as the patient or the source of the problem; assume it's a family matter requiring change on everyone's part. If an older child, perhaps a high schooler, wants individual counseling or psychotherapy, then you probably should seek help for yourself as well, and go to sessions periodically with your teenager if at all possible.

Peter T. Oas (1997) is a Niceville, Florida, psychologist who has worked extensively with families with children diagnosed as ADHD. In helping families, Oas makes clear it's not useful to think in terms of blaming the parent. Nowadays family life itself is often "hyperactive" and stressed with both parents often preoccupied with making a living. Oas observes:

> These changes in families have caused a lot of attention to be placed on working and "doing" rather than listening and spending time together. It is very difficult for people to actually consciously schedule time to sit down and talk to each other. Not just to talk, but to listen more deeply and to search for causes of problems even though the causes are not readily apparent.

This is my experience as well. The couples I work with often seem to wait all week for the session before talking with each other about pressing matters. I have to remind them every week of the necessity of making their own intimate talking time together outside of sessions.

Getting the Best Help

I believe that the best professional help can be found through a counselor or therapist who is wise and experienced with children and with schools—someone who can help to empower you as a parent in dealing with your children and with the other adults in their lives. Often it will be difficult to find a professional who does not believe in ADHD/Ritalin. You may have to search for other parents who share your views and can support your efforts in helping your child. You may have to turn to reading books about parenting and child development. Parent training seminars may sometimes provide a better route than seeking a mental health professional.

It is unlikely that medically-trained professionals—such as a pediatrician, neurologist, or psychiatrist—will be able to provide you with help in your parenting. As discussed earlier in the book, they are often limited in the amount of time they can spend with individual patients. Have your child checked by a physician for genuine medical problems but not for "behavioral" disorders. Physicians, including psychiatrists, rarely have any special knowledge about family conflict resolution, unconditional love, rational discipline, and identifying and fulfilling the basic needs of children. As a medically-trained psychiatrist, it saddens me to have to say all this, but it's the truth.

You are more likely to receive real help from a counselor, psychologist, social worker, or family therapist whose orientation is toward empowering your parenting rather than to diagnosing and drugging your child.

Form a Parent Reading Group

There are a wide variety of useful parenting books, literally shelves of them to choose from in any large book store. I favor two classics that are still readily available, Thomas Gordon's (1970) *P.E.T.: Parent Effectiveness Training* and Haim Ginott's *Between Parent and Child* (1969). Any parent can benefit from these approaches to children that emphasize conflict resolution, love, reasonableness, and gentleness. My recent book, *The Heart of Being Helpful: Empathy and the Role of a Healing Presence* (1997b) shows how we can become more helpful people in every aspect of our professional and family lives.

The more recent STEP series are already classics, including Don Dinkmeyer, Sr., Gary D. McKay, and Don Dinkmeyer, Jr. (1997), *The Parent's Handbook*. STEP stands for Systematic Training for Effective Parenting. Picking from a number of other books, you might try Peter Williamson (1990), *Good Kids, Bad Behavior*, and Adele Faber and Elaine Mazlish (1980), *How To Talk So Kids Will Listen & Listen So Kids Will Talk*. For a rather lengthy in-depth formulation of principles and practical applications, readers may want to check out Stephen R. Covey's new book, *The 7 Habits of Highly Effective Families* (1997).

Educator Michael Valentine's books (1987 & 1988) are written for teachers and counselors. However, they can also provide parents with valuable guidelines for how to establish effective communication that will achieve positive results with children. Parents may find Valentine's *How to Deal with Difficult Discipline Problems: A Family Systems Approach* (1988) especially useful.

Some of these books also provide information on locating parent training courses and workshops. As many of the authors emphasize, parenting is one of the few jobs for which there's no formal training, yet parenting is one of the hardest jobs to perform without guidance and help.

If you read a few of these books carefully and discuss them with other adults and with your children, you may develop a better background in how to parent than the average psychiatrist, family doctor, or pediatrician. Their professional training does not necessarily include any practical books on parenting.

Rather than going to a seminar on ADHD, you would be much better off creating a parent's reading group starting with the books by Gordon, Ginott, Dinkmeyer, and Valentine, bolstered perhaps by this book as well. Meeting with loving, concerned, responsible parents regularly to discuss the joys and the trials of parenting, with reading based on solid principles, should be helpful to any parent.

Words from Ginger

As I began writing this book, Ginger Breggin made some notes on her thoughts. They came unedited from the heart:

We probably all have some visions, as new parents holding our new infant, of our child's future. It is most likely stereotypical of our cultural expectations—but probably includes academic competence, if not excellence, a degree of popularity, a child moving step by step through the stages and grades of schools. We vow we will ensure our child gets a good college education if we had the same opportunity and especially if we did not. Perhaps we value athletic excellence, or dance, or music, and recognize its potential for providing an education through scholarships.

So often I've heard a person exclaim over a toddler, "You are such a big boy—I'll bet you'll be a football player." And if the boy is tall, then a basketball player. If it's a girl and she's beautiful, she may be told she can model. Some children may adore the opportunities provided by their parents. Others may be disinterested or may even hate what their parents want them to do. Spirited children may refuse in principle to pursue their parents' ambitions for them.

Very early in our child's development, we have to begin to separate out what we want for our child from what our child wants, and is inclined toward and capable of doing. We have to start to really see our child as a separate, discrete individual. And we may watch our private vision of their future as it smashes on the rock of reality. It may be that the child we hoped would excel at sports or dance or music hates anything competitive or public, and wants to work alone with computers. Or the daughter we wanted to be a model shrinks away from being the center of attention. Or the child who was going to carry on the family academic traditions only wants to "get through school" so he can go to work.

Hopefully, by the time our children are adults, especially given enough love and positive attention while growing up, we will recognize them as being our offspring. We will be able to take pride in their accomplishments, marvel at their personal interests, and enjoy their passions and their happiness. But to reach that point, our child will need the room to grow in his or her own directions, loved and supported by parents wise enough to open their hand and let the bird fly free.

Chapter 18

THE ENVIRONMENTAL
STRESSOR CHECKLIST

How to Find Out What's Upsetting Your Child

The Important Job of Being a Parent: For many years children's teachers, counselors, and day-care providers have had training to do their jobs. Yet the idea of parents needing education to become better mothers and fathers was not widespread.

This is no longer true. Society has begun to value the job of parenting more and more. After all, parents are the most important people in children's lives!

—Don Dinkmeyer, Sr., Gary D. McKay, and Don Dinkmeyer, Jr.,
The Parent's Handbook (1997)

Instead of a symptom checklist that focuses on the child's supposed "disorder," parents need a situations checklist that focuses on stressors in the child's environment to help in identifying the causes behind a child's seemingly disturbed or disturbing behavior. It is almost always best to view a child's "symptoms" as a natural or normal reaction to frustrating, humiliating, threatening, dangerous, or overwhelming circumstances. Instead of diagnosing and drugging the child, we can then focus on understanding and empowering the child, while doing our best to improve the child's circumstances in life.

Environmental Stressor Checklist for Children
I. Stressors in the Family

1. Lack or loss of love, closeness, or attention from a parent or other significant adult.

Many of the stressors in this list have much of their impact through causing a loss of love and attention in the child's life. The loss can be caused by stresses in the adult's life: emotional problems, job loss or chronic unemployment, marital problems, alcohol or substance abuse, or physical illness. School or job obligations, including military assignment, may remove the parent from the home. A parent who withdraws emotionally can have at least as devastating an impact on a child as a parent who leaves outright. Significant adults living in the household can play a major role in a child's life, including extended family, family friends, teachers, coaches, ministers and priests, babysitters, nannies, and housekeepers. Often "domestic help" become a major influence in a small child's life and end up providing more nurturing than the parents. Loss of their love and attention can also be devastating.

2. Death of a parent or parent figure.

When someone in the family dies, children need to be able to express their grief, pain, and confusion. Too often a child is left to go through bereavement without emotional support while the adults tend to take care of each other.

3. The sickness or death of a sibling or friend.

The illness or loss of a sibling can impact on the parents in ways that affect all their remaining and future children. Many of my clients date their problems to when a brother or sister became ill or died. These events transformed their parents' attitudes and even emotional stability. Not only through parental reactions but through a direct impact on the child, the death of a sibling can cause overwhelming sadness, loneliness, guilt feelings, or fright over dying. The death of a childhood friend or acquaintance can also have more importance than parents sometimes realize.

4. Death or departure of a pet.

For some children, pets become a tremendous source of shared love. Their loss can leave a lasting mark on a child's development. If the child blames the death on himself or herself, or on the parents, then the bereavement is complicated by feelings of guilt, anger, fear, and betrayal.

5. Discord, conflict, separation, or divorce of the parents.

Parents usually hope to shield a child from their conflicts but they cannot. Hostility between parents cannot be hidden and is very destructive to children. Often children feel helpless, hopeless, and alienated in the face of conflict between their parents. I have seen too many children given psychiatric drugs in the midst of acrimonious divorces. Instead, children need to feel that their own security will not be destroyed by the conflict.

6. Domestic violence.

Children feel terrified, helpless, guilty, and humiliated when one of their parents or another sibling is physically abused. Often they feel that they are to blame. Keep in mind that *witnessing* abuse can have at least as negative an impact on children as directly enduring it.

7. Physical, sexual, or emotional abuse by a parent.

The abuse of children is common but often undetected. When biological psychiatrists state that they can find no problems in many of the families of very disturbed children, this does not prove anything. Abuse can be hard to spot and it can take place outside the family.

8. Confused or contradictory parenting practices.

There is a tendency among ADHD/Ritalin advocates to believe that it takes obvious neglect, abuse, and other extreme parental misdeeds in order to adversely affect a child's outlook and behavior. In reality, children can be hurt by subtle problems in parenting. Contradictions may occur between the parents or they may stem from inconsistencies within the individual parent. Often parents pass on the abusive practices of their own parents without sufficiently questioning them. Instead of perpetuating them, we need to learn from the mistakes of our parents.

9. Physical, sexual, or emotional abuse by siblings.

Although often overlooked, older children can easily victimize younger ones through ridicule and intimidation, as well as by sexual and physical abuse. Many women whom I know personally and through my clinical practice have been sexually abused by older brothers.

Most of my clients are surprised by how easily they begin to recall episodes of severe ridicule, including unmerciful tickling, at the hands of older children. Sometimes children are given humiliating nicknames that they cannot escape. Frequently there is a pervasive style of belittling language toward children.

10. Major changes in the family structure.

Major changes in the family include the birth or adoption of a sibling, remarriage, and the entrance of another adult into a previously one-parent household, often accompanied by additional children. Many children never fully recover from these unwanted transformations in their lives. They remain resentful, withdrawn, and anxious.

11. Inattention and neglect.

There is a spectrum of degrees of abandonment with lack of attention on one end and outright rejection on the other. Parental inattention and neglect are common in modern families in which a single working parent may be the head of household or in which two parents are working or otherwise occupied outside the home. Infants and children need a great deal of loving attention, holding, and comforting.

Poverty places stresses on parents that can lead to inattention and neglect. Lack of mental stimulation during infancy and childhood may delay cognitive and social development. Sometimes one parent is much more inattentive and neglectful, and that parent's influence may sully the child's entire childhood experience.

12. Personality clashes and conflicts with a parent.

Many of the children seen by therapists are in conflict with their parents due, in part, to differences in personality and communication style. When we choose a spouse or friend, we can avoid people with whom we have "nothing in common" or with whom we can't seem to get along. As parents, we have to deal with whatever personality the child brings into the family.

13. Envy from parents and siblings.

While it has received little attention, envy frequently has a devastating impact on a child's attitudes toward success, including school achievement. Parents and siblings alike can direct withering envy at a youngster who is especially attractive, daring, bright, creative, or successful. To ward off these threats from others in the family, the envied child will often inhibit his or her own growth and development.

People are rarely aware of being envied in their own families. It is too devastating to be allowed into consciousness. Without realizing it, many people denigrate their own skills and put down their own achievements to avoid the envy directed at them as children. Often the envied child will also be envied as an adult in the family.

14. Witnessing someone else's suffering.

Although this category overlaps several others, it emphasizes that any suffering witnessed by a child can inflict emotional damage that manifests as items on the ADHD checklist or symptoms of emotional distress. Children can be exposed to suffering when living with a parent who is afflicted by a chronic, painful disease, such as arthritis or cancer. They may see emotional suffering among other children in the neighborhood or school, and they may watch it on television and in the movies. Great distress can be generated by witnessing a child or an animal being beaten up, burned, or otherwise injured. What seems to be everyday life on a farm with the routine slaughter of animals can fill a child with torment.

15. Illness in the child.

Physical illness in a child can have many adverse effects, including physical and emotional pain, loss of contact with friends, removal from the family, and fear of death. If the illness involves a physical or mental disability, it can result in labeling and stigmatization that scars the child's spirit.

16. Changing neighborhoods and schools.

Children understandably have difficulty with change. In therapy, adults often date downturns in their childhood to times when their family moved. Frequent moves during childhood can cause innumerable difficulties relating to other people and to school.

17. Family isolation.

Some families live in relative isolation, cutting off their children from normal relationships with neighbors and friends, fostering paranoia and fearfulness. Isolation is often associated with incest, alcoholism and drug addiction, and with severe emotional problems in the parents.

18. Loss of childhood.

The loss of childhood is rarely defined as a stressor but it has become commonplace in the lives of modern children. Today's child is given much less time to be child-like, to play, and to grow up at his or her own rate.

Parents also lose out when their children don't get to be children. One of the joys of parenthood is having fun playing with our children. Instead of something frivolous, play should be viewed as one of the most important and highly cherished aspects of being with our children.

II. Stressors Outside the Family

1. Institutionalization and placement.

Children are placed in a variety of potentially harmful institutional settings, including mental hospitals, special schools or other facilities for delinquents or the developmentally disabled, and jails. Foster placement, depending on the circumstances, can have similar effects. So can preschool and day care programs. Poorly run or abusive settings can lower a child's self-esteem and respect for adults. They can cause emotional suffering and teach destructive behaviors.

Summer vacations with relatives, overnight camp, school trips, and other excursions away from home are a frequent source of child abuse that parents fail to perceive. They may dismiss the child's complaints as "being spoiled" or "being homesick." My patients, to their own surprise, frequently discover that they were sexually or emotionally abused by camp counselors or relatives during summer separations from home without their parents having any idea about it.

2. Psychiatric stigmatization.

Being labeled learning disabled or ADHD, as well as being diagnosed with more severe disorders, can wreck a child's self-esteem and cause a worsening of behavior. Being removed from the mainstream in school, even for only an hour or two each day, can be humiliating. As Louise Armstrong (1993) described, psychiatric hospitalization can devastate a child.

In my initial evaluation of children, I am often able to reassure them that they have nothing wrong with them, and it always makes them joyful and more willing to learn from me and to work with their parents in improving their family life.

3. Physical, sexual, and emotional abuse at the hands of adults.

Newspaper reports make clear that adults in any position of authority—relatives, teachers, coaches, ministers and priests, day care personnel, babysitters—may take advantage of children. Out of fear, guilt, confusion, and humiliation, most children do not report to their parents even life-threatening encounters with adults. Abuse can also take much more subtle forms in how children are spoken to and looked at. Young girls, for example, are frequently exposed to disturbing leers and gestures from men.

Very often parents assume that the teachers, coaches, or ministers in a child's life would never be abusive. Unfortunately, it's untrue—authorities frequently take advantage of children emotionally and sexually. It's also easy to miss what's going on. Adolescent and adult abusers are not easy to spot. A very meek-looking man can turn out to be a pedophile.

The best way to prevent adults from abusing your child is to express obvious and unflagging interest in your child to every adult with whom your child has any contact. Abusers tend to stay away from children who have strong, involved parents. They're afraid of being found out by them.

4. Peer abuse.

Although much less recognized than abuse by adults, abuse by peers can cause severe emotional suffering. As I describe in *Reclaiming Our Children* (2000), most or all school shooters have been subjected to extreme humiliation by the peers before becoming violent. Such abuse is commonplace in our schools.

More dominant boys and girls may pick on a peer to intimidate, humiliate, and sometimes to physically and sexually abuse. Even in seemingly well-supervised schools, children will frequently gang up on an isolated child who seems vulnerable or who makes them feel jealous. The harassment can make a child's life seem unbearable. Out of humiliation, fear, or hopelessness, children rarely communicate about these threats to adults. When alerted to them, adults too often dismiss the report as "kid stuff."

5. Conflict with teachers, tutors, and coaches.

Even brief exposures to suppressive or disturbed teachers, and other educators, can harm a child. Often the child will hide the experiences from parents. Children always tend to feel humiliated, to blame themselves, and to become secretive when they have been abused.

6. Stressful schooling experiences.

This general term—stressful schooling—is meant to cover the spectrum of the frustration and suffering that seems endemic to schooling in America, including overworked and overwhelmed teachers, inadequate instructional materials, too large classes, undisciplined and dangerous classrooms, and lack of individualized attention. For many, if not most children, the school experience is a chronic stressor. Most adults can easily recall school experiences—often with particular teachers, coaches, or peers—that still evoke shame or anxiety years later. Sometimes these memories, when openly faced, can help us to be more sensitive in dealing with the school experiences of our own children.

7. Religious terrors and scruples.

Most religions teach love for children. They view children as divine gifts and treasures. Nonetheless, some expressions of religious devotion can frighten children and make them feel unnecessarily guilty. Children often take what they hear very concretely or literally. In my clinical practice, I have worked with adults who were terrified as children that momentarily they would be swallowed up into hell for having a "bad" thought. Keep in mind that children are very impressionable and easily overcome with anxiety, shame, and guilt.

8. Terrifying "entertainment."

Recently, the movie "Jurassic Park" and its sequel were criticized for exposing small children to dinosaurs devouring people. At least as far back as the original "Wizard of Oz," small children have been terrified by movies created for their entertainment. Even the movie "ET" about the charming visitor from Outer Space can cause terrors and nightmares for preschoolers. These experiences can be very traumatic, in part because the child encounters them in an open and vulnerable state with the expectation of having fun. The child may also be unable to draw a line between a movie and real life. The effects of even a single traumatic movie can last for months and, to some degree, for years. Constant exposure to violence, racism, and sexism on TV and in the movies can have a damaging effect on people of any age but especially on the young.

9. Catastrophic events and accidents.

War, genocide, epidemics, floods, hurricanes and tornadoes, and other catastrophic events directly traumatize a significant portion of the world's children. Others are traumatized through exposure to them on television. In America, many children are exposed to terrifying automobile accidents and to street violence in urban areas. In general, modern children are exposed to much more real life violence than in prior decades. They often know other children who have been killed or injured. Many also experience near-drowning, severe burns, and other accidents.

Many others have an acute awareness of the ever-present dangers portrayed in the media—everything from environmental disasters to terrorist bombings. Much more than past generations of children, the modern child has a global awareness and hence global fears. Remember, children live in the same world as we do and often share our fears.

10. Unsafe communities and exposure to violence.

More and more commonly, even outside the inner city, children grow up with intense exposures to violence. Violence and fears of violence can foster post-traumatic stress disorder with ADHD-like symptoms.

11. Racism, sexism, pedism, and religious persecution.

All children are chronically exposed to pedism—prejudice against children.[1] They are also vulnerable to racism, sexism, and religious persecution. Children are often taunted for membership in minority groups and religions. Often they will not report these experiences to their parents or to anyone else.

12. Poverty.

One-quarter of America's children are estimated to live in poverty, increasing the likelihood of their exposure to almost all the family and community stressors in this list, plus substandard education and health care, and alienation from the larger American community. The richest nation in the western world, we are the poorest in terms of the support we provide to children, and to families with children. Many children lack adequate health care, nutrition, and education. It would be immoral to provide more psychiatric drugs to the children of the poor rather than addressing the deplorable conditions under which most of them now grow up.

III. Pharmacological and Medical Stressors

This heading is a reminder to evaluate a child for medical problems, prescription and non-prescription drug effects, and substance abuse whenever there is a significant worsening in the child's outlook or behavior, or increasing conflict at home or in school. Chapter 13 lists many prescription and illicit drugs, as well as physical disorders, that can cause ADHD-like symptoms.

You may think your child is too young to be "experimenting" with drugs. Think again. Nowadays, if children are in elementary school, they can be in danger of being exposed to and being enticed into trying drugs.

Responding to the Environmental Stressor Checklist

In making use of the environmental stressor checklist, a number of principles may be useful:

First, children are not likely to spontaneously inform an adult about stresses they have undergone. Typically, if the stressor is brought to light, the child will deny its existence or not realize its importance.

Second, children need a great deal of encouragement to talk about stressful or traumatic events. Young children may have to be approached indirectly, through play, making up stories, or other imaginative techniques. A very simple technique is to draw pictures with a child or to make up stories, and then to talk about them.

Third, look for changes in the child's personality, attitudes, or behavior that coincide with a stressor.

Fourth, be alert to any changes in your child's life, from new friends to a new teacher, and try to be aware of your child's feelings about the changes.

A glance through this list of stressors is likely to leave parents feeling somewhat discouraged and wondering "How can we, as parents, keep our children safe?" The unfortunate answer is that we can't. However, we can do our best to maximize the safety of our children without frightening or isolating them. Parents will also wonder, "How can I find out what's upsetting my child?" Once again, the answer isn't reassuring. Often we cannot figure out what's bothering or even terrifying our children. The truth is that our children, like most, will grow up dealing with an infinite variety of stressors that they can't identify for themselves or that they will consciously hide from us.

What More Can Parents Do?

Most importantly, be a presence in your child's relationships with older children and with adults. Get to know the babysitter. Get to know the babysitter's mother and father. Get to know the teacher. Make clear to the teacher that you have a close relationship with your child. If your child goes away from home on a visit or vacation, talk a great deal in advance with the responsible adults about how closely you plan to stay in touch with your child. While by no means a complete protection, it is very helpful to let everyone who deals with your child know that you're involved with your child and that you're someone to be reckoned with.

Notice the changing expressions on your children's faces from day to day. Listen not only to their words, but to the tone of voice and the inflection that signals something is amiss. Don't be put off when your child acts like he or she doesn't want to be asked about what's going wrong. Ask as gently as you can, persist in asking and observe more closely if the suffering seems to persist. Especially with younger children who won't be humiliated by a parental intervention, be a "private detective" on your child's behalf—find out what's going on from other children or adults.

If you discover that your child is being hurt or frightened by someone, it is almost always wrong to let the youngster try to handle it without parental intervention. Children should not be left to struggle alone with an intimidating babysitter, a school bully, an abusive older sibling, or an insensitive teacher. If your child is old enough and mature enough to discuss why he or she doesn't want you to intervene, by all means listen to your child's viewpoint. But make an adult decision about whether or not you need to intervene.

Our goal should be to provide our children with as ethical and as loving a relationship as possible. If we can develop a close and trusting way of being with our children, they are more likely to share their fears and upsets with us, and to accept our advice, direction, or help. Even if they don't open up with us, they will gain strength from knowing that they are respected and loved by us as their parents. Hopefully, they will also find us useful as models for how to handle stress without becoming overwhelmed and without losing track of ethical, loving conduct. Once again, regardless of the intensity of the stressors in their lives, our children need us to be as good parents as we can be. Our children need us—lots of us.

Chapter 19

MAKING OURSELVES READY TO HELP OUR CHILDREN

Love is born when the child rests in its mother's arms. From this beginning, love grows until it includes the love of family and friends, of school and country, and ultimately of all the world... Love is all of one piece—from the love of mother and child to the love of sweethearts, husbands and wives, and friends. It is present, too, in the laborer's devotion to his work, in the teacher's solicitude for her pupils, in the physician's dedication to his art. All that heals, cultivates, protects, and inspires—all this is part of love.

—Smiley Blanton, psychiatrist (1956)

There is one single most important guiding principle in helping a child: To create a loving relationship with the child.[1] Whether we are trying to be good parents, teachers, coaches, or older brothers and sisters, the caring relationship is the essential ingredient. Everything else flows, or fails to flow, from the quality of the relationship between ourselves as adults and the children we are trying to help. Compared to a positive relationship, everything else pales in importance. Without a loving relationship, nothing else can succeed.

The existence of a loving relationship can never be taken for granted. Often I hear adults dismiss the importance of love by assuming that parents or teachers have a caring, treasuring relationship with the children in their care. Despite the best of intentions, it often isn't so.

How do we know if we've succeeded in creating a caring relationship? Accept that we never quite succeed. An adult's relationship with a child is always a work in progress. We can best measure our success by the child's response to us and to life.

What Is Love?

This chapter begins with an eloquent quote about love from Smiley Blanton, a psychiatrist who worked closely with the famous minister Norman

Vincent Peale. Blanton believes, as I do, that love inspires the successful work of parents, teachers, and physicians alike.

Love is the central principle of relationship and healing. I have defined love as a *joyful awareness* that generates *reverence, treasuring,* and *caring*.[2] When we remain joyfully aware of children, and treat them with reverence, treasuring, and care, we are at our best. This kind of love is unconditional. It can be regenerated throughout the ups and downs of parent-child relationships. Its regeneration is a parent's key task when undergoing frustration and difficulty with a child.

Is Love Enough?

ADHD/Ritalin advocates frequently contend that love is not enough. They assume that most children have enough love and that more is not needed. While there's more to parenting than expressing love—without love, nothing else is going to make much difference. Being loved is the foundation of a child's life. Giving love is the essential starting point of parenting. Beyond that it helps for a parent or teacher to have solid principles and skills for carrying out the difficult jobs of parenting and teaching.

Beginning with Ourselves to Help a Child

Instead of trying to *do* something to children, we should try to *be* something to them. We must find the resources within *ourselves* to *invite* that child into a relationship. Sometimes this will require creating a new relationship, sometimes improving an old one. But the efforts will be fruitless unless the child embraces the relationship and thrives within it.

That is the art of being a parent, teacher, or other significant adult in the life of children—learning to welcome vulnerable children into meaningful relationships, and understanding how the world affects them for better or worse. As parents, we should, whenever possible, seek help for ourselves rather than for our children. Especially when a child is preadolescent, we can do much more than any other person to improve our child's life. If we don't feel competent for the task, we may need to involve other adults directly in our child's life in the form of, for example, another relative, a volunteer Big Brother, or a therapist. But whenever we seek advice or help, we must make sure to keep our child's best interests as the main criteria.

Changing Ourselves to Help Our Children

Parents should be cautious about placing a preadolescent child in individual psychotherapy. While sometimes beneficial, placing a child in individual therapy can distract from the fundamental need to improve the quality of parenting and teaching in the child's life. Focusing on the child as the patient makes the child feel responsible for the family crisis. It can encourage lifelong dependence on therapy.

Often children are sent to therapists to improve their self-esteem or to provide them with a supportive relationship, roles that properly belong to a parent. While the parent may feel relieved and grateful to have the help, the parent's identity is chipped away.

As a therapist and psychiatrist, I try *not* to become the central helping person in the child's life. Instead, I help the parents and the teachers in their efforts to relate to the child. Children can gain much more from the adults with whom they live, learn, and play than from periodic meetings with a therapist. This cannot be said enough: All adults in a troubled or troubling child's life need to revitalize their personal commitment to parenting and to teaching rather than to finding fault with the child. The first step is recognizing the necessity of changing ourselves rather than the child—a major task for us as parents and teachers when we feel frustrated, harassed, angry, and overwhelmed.

Treasuring the Child

Remember my definition of love: a *joyful awareness* that generates *reverence, treasuring,* and *caring.* When we set out to create a helpful relationship with a child, we must focus with all our heart on the child's emotional, spiritual, and educational needs rather than our own. All children need to feel treasured by at least one adult in their lives; preferably, by several.

If your child is troubled, first tend to your relationship with the youngster. If you can remember and implement this principle—that everything beneficial begins with creating or improving a relationship—you will start in the right direction. If you don't know how to begin anew, then get help from a friend, relative, or counselor—but not from a physician armed with diagnoses and drugs.

The books described in chapter 17 can also be useful in helping parents to focus on principles of conflict resolution rather than domination and control. My own book, *The Heart of Being Helpful,* emphasizes how to change ourselves in order to become a healing presence for the people in our lives.

When to Discipline

Once you have begun to renew or to develop your relationship with your child, you can begin to discuss issues of discipline and responsibility with the child. In the absence of a relationship with you that is meaningful to the child, efforts to impose discipline will be experienced as unfair punishments that only breed more antagonism and resistance.

You can negotiate the necessary limits or boundaries that all children need by approaching the child in a rational, open-minded fashion. While you hold the ultimate decision-making power as a parent, you can learn to develop more democratic means of arriving at mutually agreeable solutions. It is astonishing how often children will respond to a parent with rational suggestions of their own about discipline and setting limits.

Probably you will find that your child needs fewer limits, rules, and regulations than you have thought a good parent should implement. But you will also find that your child needs a *few basic principles* implemented consistently. These principles begin with showing mutual respect for each other—parents toward children, and children toward parents. Respect is at the root of discipline. The first thing I teach to couples and families is the necessity of treating each other with respect. Individuals of any age only feel safe and imperative when they are treated with respect. Other essential rules have to do with health and safety.

Begin with discussion and negotiation. Emphasize the importance of mutual respect and a few rules pertinent to safety and to health. Beyond that, be patient. A child who feels loved will eventually prosper.

ADHD/Ritalin approaches sometimes emphasize teaching parenting skills to parents. But they almost always focus on getting a child to change behavior, especially in regard to issues of discipline. It's far better to begin with creating a more loving environment in which mutual respect is encouraged.

Rewards and punishments? Punishments are generally counterproductive in raising children. They achieve the opposite result of what's intended by causing fear and resentment. Punishments encourage children to hide their angry feelings and their misdeeds. A child who lies or manipulates a lot is a child who is afraid and distrustful. The goal is not to punish but to overcome the child's fear and distrust through a more loving, safe relationship.

Children sometimes rebel even more against rewards than punishments because they realize that the rewards are contrived and that they replace a genuine relationship. In their outrage at not feeling loved, spirited or proud children will fight, kick, scream, and defy adults even at the risk of being beaten to death. Kids see through behavioral tactics right away. They see the same lack of relationship. The job of parenting is much more the job of relationship building than punishing and rewarding or otherwise "controlling the child."

Entrenched Conflicts between Adults and Children

By the time parents feel desperate enough to turn to doctors and to drugs, something has gone desperately wrong with their relationship to the child. The adults usually feel like failures, at least around the sources of conflict. In this vulnerable state, parents can easily be manipulated by professionals who promise to exonerate them and to provide quick or easy cures. They may be tempted to accept an explanation that finds the fault or defect in the child.

The answer is not to do something to the child but to reaffirm our dedication as a parent or teacher to building a meaningful relationship with the child—a relationship that begins with respectful relating and progresses to unconditional love and treasuring.

If the child is identified as the sole cause of the difficulty, all is lost. Harmful things will be done to the child, including psychiatric diagnosis and drugs.

For All Children

It makes no essential difference whether the children we are trying to help are so withdrawn that they have been diagnosed "autistic," or so angry and rebellious that they've been labeled "oppositional defiant disorder," or so inattentive, hyperactive, and impulsive that they've been labeled "ADHD." If anything, the more seemingly disturbed and disturbing a child has become, the more the child needs, *above all else*, to have a mutually respectful, caring relationship with a mature adult.

Many parents and professionals have come to a similar conclusion in regard to autistic children.[3] There are also many clinical reports and some controlled research projects showing that patients labeled schizophrenic do better without psychiatric drugs in a safe, loving, rational environment.[4]

When children do suffer from brain disorders affecting their ability to learn, these principles become even more important. Parents of children who have impaired brain function are very susceptible to pressure from professionals to medicate or to institutionalize them. One of my friends has a child with Down's syndrome. With loving care and careful guidance, this child has become bilingual and graduated from high school. He can even use a computer! Knowing that psychiatric drugs could only further impair his already compromised brain function,[5] the parents rely entirely on psychological, social, and educational approaches.

Even youngsters with known brain disabilities and with the most serious diagnoses can benefit from psychosocial and educational approaches without drugs. Certainly children labeled ADHD deserve the same drug-free caring human approaches to their conflicts and difficulties at home and in school.

The vast majority of children labeled ADHD are simply in conflict with their parents and teachers. They aren't seriously disturbed children. Often they aren't even seriously disturbing. If their present conflicts can be resolved, the likelihood of their developing new and more severe ones in adulthood is greatly diminished.

Talked out of the Truth

Mental health specialists have talked teachers and parents out of the timeless truths of parental and community responsibility for the quality of life of their children. They have instead created diagnostic categories of children who are then seen as incorrigible, that is, as untouchable by ordinary human means. This is good for the business of doctoring and the business of selling drugs. It may make life easier for some parents and teachers. But it is very bad for children.

Often parents are talked out of the truth because they don't know how to implement their intuitive knowledge about the importance of their way of relating to their children. Creating a relationship or improving a relationship with a child is a matter of rational *conflict resolution* within the context of a safe, mutually respectful relationship. The next chapter will deal more specifically with resolving conflict between parents and children.

Chapter 20

WHEN ADULTS ARE IN CONFLICT WITH
THE CHILDREN THEY LOVE

Good families—even great families—are off track 90 percent of the time!
They key is that they have a sense of destination. They know what the
"track" looks like. And they keep coming back to it time and time again.

—Stephen R. Covey, *The 7 Habits of Highly Effective Families* (1997)

It comes as a revelation to parents, locked in by tradition to… the "win-
lose" power methods of resolving conflicts, that they do have an alternative. Almost without exception, parents are relieved to learn that there is
a third method.… The alternative is the "no-lose" method of resolving
conflicts—where nobody loses.

—Thomas Gordon, *P.E.T.: Parent Effectiveness Training* (1970)

Conflict, even serious conflict, is a part of family life. Parental efforts to
stifle conflict lead to much that goes wrong in families. Severe conflict is a sign of unmet needs. As I describe in *Beyond Conflict* (1992), conflict resolution is always best achieved by finding mutually beneficial ways of
meeting everyone's needs.

Conflict Is Normal

Children and adults routinely come into conflict with one another. Any
parent who tries to run a scout troop, coach a team, or assist on a class out-
ing knows how hard a task it is to manage even a small group of children.
Parents with several children, or parents who routinely help out with other
children, face the same challenge. Parents with an especially active, energetic, demanding, creative, or independent child may also feel their personal resources tested on a daily basis. They may feel, "My child's like a mob of
children."

From toddlers to teenagers, children and youngsters in groups quickly
become bored and restless, and sometimes antagonistic. Feeling ill or hungry,
having to go to the bathroom, and missing their parents are among their

numerous and sometimes unexpected needs. The adult in charge will often feel tested by the need to be a combination of loving parent, stern disciplinarian, ideal teacher, and recreation director.

The ADHD/Ritalin movement tells us that when adults are having a difficult time with a particular child, it's time to evaluate and to treat the child. But there's a better model—a more effective paradigm or lens—with which to examine the overall situation. When having difficulty managing, teaching, or raising a child, it's useful for adults to think in terms of resolving *conflicts* rather than enforcing compliance.

As adults, it's our job to figure out the cause of the conflicts we have with children. Usually, we will have to find new approaches to meeting one or more of the child's basic needs for unconditional love, rational and consistent discipline, inspired education, and play.

Born to Be a Good Child?

Happy, well-functioning children aren't born that way. They are nurtured with careful discipline, loving care, and proper education. The infant requires the attention of adults, ideally in an extended family, in order to mature into a small child who is recognizable as a functioning human being. The small child needs additional help from parents, teachers, older siblings, peers, and a wide variety of adults. No child has ever traversed the normal developmental stages without continued help from adults.

Born to Be a Good Parent?

Similarly, no one is born into being a well-functioning parent. It requires enormous energy, thought, self-discipline, patience, and love to successfully raise a human being through infancy and adolescence into young adulthood. Parenthood, like childhood, is a process.

Hopefully we mature as we grow older. Learning to handle conflict in a more rational and loving manner is the essence of maturity. But just when we think we've got it down pat, our children and their emerging lives present us with new challenges. For many of us, the challenge nowadays persists long after the anticipated period of childhood. Our young adult children continue to require our guidance and, often, our economic support.

Unfortunately, very few children or adults receive any formal training in parenting or in conflict resolution. Most adults stumble blindly into the hardest job they will ever undertake. The average mother devotes much more time to prenatal care than to preparing to be a mother to a living child. Similarly, the average modern father spends more time in birthing classes learning to help mom breathe during labor than he does in classes learning how to raise the child once it's born. This is not the fault of the parents—it's built into the society. Parenting is taken for granted when in reality it requires more effort than any other task or responsibility.

Surveys have shown that more than 50 percent of new parents leaving the hospital don't feel competent to raise their first child. Later on, more than 50 percent feel stressed and "worn out" by the time the child is three. Half of parents worry about doing something wrong and wonder if they are being good parents.[1] No wonder parents are often so quick to turn to experts when they are having trouble relating to their child. No wonder they are so seemingly eager to accept medication shortcuts.

What Should We Expect of Children?

Usually children are diagnosed and drugged because they are creating difficulties. Every one of the "behaviors" listed in the ADHD diagnosis are associated with children who seem to be making it harder for parents or teachers to carry on as they wish. Much of it comes down to conformity or compliance.

To what degree should we expect children to be docile and submissive? The answer depends on many factors: the purpose of the group, the length of time that we expect them to remain quiet and still, the time of day, the size of the group, the physical comfort of the chairs, the physical comfort of the room, the age of the children, the quality of the activities provided to them, the quality of the adult supervision, and the number of disturbing or disturbed children and adults in the room.

We also need to know about the individual children before deciding if they should be able to sit still and silent for a lengthy period of time in a group. How old are they? Are they near to each other in age and in their level of maturity? Do they have any illnesses or physical disabilities? Are they used to this kind of enforced group silence and stillness? Do they see it as a punishment or welcome it as an opportunity to concentrate? Are they hungry? Are they anxious? Do they have to go to the bathroom? What has their day been like? Have they already been given opportunities to play spontaneously with each other, to visit together, and to burn off physical energy? What can they look forward to for the rest of the day?

We also need to know about the adults who are in charge of the children. Are there enough adults to easily and effectively handle this size group of this age children? Are they experienced and do they have a good activity plan? What's the mental state of each of the caretaking adults? What sort of "vibes"—emotional messages—are they giving off to the children? Do they like what they are doing? Do they love children? Are they experienced in these situations? Do they have a clear enough purpose and the skills and materials to fulfill it? What sort of back up resources do they have if they need help in dealing with the group?

These questions have real meaning. An adult who is planning or running a day care center, summer camp, school, sports team, or class must address these questions if the project is to serve the real needs of the children.

We need an enormous amount of information about the entire situation, as well as about the adults and each individual child, before deciding that a "disorder" in the child is causing a child to make noise or to otherwise require adult attention. It is usually impossible to diagnose the nature or causes of a child's behavior without regard for the child's circumstances.

We should also ask a larger question: Is it necessary or valuable to enforce the kind of docility suggested in the ADHD diagnostic standards? Many enlightened educators and schools reject making children sit still while they learn rote materials as a group. Why do we see silence and stillness in a group as the ideal behavior for a child? Why are adults in general seemingly so often reluctant to provide more individual attention to the children in their care? It is as if we have carried to an extreme the old axiom, "Children should be seen and not heard." Worse, children who *are* seen and heard are defined as mentally ill.

Is It Ever Justified to Medicate a Child's Brain for the Control of Behavior?

I am often asked, "Aren't there any circumstances when you would give a psychiatric drug to a child?" One comes to mind.

There is a scene in the movie "Exodus" in which a group of young Israeli children must be carried over a mountain under cover of dark in order to escape danger during an attack on their frontier settlement. One child's cry could alert their enemies and expose them to possible slaughter. Reluctantly, the adults drug the children into stupor and sleep. This is an example of when it might be justified to drug children into being still and silent.

In America, we are all too eager to drug children into silence and stillness while we "educate" them. Too often it seems more like "brainwashing" than like genuine education. Reconsider the scene described by CHADD in which the adult walks "through places where children are—particularly those places where children are expected to behave in a quiet, orderly, and productive fashion."[2] Presumably, the adult could simply dispense Ritalin to every child who wasn't sitting down and shutting up, and the problem would be solved. To a great extent, this is what is being advocated—what is being done!—throughout America's schools. Ritalin and other stimulants are used to control conflicts between children and adults by medicating the children into submission. While many excellent teachers want to meet the genuine educational needs of their children, they are being hamstrung by school systems that enforce conformity instead of educating.

What If We Diagnosed the Situation?

Whenever we talk about "children with ADHD" we focus on the child. If, instead, we recognize that the life experiences of children shape how they conduct themselves, we might then ask, "What life experiences and what situations cause children to behave with extremes of inattention, hyperactivity, and impulsivity?" Instead of diagnosing the children, we would diagnose the environments created for them by adults.

The list of "ADHD-inducing Life Experiences and Situations" includes:

(1) Environments that don't meet a child's basic needs for positive involvement with life, including unconditional love from attentive adults, supervision by caring adults who know how to recognize and to meet the needs of children, interesting and creative activities, fun, physical activity, and contact with nature.

(2) Environments that don't meet a child's basic needs for rational and consistent discipline, reasonable principles of conduct, and firm but loving limits on negative behavior.

(3) Environments devoid of older children and adults who can provide models for rational, moral, and loving behavior.

(4) Environments created for the convenience of adult managers rather than for the growth and development of children.

(5) Environments with excessive expectations for silence, stillness, and docility.

(6) Environments with impossible expectations, such as "Stay alert while sitting still for long periods of time," "Act very interested despite boring and confusing materials," and "Set aside your own natural curiosity and imagination in order to stay on task with thirty other children."

(7) Environments charged with adult tension, impatience, and stress.

(8) Environments that feel or are unsafe because of the presence of angry or upset adults and peers. Children are increasingly exposed to realistically dangerous situations at home, on the way to school, in school, at school events, at parties, and almost everywhere they go.

(9) Environments that aren't fun.

A Good Use for the ADHD Checklist

When I work with groups of children, teach students, or give lectures and workshops, I keep a careful eye on the participants to see if any of them seem disinterested, distracted, inattentive, restless, or fidgety. I'm not only listening to the feedback that I get, I'm observing more subtle body language. If I notice even one or two in a large group showing ADHD-like behaviors, I assume I'm not reaching them. I try to catch their eye to engage them, I try to figure out when I lost them, or I try to say something that grabs their attention. I might even ask the group if I've lost or bored some of them. If I can't read the feedback I'm getting—perhaps I can't tell if my audience is upset or confused by what I'm saying—then I stop for a moment and ask them how they're reacting. In evaluating the responses to me, I'm using an informal list that's quite similar to the ADHD checklist, but I use it to monitor the success of my teaching or lecturing, not the "disorders" in my audience.

Almost all effective teachers routinely do something similar to what I do when I lecture. They observe their students' behavior to monitor whether or not the material is getting across to them in an interesting, engaging manner that's appropriate to the ability of each of the children. Parents can use a similar checklist to make sure that they're providing their children with rational discipline, a sufficiently stimulating environment, and sufficient love and attention.

This cannot be over-emphasized: If we see ourselves as responsible for the behavior of the children in our care, we will use the "symptoms of ADHD" as indicators for when we need to give more and better attention to the children.

The Responsiveness of Children to Adults

Children respond in a most remarkable fashion to the adults and to the environment around them. If one adult, by his or her mere presence, can calm and delight children, then another adult by his or her mere presence, can upset or unnerve children.

I have a friend who loves children and feels very comfortable with them. When we walk into a restaurant, children turn around and smile at him. The other day I was having lunch with him and I happened to look across the room. A five-year-old boy was adoring him from a distance without my friend even taking notice. He was too busy chatting with me in his usual animated fashion. Once I happened to be walking with him through a store when we passed by a child who was crying in his mother's arm. My friend smiled, the child instantly stopped crying, smiled back, and then reached out to him. The mom, who had been considerably embarrassed by her son's public display, was grateful.

Teachers in the same school often have very different classrooms. One teacher may have a relatively relaxed style that allows for considerable interplay among the children while nonetheless getting the necessary work done and stimulating them educationally. Another teacher may have a more disciplined style, requiring greater concentration on specific educational activities, while nonetheless engaging the interest of the children. While their styles differ, both teachers are doing a good job. Yet another teacher in the same school will not be able to develop any kind of consistent discipline. There will be constant conflicts among the children, and between the children and the teacher, and it will be difficult for the children to learn anything.

Similar observations can be made about religious observances, scout meetings, team sports, and birthday parties. One minister, scout leader, coach, or parent will be able to take charge of these group activities in productive ways while minimizing distraction, frustration, and conflict. Yet another wouldn't be able to handle the same groups without boring everyone and stirring up discontent and conflict.

Transformed in My Office

The majority of children labeled ADHD do fine when the setting meets their needs with an appropriate combination of discipline, love, and engaging activities. Nearly every "hyperactive" or "inattentive" child who has come into my office has been fully able to cooperate in a mutually respectful and productive fashion. As already noted, this is such a frequent occurrence in many doctor's offices that it's mentioned in the official American Psychiatric Association's (1994) *Diagnostic and Statistical Manual.*[3]

When I'm alone with an "ADHD child," the youngster almost always calms down and engages me in animated, focused conversation. I'll be able to start a mutually interesting exchange about various curious objects in the office. Or I might bring in Blue, our aging Shetland sheepdog who still loves to help me out in sessions.

Often the "ADHD child" who "shows no interest in school" will eagerly ply me with questions about all the books that line and litter the space in my office. The child will wonder, "Why do you have so many? Do you read them all? What's in them?" We may talk about the controversy surrounding the ADHD diagnosis or the use of stimulants. We may even end up talking about how his friends are selling Ritalin to each other. Often these supposedly "out of control" children are able to relate to me, to the fun stuff in my office, and to my animals in very respectful and caring ways. They frequently become models of good behavior when they visit with my wife, Ginger, in the house or garden while I talk alone with the parents.

Even if they start out anxious, upset and inattentive, once children realize that their thoughts are being taken seriously, they almost always settle down to highly focused family discussions. When talking openly about conflicts in the family and at school, they frequently display more sustained attention than their parents.

Some children are so deeply disturbed that they cannot be reached within minutes by a caring adult. Children who get labeled autistic, for example, may require the active intervention of an entire psychosocial, educational program. But the great majority of children labeled ADHD are not that emotionally injured. They are, as the *Diagnostic and Statistical Manual* admits, failing to meet our expectations and standards for ordinary behavior in relatively stifling settings. Their diagnosis usually has more to do with the environment than with the individual child. Therein lies the essence of how we should approach these children: by providing them with improved adult attention and improved child-oriented homes and schools. We may have to change our standards in order to meet the real-life needs of children with energetic young bodies and active minds.

Healing Conflict

How to handle conflict within a family is a large subject that is addressed in a number of good books that are mentioned in chapter 17. First we must realize that most problems between children and adults can be viewed as conflicts rather than as problems located within the isolated child. This approach requires treating the child with sufficient respect and love to work out the conflict in a way that meets the child's basic needs.

Whether the youngsters are seen as hyperactive, impulsive, or inattentive, nearly all children labeled ADHD are best approached as children in conflict with parents and teachers. They are failing to conform to our expectations and causing conflict in the classroom or home. In the extreme, the child is engaged in outright rebellion. Anger, outrage, threats, and even violence may be emanating from the child as well as from the parents. As adults, the parents must take charge of defusing this conflict with unconditional love, rational discipline, and a commitment to recognizing and meeting the child's underlying emotional needs.

ADHD "symptoms" are often best understood as signals of conflict between children and the adults in their lives. Instead of diagnosing and treating the children in our care, adults should take the lead in resolving the conflicts with them. Motivated by love and responsibility, we should resolve these conflicts in favor of their needs as children rather than our needs as adults.

Drugging the most vulnerable, immature, and powerless member of the conflict—the child—is not the most effective or ethical solution to a conflict. Healing begins with a responsible adult creating a *respectful* and *loving* relationship with the child. While children need more than love, without love nothing else good can take place. With love, most other good things will follow.

Chapter 21

What to Do When the Teacher Says Your Child Has ADHD

One survey found that 40% of public school teachers would not go into teaching if they had to choose a career again. According to the federal Department of Education, 30% of new teachers leave the classroom within the first three years.

—Steve Wulf, journalist, *Time* (1997)

Researchers have concluded that there exists no evidence of any beneficial effects of Ritalin on learning or academic achievement. Ritalin, at least for the short term, simply suppresses motor behavior resulting in a more docile and ultimately more manageable child. Rather than altering the chemistry of children's brains, support should be provided to parents and teachers. Schools must involve the family in the design of their child's education program.

—John George, educator (1993a)

The not so good news is that the 8th graders were still below the international average. And not surprising, is it, because that's when a lot of problems hit kids in adolescence. And a lot of our middle schools are still organized for those Ozzie and Harriet days that are long gone. A lot of them are just too big and unwieldy to do right by the kids.... [W]e have to stop making excuses for ourselves for failing these children, and making excuses for them for not learning.

—President Bill Clinton (1997)

The calls are anguished:

"The school is telling me I have to give my child Ritalin," the parent explains. "Can they do that?"

"Not legally," I explain.

"The teachers say they can't teach him unless I put him on Ritalin. Otherwise they'll recommend him for special classes."

Now the answer becomes more complex. Yes, the school can determine that a child is too "emotionally disturbed" for mainstreaming. Then the parent can be caught between two choices—mainstreaming the child on drugs or having the child forced into special education classes.[1] What can a parent do under these circumstances?

Millions of Americans are being confronted with painful choices surrounding the school pressure to drug their children. We need legislation and legal precedents to outlaw this kind of harassment. In the meanwhile, the problem grows, and must be dealt with.

Teachers Are Feeling Pressured, Too

Before we become too confrontational with our child's teacher or school, it is important to remind ourselves that teachers are feeling pressured, too. While parenting in modern society is unimaginably challenging, teaching can be a close rival in degree of difficulty. Teacher education, as described in chapter 15, is being criticized by educators for failing to prepare teachers for the realities of the contemporary classroom and the needs of today's children. Classroom conditions often make it close to impossible to teach in an effective manner.

Both parenting and teaching are high stress, potentially overwhelming roles that receive too little social support or recognition. When crises arise, parents and teachers alike can feel isolated and abandoned.

Indeed, many teachers are also the parents of young children. They are working parents! Faced with the *two hardest jobs in the world*, they surely deserve our patience and understanding.

Schools Are Also Feeling Pressured

All of the difficulties that impinge on the family and parents have been transferred to the schools. Schools are increasingly forced to pick up where the family has left off. They are expected to provide moral guidance in a world that seems to lack morality; they are expected to discipline the undisciplined. It is no wonder that teachers are tempted to single out one or two, or even more, of their difficult, needy, or demanding children for medical management.

Furthermore, schools and teachers are subjected to an enormous amount of propaganda in favor of diagnosis and drugging children. The pressure comes not only from the media but from many other influential institutions, including federal agencies such as NIMH and the Department of Education.[2]

Meanwhile, most schools have been unable to keep up with modern teaching technology. Their instructional materials can be boring compared to the videos and computers to which the minds of modern children are attuned. Their classrooms are much too large and structured for children accustomed to more self-expression and freedom in their early years at home and in preschool. These volatile conditions have been exacerbated by the breakdown of authority in the family and in school. When some of us went to public school, getting caught chewing gum in class was a major offense. Now schools have metal detectors to screen out knives and guns. It was a big deal in the old days to get caught smoking your first cigarette on the hill behind the schoolyard. Now even elementary school children are trying street drugs. There are routine searches for narcotics hidden in student lockers inside our middle and high schools. Verbal expressions of disrespect that would have previously earned expulsion are now accepted as inevitable.

As parents, we should approach teachers with respect as well as with concern for the difficulty of their tasks. This insight leads directly to the first principle we need to implement when faced with a potential conflict with the school:

First, build rapport with your child's teachers and any other resource people in the school.

When a school urges parents to have their child evaluated for stimulant treatment, parents can understandably become incensed. Don't shoot from the hip. Instead, get to know the teacher in as sympathetic a fashion as possible. Making your presence known, showing an interest in both the teacher and your child, and asking for more information, may suffice to calm down any urgency the school may feel. Early on, you can communicate your concerns about the ADHD diagnosis and Ritalin while you show as much interest as possible in working out more child-oriented solutions. Remember that these people have probably been bombarded with ADHD-Ritalin propaganda. Talk to them about it. Show them alternative publications. Try to use the conflict resolution model—finding mutually satisfying, win-win solutions. Try to help your teacher work out conflicts with your child in a way that's in everyone's best interest.

Second, listen carefully to the teachers in order to understand their concerns about your child.

If the teacher believes that your child has a behavior or learning problem worthy of serious attention, take your time finding out what the teacher means. But don't believe there's anything genetically, biochemically, or inherently wrong with your child. By patiently asking the teacher questions about the problem, you may help the teacher figure out the roots of the difficulty. Or you may be able to come up with perspectives the teacher isn't aware of. But *never* accept the ADHD diagnosis for your child. Never!

Third, avoid starting down the path of psychological and psychiatric evaluation.

It is usually a bad idea to give permission to have your child tested in any way other than the standardized tests given to *all children* periodically by state law in order to evaluate their level of *academic* achievement. Psychological tests and tests aimed at diagnosing ADHD, dyslexia, or other "learning disorders" open the door to labeling your child for life.[3] Any specialized test for your child, rather than for every child in the class, should be avoided.

Try to avoid going down the path that leads to "team meetings" involving a school psychologist concerned with disabilities or disorders. If a school counselor has a genuine concern about your child's emotional well-being, it could be beneficial to have a consultation—but not with a "team" that has a mental health orientation and not with the aim of making a diagnosis that will justify special interventions. Meeting with a team of teachers is fine but unless you have a lot of confidence in the psychologist, I wouldn't let the school involve one on the team. If a psychologist is involved, explain that you do not want your child psychiatrically or psychologically evaluated by the school. Explain that if you decide it's necessary or valuable to have your child evaluated psychologically, you'll have it done privately.

Schools can usually obtain sufficient information from classroom performance and standardized tests of academic achievement to evaluate your child's educational strengths and weaknesses. If you feel the need for something more refined, you are much better off going to a private resource who will not share the records with the school without your permission.

Fourth, if at all possible, have a family member go to school to observe and to help out.

Especially if the teacher describes a problem in class—such as daydreaming, not paying attention, failing to heed instructions, asking too many questions, or disturbing other children—urge the school to let you or another family member come to class to observe. If you have the time, and the school is willing, volunteer to assist the teacher.

Explain that you need to know more clearly the nature of the problem so that you can discuss it with your child, as well as with your family and any professional from whom you might seek help. You might also suggest that your presence in class will make clear the importance of the problem to your child and hence encourage improved behavior. I have known parents who have turned their children's school careers around by being present in class for a period of time.

Remember, don't accept the idea that there's something inherently wrong with how your child thinks, learns, or acts. Encourage the viewpoint that teaching good behavior and good learning skills requires the combined efforts of family and the school. Remind yourself that *all* children have "learning problems"—that's why they need teachers and parents.

Fifth, pay special attention to the improvement of your child's reading skills and enjoyment.

The vast majority of academic problems in preschool and early elementary school children can be corrected through improved reading skills. As a parent, you may not feel competent to help your child learn some of the latest materials in their curriculum even in the early grades. Much of it may simply look unfamiliar to you. But if you can read this book, you can make the single most important educational intervention in the life of your children. You can read to them! In addition to interesting them in reading and helping them learn to read, reading with your child will help to develop their attention span, focus, or concentration. Most important of all, as the research literature confirms, it will help you bond with them.[4]

Parents who read with their children tend to have stronger bonds with their children. Reading together with children is one of the single most important activities for cementing meaningful relationships and for encouraging the mental development of the child. The concept of reading should also be expanded to include parents taking children to the library, theater, museum, and other places that communicate in multiple ways about myriad things.

Sixth, consider obtaining tutors for your child.

When was the last time you heard a private school or educational service brag, "We teach in large groups. The more the merrier." Almost everyone learns better in small groups and one-to-one than in groups the size of typical classrooms. In fact, small, well-taught classes are a "cure" for most of the problems labeled ADHD. The vast majority of academic problems can be overcome with the use of skilled, sensitive tutors. Tutoring doesn't have to be expensive. It can often be done by nonprofessionals, including older or more successful students. Local graduate schools are a plentiful soure of good tutors. They should be among your first alternatives when your child is having any kind of academic problem, including problems organizing materials or settling down for homework.

What Teachers Can Do for Difficult Children
Straight, Realistic Talk

Educator Michael Valentine (1988) bases discipline on sound principles of communication. Valentine begins with the idea that our beliefs about children determine what we will say to them. He makes a seemingly simple point but one that could transform homes and classrooms:

> A ... basic tenet of this model is that the child is seen as being capable of doing what he is requested to do. The child's behavior isn't seen as sick, crazy or emotionally ill, or incapable. ... The child's behavior is simply seen as *inappropriate* behavior that needs to be stopped. The behaviors that the schools require of students, especially in the discipline areas, are relatively simple and well within the ranges of the child's capabilities (e.g., don't talk when the teacher is giving instructions, line up to go outside, don't hit anyone, raise your hand and get permission before you,... and so on).[5]

Using specific examples, Valentine shows teachers and parents how to develop reasonable expectations and then how to communicate them effectively to children. This is one of the most important communication principles for parents and teachers: Develop reasonable expectations and then learn how to communicate them with clarity, simplicity, and conviction.

Classroom Strategies from the Department of Education

Teachers are encouraged by the U.S. Department of Education and other resources to take a variety of measures with "ADHD children."[6] These techniques are so basic that they should already be a part of every child's school experience. As a parent, awareness of these approaches may help you to evaluate your child's classroom and to make suggestions to the teacher.

Under the heading, "Classroom Strategies for a Class with Students with ADD," the Department of Education suggests:

(1) "a structured classroom—one where expectations and rules are clearly communicated to them, and where academic tasks are carefully designed for manageability and clarity."

(2) "teachers can break down assignments into smaller, less complex units, and build in reinforcement as the student finishes with each part."

(3) "pairing a student with ADD with another student or dividing the class into cooperative groups can be an effective way to encourage the student to concentrate on work."

(4) "maintaining eye contact with students; using gestures to emphasize points; and providing a work area away from distractions."

(5) "students may need both verbal and visual directions."

(6) "help students shift from one task to another by providing clear and consistent transitions between activities or warning students a few minutes before changing activities."

(7) "when you ask a student with ADD a question, begin the question with the child's name and then pause for a few seconds as a signal to the child to pay close attention."

Strengthening Basic Teaching

The DOE pamphlet describes additional ways of giving special attention to children diagnosed as ADHD. For example, the teacher can have the children write down assignments and then the teacher or an assistant can check them for accuracy. The teacher can repeat assignments at the end of class "out loud as a reminder." Parents can then use the written assignment to ensure the child completes the homework.

The teachers can help the students learn to study and organize their work more efficiently. They can provide lessons that "include focusing on listening skills, outlining structure, task structuring, and notebook organization. Teach students techniques for taking notes from both lectures and textbooks."

These are good suggestions, of course. If you are a parent, you might try to find a tactful way to encourage the teachers to use them. If you feel the teacher may be offended by your suggestions, perhaps the guidance counselor, resource teacher, or assistant principal can act as an intermediary.

The Department of Education pamphlet also makes recommendations on "How to Manage ADD Behavior":

> You can help children with ADD behave in a disciplined manner in the classroom by establishing a few rules which result in immediate consequences if they are broken. Give the child specific rules that are phrased positively in terms of what the child should do. When you praise the child for good behavior and punish for inappropriate behavior, the child can see you apply the rules fairly and consistently.

Exceptional Public Schools

Many communities and school districts have exceptional schools, often called magnets, that provide more individualized education. Often they specialize in music and art, math and science, or some other discipline, and make use of modern technology. Sometimes they encourage racial integration and provide opportunity to neglected communities.

In Montgomery County, Maryland, there is a wonderful public school called Phoenix I, founded and directed by Brian Berthiaume, that serves high school students with drug and alcohol addiction problems. It is based on therapeutic, twelve-step program principles. This successful program should be adopted throughout the country. I have described it in more detail in *reclaiming Our Children* (2000).

If a parent is dissatisfied with the local public school, it's worth exploring other alternatives in your school district. Sometimes excellent alternatives remain relatively unknown within the community.

Home Schooling: No Longer Exotic .

Thirty years ago, few children were home-schooled. Most Americans looked upon it suspiciously as an exotic and even harmful alternative. Since 1990, home schooling has jumped from 300,000 to 900,000 children, according to the Home School Legal Defense Association. The escalating growth of home schooling, like that of the ADHD/Ritalin movement, reflects the failure of our public and private schools to meet the basic needs of parents and children. Standardized tests and other measures show that as a group home-schooled children do as well or better than children in public schools. Home schooling encourages more parent interaction and quality time, factors known to enhance academic achievement. These factors are known to reduce the risk of drugs, premature sexuality, and violence.[7] The parents as a group have some college education and earn $25,000–$50,000 per year. States have varying requirements for home schooling. Most colleges accept home-schooled applicants.[8]

Home schooling parents vary across the spectrum of American values from atheism to fundamentalism, from libertarians who resist government intrusion in their family lives to parents who simply want to protect their children from drugs and violence. Some children are home-schooled when they travel abroad with their parents or participate in activities, such as acting and athletics, that keep them away from their school district.

Some parents make the decision when their children become bored and begin to hate school. As one mother put it, "Because her needs weren't met, she went from self-assured to withdrawn. I felt I could do better."[9]

Home schooling programs also vary enormously from those created and taught by parents, to religiously-based programs, to formal university-run programs.

Indeed, they vary so much that the reader should not assume a familiarity with "home schooling" on the basis of the experience of a few friends or families.

"Delight Centered Education"

Susan Martino is a physician in a small midwestern city who became increasingly concerned about the way her two boys were being treated in school. The teachers seemed unable to respond to the "inner time table" of her two children, instead forcing them to march lock-step with the other children. She felt her boys were being demeaned by having their behavior forced into conformity all day long in large regimented groups. She watched her older child lose his joy over learning and begin to hate school.

The public school was feeding her children "predigested material, never allowing them to think; never encouraging them to discover what anything means to them." Her children were "not learning how to search out the truth for themselves."

When the city's best private school turned out to be run on the same conformist principles as the public schools, Dr. Martino and her husband had a serious talk about how to educate their children. He was in transition between jobs. She suggested he consider a new job—raising and educating their children four days a week. She would take off one day from her practice for the fifth day. It would mean a drastic decline in their material standard of living but an enormous uplift in their spiritual standard.

The Martinos determined to raise their children with "delight centered education" without any set curriculum. The orientation was not to learning specific subjects but to "learning to learn." With the exception of math, for which they obtained a tutor, the parents did all the teaching themselves, often turning to community resources, such as the planetarium, zoo, library, and theater center.

They now have three children, two boys age seventeen and fifteen, and a girl age ten. Their oldest boy's main interest became music. He started his own band and found instructors in the community to help him develop his talents. He is now looking for a small college compatible with his desire to continue designing his own kind of education. There are a number that are well-known for this. The two younger children have never known what it is to "hate school." They love learning. The family is close-knit and has suffered from few of the problems that plague most modern families whose children grow up going to suppressive schools amid peer pressure for sex, drugs, and rebellion against authority.

Coming Home in Tears

Jessica Brown came home in tears at the end of the first week of middle school. At thirteen, she'd been eagerly looking forward to moving on from elementary school and "growing up" to be a teenager. Instead, she'd been yelled at in two of her classes for daydreaming. "They were boring, mom, boring!" she complained. In another class, the teacher was so nervous that it made Jessica anxious. On top of that, two different girls had offered her drugs during lunch breaks and an older boy had "come on" to her while waiting for the school bus. She couldn't get away from him without missing the bus.

That night Jessica's mom and dad had a long talk between themselves. They agreed that it would be cruel and destructive to tell Jessica she had to put up "with real life." It was radical for them to consider alternatives to public education, but they felt deeply sympathetic with their daughter's plight. With more open minds about alternatives, they got together with their daughter.

The Brown family couldn't afford private school, but they knew another parent who was home schooling. Would it isolate their daughter? Would it leave her unprepared for the real world? Jessica also had doubts about it. The family decided to hope for things to get better at school. Jessica was determined to show she could "make it" in public school.

Two months later Jessica's parents were called to school for a conference with the teaching team. Jessica's five teachers were present, as well as the school psychologist and the assistant principal. It was a formidable group. Jessica was so intimidated, she asked and received permission to leave the room. Three of the teachers felt that Jessica had a problem. The two teachers whom Jessica found boring thought Jessica displayed signs of "inattention." The third teacher thought Jessica was "borderline Attention Deficit-Hyperactivity Disorder." It was astonishing with what facility the tongue-tying phrase spilled from her lips. This was the teacher who made Jessica anxious. The other two teachers seemed to think Jessica was charming, well-behaved, and intelligent. One of them said, "She's a delight to have in my class," but she clearly wanted to stay out of the controversy. Everyone agreed Jessica was achieving above grade level.

The school psychologist favored testing for ADHD with a probable recommendation for Ritalin. That night, after another family conference, Jessica and her parents decided to look into home schooling.

Jessica's parents wanted her to have a traditional academic education. They chose the University of North Dakota program which provides a complete off-campus high school curriculum with academic standards that exceed most public schools. Supervised exams are administered by an authorized adult and faxed or mailed to the university for grading. Again by means of fax or mail, teachers at the university grade and comment on the student's work. The cost? A small fraction of the expense of going to a traditional private school.

The North Dakota program provides teachers and tailors its curriculum so that it can be learned with long-distance guidance from its own instructors. But Jessica and her parents decided to hire two local graduate students to act as additional tutors. When Jessica decided that one of these tutors didn't inspire her, her parents let the tutor go and found another. It was a remarkably refreshing change from being "stuck" with the public school teachers regardless of their ability or enthusiasm. Jessica spent an average of two hours three days a week being tutored and worked on her own the rest of the time. She got A's in courses that were much more demanding than those at her public school.

Worries about Home Schooling

Jessica's parents were at first worried about her social life but Jessica continued her relationship with several school girlfriends and made some new ones at a dance for home schoolers in her community. She supplemented her schooling with weekend art and poetry classes sponsored by the county. There she made friends with one of her teachers. The young woman writer became a mentor and model for her. Jessica's parents began to feel that home schooling actually opened up the community and increased their daughter's opportunity to meet creative, successful young adults.

Critics fear that home schooling isolates a child from community and peers. While this could happen, there are enormous resources for children and parents to utilize. Many communities have home schooling networks for sports, music, recreation, and socializing. Community centers and religious institutions can be valuable resources. For many young people with drug- and alcohol-related problems, twelve-step programs provide opportunities to learn from adult sponsors and to be with other youth.

Parents who opt for home schooling should ensure that their children have plenty of opportunity to make friends with other youngsters, as well as opportunities for interesting and exciting activities outside the home. This is not usually difficult.

What's Real?

Critics also fear that home schooling won't prepare children for "real life." It used to strike me as "unnatural" to home school a child but I've changed my mind. Few public schools reflect adult life in the community or workplace. With rare exceptions, such as some magnet schools, most of them stifle individual initiative.

Real life? How many adults will be asked every day to sit silent and still on hard chairs in a room of thirty peers through hour after hour of lectures and rote exercises by single instructors of varying ability? How many will have to raise their hands before being able to go to the bathroom? How many will be unable to leave the room at all during the entire day simply to take a break, get a snack, or call home? How many will be plied with drugs, threatened with violence, or sexually and racially harassed on a daily basis in the hallways at work? How many will have to contend at work with openly hostile cliques that exclude anyone who seems at all different?

With increasing numbers of computer-based jobs, often through a solo consultation practice or a home-office, home schooling has become more real-world than public school.

In *The Myth of the A.D.D. Child*, Thomas Armstrong (1995) encourages parents to let their child know that "the kinds of traits he possesses are valuable out there in the workplace. In terms of the characteristics associated with A.D.D.-like behavior—need for novelty, change, imagination, movement, and spontaneous expression—there are many work roles that fit the bill...." He then lists more than two dozen options, from self-employed businessperson and traveling salesperson to family-practice physician, fashion model, and public relations consultant. In this computer age, opportunities for independent, creative work are limitless.

In my own varied professional activities—psychiatrist and therapist, university teacher, workshop leader, forensic expert, researcher, center director, and author—none of my real world looks anything like spending a day as a pupil in a public school classroom. I have tried to encourage my children and my patients to create their own real worlds in terms of occupations, relationships, and recreational activities that they value and truly enjoy. If you give up the concept of ADHD and the resort to medication, you can do the same for your children.

Alternative Private Schools

Not all educators have adopted the ADHD/Ritalin party line but resisters seem to be in the minority. Arthur Allen (1997) speaks with admiration of Principal William Patterson, the former head of a small school for the learning disabled in Silver Spring, Maryland:

> Patterson is an anomaly, and something of an embarrassment to his staff at the Chelsea School. He has the nerve, in this era of the biologization of everything, to think that giving children psychoactive pills is a bad idea. Patterson actually believes he can teach children to control their behavioral problems. At his previous job as a headmaster of a boarding school for dyslexics in Massachusetts, he saw to it that Ritalin was banned from the premises.

Allen quotes Patterson, "There's no way that I or anybody else can stem the tide of drugs." But the school principal adds, "What are we telling kids? Take a pill and it will be all better? How about a little heroin?"

What's Really Needed

This is worth repeating: Knowing that a child fits into the diagnosis called ADHD gives us very little useful information about the child's inner life or about the child's home and school life. That the child fits the ADHD category tells us next to nothing about the child's real needs. To recognize each child's needs and to respond to them requires time, effort, patience, wisdom, and love. Even if a child displays the whole range of ADHD symptoms to a severe degree, it tells us nothing about what to do next except to carefully evaluate the source of the child's problem.

What's needed is a careful, informed, and loving evaluation of each individual child's needs. The following vignettes or sketches are very simplified but they reflect reality:

- The "over-active" or "hyperactive" child who may have more abundant energy than other children, and who needs more challenging outlets for physical and emotional self-expression;

- The "rebellious" or "negative" child who may have more autonomy and determination than most kids, and who needs a strong guiding hand that doesn't crush that gift;

- The "impulsive" child who may be unusually exuberant and daring, and who needs consistent discipline combined with imaginative guidance to channel all that vitality;

- The "day-dreamer" child who has a poetic soul and who needs especially creative nurturing and artistic outlets;

- The "sensitive" child who is shy and somewhat fearful, and needs an adult who is sensitive enough to respond to the child's needs in an empowering fashion;

- The "undisciplined" child who has a great deal of potential but lacks the patience and discipline to master it, and who needs a kind but firm role model of discipline;

- The "bored" child with a restless spirit who is especially bright and creative, and who needs more inspired learning opportunities;

- The "slow" child for whom ordinary expectations are frustrating and sometimes overwhelming, and who needs patience and more individualized educational opportunities;

- The "immature child" or "late bloomer" who is taking his or her time growing up, and who needs acceptance along the way;

- The "troubled child" who is undergoing a great deal of stress in a conflicted or disorderly home, and who needs his parents to get help for themselves;

- The "learning disabled" child who has difficulties with specific aspects of the school program, and needs individualized educational help, perhaps including tutoring, and a lot of reassurance that there's nothing wrong;

- The medically ill child who suffers from the effects of an old head injury, lead poisoning, thyroid disorder, medication side effects, or some other physical problem, and who needs a real medical evaluation, rather than a concocted diagnosis of ADHD;

- The severely abused or deprived child who suffers from an extreme lack of nurturing, abandonment, various kinds of abuse, or malnutrition, and who needs a social service intervention by appropriate agencies.

To these groups we may add "all school-age children," because all children need small classrooms, interesting educational materials, inspired teachers, and devoted parents. They all need a carefully balanced mixture of unconditional love, rational discipline, inspiring educational activities, and play. They all need good role models.

These are the types of children who get diagnosed as suffering from ADHD and who get subdued with stimulants and other medications. Do we *really* believe that drugs are the solution to the challenges that they present us, our families, and our schools?

Parents and Teachers United for Children

If teachers find that their classrooms and schools are incompatible with a high level of teaching, then they should spend more time on picket lines or in political action groups. If parents find themselves tempted to medicate their children in order to make them conform to the "realities" of school, they too should devote themselves to educational and political reform. It is flat out wrong to go along with a system that tells a parent or teacher to drug a child rather than to make the necessary changes in the child's educational or family environment. This is not an impractical, idealistic vision—it is the only moral and effective one. As long as we drug our children, we won't improve the schools or our homes. As long as we drug our children, we fail to provide them what they need.

Individual teachers and parents cannot change the schools by acting in isolation or on their own. What's needed is a coalition of parents, teachers, and all adults concerned for the well-being of children. One approach to ending the over-promotion of ADHD and Ritalin is found in the new class action suits against the manufacturer of Ritalin, Novartis, as well as against the parents' group CHADD and the American Psychiatric Association (chapter 1). The International Center for the Study of Psychiatry and Psychology (Appendix B) offers an organized effort against the drugging of children and for making our institutions and ourselves more focused on their real needs.

The situation in our schools will not improve without widespread protest from outraged Americans. Has our society forsaken its children? Will we sit by idly while a large percentage of our children are drugged into conformity with poorly trained teachers and outmoded schools? Have common sense, ethics, and love for our children been crushed beneath the ADHD/Ritalin avalanche? A great deal depends on us as individuals—whether we are willing to band together and to speak out in public against the ADHD/Ritalin movement and for a more child-centered America. It also depends on us as individuals to protect, to love, and to meet the needs of the children in our care.

Appendix A

STIMULANT DRUG INFORMATION
SUMMARY

Summarized from *Talking Back to Ritalin*
by Peter R. Breggin, M.D.

- Several million children, probably 15% or more of boys, are being treated with Ritalin and other stimulants on the grounds that they have attention deficit-hyperactivity disorder (ADHD) and suffer from inattention, hyperactivity, or impulsivity. The stimulants include:

    —Ritalin (methylphenidate)

    —Metadate ER and Concerta (long-acting forms of methylphenidate)

    —Dexedrine and DextroStat (dextroamphetamine or d-amphetamine)

    —Adderall (d-amphetamine and amphetamine mixture)

    —Desoxyn (methamphetamine)

    —Gradumet (long-acting form of methamphetamine)

    —Cylert (pemoline)

Except for Cylert, all of these drugs have nearly identical effects and side effects. Ritalin and the amphetamines like Adderall can for most purposes be considered one type of drug.

When parents are reluctant to have Ritalin prescribed to their children, some doctors offer Adderall as an alternative. Parents should know that Adderall is a new packaging of amphetamines, drugs that are at least as dangerous as Ritalin. Animal research shows that small, short-term doses of amphetamines like Adderall can cause permanent brain damage.

- The number of children being drugged has escalated ten-fold in the last decade. There has been a several-fold increase in drugging preschool toddlers.

- Ritalin and amphetamines such as Adderall have almost identical adverse effects on the brain, mind and behavior, including the production of drug-induced behavioral disorders, psychosis, mania, drug abuse, and addiction.

- Ritalin and amphetamines such as Adderall frequently cause the very same problems they are supposed to treat—inattention, hyperactivity, and impulsivity.

- A large percentage of children become robotic, lethargic, depressed, or withdrawn on stimulants.

- Ritalin and amphetamines like Adderall can cause permanent neurological tics including Tourette's syndrome.

- Ritalin and amphetamines like Adderall can retard growth in children by disrupting the cycles of growth hormone released by the pituitary gland, as well as by suppressing appetite.

- The recent finding that Ritalin can cause cancer in some animals was not taken seriously enough by the drug company or the FDA.

- Ritalin and amphetamines like Adderall routinely cause gross malfunctions in the brain of the child. There is research evidence from controlled scientific studies that Ritalin can cause shrinkage (atrophy) or other permanent physical abnormalities in the brain. Amphetamines, including Adderall and Dexedrine, cause cell death in animals in relatively low doses.

- Withdrawal from Ritalin, Adderall, Dexedrine and other stimulants can cause emotional suffering, including depression, exhaustion, and suicide. This can make children seem psychiatrically disturbed and lead mistakenly to increased doses of medication or the prescription of new medications. Thus the stimulants become a gateway drug to other psychiatric medications, and the child ends up on multiple unnecessary, harmful drugs.

- Ritalin and amphetamines like Adderall are addictive and can become gateway drugs to other addictions. Stimulants are common drugs of abuse among children and adults.

- New research shows that children who receive prescription stimulants such as Ritalin and the amphetamines will be more prone to cocaine abuse as young adults.

- ADHD and Ritalin are American and Canadian medical fads. The U.S. uses 90% of the world's Ritalin. Ciba-Geigy Corporation, a division of Novartis, is the manufacturer of Ritalin. It is trying to expand the Ritalin market to Europe and the rest of the world.

- Ritalin and amphetamines like Adderall "work" by producing malfunctions in the brain rather than by improving brain function. This is the only way they work.

- Ritalin, Adderall, Dexedrine and other stimulants suppresses creative, spontaneous, playful, and social activity in children. This makes the children more docile and obedient, and more willing to comply with rote, boring tasks, such as classroom school work and homework.

- Ritalin, Adderall, and other stimulants have no positive effect on a child's psychology or on academic performance and achievement. This is confirmed by innumerable studies and by many professional reviews of the literature.

- Longer-term, beyond several weeks, stimulants have no positive effects on any aspect of a child's life.

- Labeling children with ADHD and treating them with Ritalin and amphetamines like Adderall and Dexedrine can keep them out of the armed services, limit their future career choices, and stigmatize them for life. It can ruin their own self-image, subtly demoralize them, and discourage them from reaching their full potential.

- There is no solid evidence that ADHD is a genuine disorder or disease of any kind.

- There is a great deal of research to confirm that environmental problems cause ADHD-like symptoms.

- A very small number of children may suffer ADHD-like symptoms because of physical disorders, such as lead poisoning, drug intoxication, exhaustion, and head injury. Physical causes may be more common among poor communities in the United States and elsewhere in the world.

- There is no proof of any physical abnormalities in the brains or bodies of children who are routinely labeled ADHD. They do not have known biochemical imbalances or "crossed wires."

- ADHD is a controversial diagnosis with little or no scientific or medical basis. A parent, teacher, or doctor can feel in good company when utterly dismissing the diagnosis and refusing to apply it to children.

- Ciba/Novartis spends millions of dollars to sell parent groups and doctors on the idea of using Ritalin. Novartis helps to support the parent group, CHADD, and organized psychiatry.

- The U.S. Department of Education and the National Institute of Mental Health (NIMH) push stimulants as vigorously as the manufacturer of the drugs, often in even more glowing terms than the drug companies could legally get away with.

- Class action suits for fraud and conspiracy to over-promote Ritalin have been brought against Ciba/Novartis, CHADD, and the American Psychiatric Association. The class action suits were inspired by *Talking Back to Ritalin*.

For more information read *Talking Back to Ritalin* by Peter R. Breggin, M.D. or find Dr. Breggin's web site at www.breggin.com.

Appendix B

ICSPP

*International Center for the
Study of Psychiatry and Psychology*

4628 Chestnut Street
Bethesda, MD 20814
301 652 5580

I CSPP is a reform-oriented international center for professionals concerned with ethical and scientific issues in human research and services. It is the only professional organization that has taken a firm public and professional stand against the massive psychiatric drugging of America's children. However, it focuses on the entire field of child and adult mental health, including the biological and social sciences.

The Board of Directors, Advisory Council and membership include hundreds of professionals in many fields spanning psychology, counseling, social work, psychiatry and other medical specialties, neuroscience, education, religion, and law. Former members of the U.S. Congress and other community leaders also belong.

Founded in 1971 by its director, Peter R. Breggin, M.D., ICSPP began its successful reform efforts with opposition to the international resurgence of psychosurgery. In the mid-1990s, ICSPP organized a campaign that caused the U. S. Government to withdraw its "violence initiative," a proposed government-wide program that called for intrusive biomedical experiments on inner-city children in the hope of demonstrating biological and genetic causes of violence.

ICSPP's most recent reform efforts are directed at the growing trend to psychiatrically diagnose and medicate children. Because of its many successful efforts on behalf of truthfulness and justice in the psychosocial and biomedical sciences, ICSPP has been called "the conscience of psychiatry."

ICSPP offers a general membership. It publishes a newsletter and periodically distributes news releases and press packages about contemporary issues in the human sciences. ICSPP hosts international conferences open to the public and to professionals.

In 1999, ICSPP began its peer-reviewed journal, *Ethical Human Sciences and Services: An International Journal of Critical Inquiry*, published by Springer Publishing Company. In keeping with ICSPP's goals, the journal gives priority to scientific papers and reviews that raise the level of ethical awareness concerning research, theory, and practice.

ICSPP general memberships are $25 (US) in the United States and $35 (US) internationally. Members receive the newsletter, a discount on the journal, and announcements of activities, including international conferences.

Further information about ICSPP membership and activities can be obtained on its web sites at www.icspp.org and at www.breggin.com.

Appendix C

ETHICAL HUMAN SCIENCES AND SERVICES

An International Journal of Critical Inquiry

The mandate of *Ethical Human Sciences and Services: An International Journal of Critical Inquiry* (EHSS) is to understand and to address the genuine needs of human beings in an ethical and scientific manner.

EHSS publishes scientific research, literature reviews, clinical reports, commentary, and book reviews that draw on broad ethical and scientific perspectives, including critiques of reductionist theories and practices in various schools of thought and ideology. It spans the fields of psychology, counseling, social work, nursing, sociology, education, public advocacy, public health, and the law, as well as medical fields such as psychiatry, pediatrics, and neurology, and biomedical sciences such as genetics and psychopharmacology.

This peer-review journal seeks to raise the level of scientific knowledge and ethical discourse, while empowering professionals who are devoted to principled human sciences and services unsullied by professional and economic interests.

The co-editors are psychiatrist Peter R. Breggin, M.D. and professor of social work David Cohen, Ph.D. EHSS is the official journal of the International Center for the Study of Psychiatry and Psychology. On the editorial advisory board are more than fifty international ICSPP members, including Fred Bemak, Ed.D.; Phyllis Chesler, Ph.D.; Graham Dukes, M.D., LLD; Alberto Fergusson, M.D.; Giovanni de Girolamo, M.D.; James Gordon, M.D.; Thomas Greening, Ph.D.; Richard Horobin, Ph.D.; Lucy Johnstone, Dip.Clin. Psych.; Bertram Karon, Ph.D.; Kate Millett, Ph.D.; Loren Mosher, M.D.; Dorothy Rowe, Ph.D.; Thomas Scheff, Ph.D.; Clemmont Vontress, Ph.D.; Lenore Walker, Ed.D.; and Wolf Wolfensberger, Ph.D.

The journal welcomes the submission of unsolicited manuscripts. Please send manuscripts and direct editorial inquiries to the editorial office: Peter R. Breggin, M.D., 4628 Chestnut Street, Bethesda, MD 20814. Office phone: 301 652-5580. Fax: 301 652-5924.

Domestic subscription rates are $44 individual and $88 institutional. Outside the United States, rates are US$52 individual and US$100 institutional. To order a subscription, contact Springer Publishing Company, 536 Broadway, New York, NY 10012-9904. Telephone: 212 431-4370; fax: 212 941-7842.

NOTES

Chapter 1: The Tide Is Shifting

1 Marshall (2000) reports on the data from studies in Virginia and in North Carolina. The 20% figure for fifth grade boys is cited in an editorial (*USA Today*, 2000, August 15) and is taken from the Virginia study. I have been informed by a professional involved in the Virginia study that 17% of all white boys were being given stimulants in the several grades studied. In response to inquiries from my researcher, the North Carolina study has refused to release figures for boys separately from girls. In news reports on September 19, 2000, the office of the Surgeon General was quoted as stating that 17% of white boys suffer from ADHD. See further discussion in chapter 16.

2 Feussner (1998) from the DEA describes an eight-fold increase between 1990 and 1998.

3 Henry, August 22, 2000.

4 See Breggin, 2000d for the text of my formal presentation which differed from my live presentation. The entire hearing was filmed by C-Span. Information on how to purchase the film can be found at U.S. House of Representatives, 2000. Presenters included myself representing the International Center for the Study of Psychiatry and Psychology, psychiatrist David Fassler representing the American Psychiatric Association, neurologist Fred Baughman, Patrician Johnson of the Colorado State Board of Education, and Patricia Weathers who is a parent.

5 Drug Enforcement Administration, 1995a&b.

6 Thomas, August 8, 2000.

7 USA Today, August 15, 2000.

8 Jensen, August 15, 2000. Jensen has become the nation's most outspoken and visible proponent of drugging children.

9 For discussions of tardive dyskinesia, see American Psychiatric Association (1992), Breggin (1997a) and Breggin and Cohen (1999). This very common disorder is produced by all of the neuroleptic or antipsychotic drugs, such as Thorazine, Haldol, Prolixin, Navane, Risperdal, Seroquel, and Zyprexa.

10 Anyone interested in joining the class action suits, or in obtaining more information, can contact attorneys C. Andrew Waters and Peter Kraus at Waters & Kraus, 4807 West Lover's Lane, Dallas, Texas 75209 (phone 214 357 6244). I was a paid consultant to the original suit but I'm not at present serving in that capacity for any of the Ritalin class action suits. More information concerning the suit can be obtained on the web site of the above-mentioned attorneys, www.Ritalinfraud.com or on www.Breggin.com.

11 Locy (2000).

12 Long and Barrett (2000, May) and Schmitt (2000, September) in the *Wall Street Journal*; Meier (2000, September) in the *New York Times*; and Locy (2000, September) in *USA Today*.

13 Lambert (1998), p. 198.

14 Feussner (1998), p. 202.

15 Feussner (1998), p. 203.

16 Feussner (1998), p. 204.

17 Carey (1998), p. 35.

18 Joseph Biederman, a Harvard professor of psychiatry, cited his own badly flawed research as evidence that stimulants do not cause growth retardation (Spencer, Biederman, et al. 1996). Spencer, Biederman, and their colleagues based their study on one measurement of height and weight during the child's lifetime. Even so, they had to use badly flawed statistical methods and a control group that was quite unlike the study group. For a more detailed evaluation of the study see Breggin (1999).

19 Child neurologist Frederick Baughman, Jr. of San Diego.

20 Swanson (1998).

21 Jensen (2000), p. 195.

22 Jensen (2000).

23 I first described the Psychopharmaceutical Complex in Toxic Psychiatry (1991).

24 The quotes from the White House Conference are taken from a transcript provided by Office of the Press Secretary (The White House, 1999). Details of the conference are discussed and further documented in Breggin (2000), *Reclaiming Our Children*.

25 Reviewed in Breggin (2000), *Reclaiming Our Children*.

26 Koplewicz (1996), pp. 6–8.

27 I have reviewed some of the research in *Beyond Conflict* (1992) and *Reclaiming Our Children* (2000). Also see chapter 12.

28 U.S. Department of Health and Human Services (1999).

29 Breggin, P. (2000, February 28).

30 See chapter two of this book.

31 Zito et al. (2000), p. 1028.

32 Coyle (2000), p. 1059.

33 Coyle (2000), p. 1060.

34 Begley (2000, February 28). The studies were based on brain scans. This is an example of the legitimate use of that technology, in contrast to the brain scan scam described in this chapter.

35 Pear (2000). The reporter is paraphrasing a comment attributed to Hillary Clinton.

36 Grinfeld (2000).

37 Pear (2000). Hyman even suggested that in some communities, children were being under-medicated.

38 Quoted in Grinfeld (2000), p. 7. Greenhill is professor of psychiatry at Columbia University's College of Physicians and Surgeons, and a research psychiatrist at the New York State Psychiatric Institute. He is overseeing the NIMH clicial trials involving preschoolers.

39 Associated Press (2000, April 16).

40 Michael Mosher, attorney, 50 North Main Street, Paris, Texas 75460, telephone 903 785 4721.

41 Janofsky (1999).

42 Chronis (1999).

43 See Karlin (2000) for an excellent news story about parents in New York State coerced into giving psychiatric drugs to their children. http://www.timesunion.com.

44 Vigue (2000).

45 I devoted chapter 7 of the original edition of this book (1998) to describing the case of a father who lost health custody over his child because of his opposition to Ritalin. Since then, the press has covered a variety of similar cases.

Chapter 2: Ritalin Is Not Candy for the Brain

1 Bradley, 1937.

2 Tucker, 1997. Cylert had 7–9% of the market.

3 *Physicians' Desk Reference* (2000), in the entry for Adderall.

4 Whalen and Henker, 1997, p. 327

5 Breggin, 1998d; Breggin 1999a,b&c; Breggin, 2000c).

6 Citations listed on the bottom of the table.

7 P. 2307

8 Burgess, 1985.

9 Pp. 165–176.

10 Burgess, 1985.

11 Dunnick and Hailey, 1995; National Toxicology Program, 1995. Estimated doses of 50–60 mg/kg.

12 Neergaard, 1996.

13 National Toxicology Program, 1995, p. 11.

14 Associated Press, 1996b. Also see 1996a

15 The FDA points out that adverse reaction reports by themselves do not prove a causal relationship. I have examined how to go about determining if an association is causal (Breggin 1997a and 1998a). Only a tiny (but undetermined) fraction of adverse reactions get reported.

16 Knapp et al., 1995.

17 This is not a particularly large number compared to some other psychiatric drugs, such as Prozac. Ritalin has been on the market since the mid 1950s, making professionals see less need to send in adverse reaction reports. The assumption, although incorrect, is that all the important adverse reactions have been identified in older drugs. In addition, only a tiny fraction of serious adverse drug reactios ever gets reported to the FDA.

18 Bloom et al., 1988; Lucas and Weiss, 1971; reviewed in Scarnati, 1986.
19 Rosenfeld, 1979.
20 Koek and Colpaert, 1993; Lieberman et al., 1987.
21 Koek and Colpaert, 1993; Kosten, 1990; Schiorring, 1981.
22 Flaum and Schultz, 1996.
23 Hall et al., 1996.
24 Rapoport et al., 1978. The dose was 0.5 mg/kg.
25 Discussed in Dackis and Gold, 1990.
26 Schleifer et al., 1975; Whalen et al, 1979; and others.
27 Blum et al., 1996.
28 Brown and Williams, 1976; Joyce et al., 1986; reviewed in Dulcan, 1994, and in Jacobovitz et al., 1990.
29 Shaywitz et al., 1985.
30 Pizzi, Rode, and Barnhart, 1986.
31 Klein and Mannuzza, 1988; Levin, 1995.
32 Safer, Allen, and Barr, 1975.
33 Mattes and Gittelman, 1983.
34 Gualtieri et al., 1981; Joyce et al., 1986.
35 Shaywitz et al., 1985.
36 Ascoli and Segaloff, 1996.
37 Associated Press, 1997b; Gong, 1997.
38 Emonson and Vanderbeek, 1995.
39 Markowtiz and Patrick, 1996.
40 Grob and Coyle, 1986.
41 *Drug Facts and Comparisons*, 1997.
42 Billing et al., 1994; Cernerud et al., 1996.
43 Thadani, 1995.
44 Vorhees, 1994.
45 Mendelson et al, 1995.
46 Neurological Drugs Advisory Committee, 1977, p. 102.
47 Pleak, 1995.
48 Rosse and Licamele, 1984.
49 Neuropharmacology Advisory Committee, 1974.
50 Food and Drug Administration, 1995. I analyze FDA procedures in regard to ascertaining safety in Breggin, 1997a and 1998a.
51 Food and Drug Administration, 1995 & 1996.
52 Food and Drug Administration, 1997a.
53 Suplee, 1997.

Chapter 3: Gross Brain Malfunctions and Cell Death Caused by Stimulants

1 Breggin 1999 a,b & c; Breggin, 2000c.
2 During et al., 1992.

3   For example, amphetamine acts by releasing newly synthesized dopamine or nor-
    epinephrine into the synapse while Ritalin releases the neurotransmitters from
    synaptic stores (see Joyce et al., 1984).

4   Reviewed in Kosten, 1990, and Hyman and Coyle, 1994. For details of the
    anatomy of dopomine pathways, see Alheid et al., 1990.

5   Reviewed in Hyman and Coyle, 1994; for details of the anatomy of norepineph-
    rine pathways, see Pearson et al., 1990.

6   Kosten, 1990. Also, Hyman and Coyle, 1994. For anatomic details of serotonin
    pathways, see Tork and Hornung, 1990.

7   See chapter 2 of this book.

8   P. 245.

9   Giedd et al., 1994; Hynd et al.,1991; Lou et al., 1984.

10 Mostofsky et al., 1998.

11 Clonidine is approved for the control of hypertension in adults. It is given to chil-
    dren because of its marked sedative effect. Especially in combination with stim-
    ulants, it is a danger to the heart.

12 Castellanos et al., 1996; Giedd et al., 1994.

13 For example, Giedd et al, 1994.

14 Hynd et al., 1991.

15 National Institutes of Health, 1998, p. 2. The original draft was handed out at
    the conference and initially put on the NIH web site. A later heavily edited ver-
    sion is now on the web site.

16 Huang et al., 1997.

17 Wagner et al., 1980; Juan et al., 1997.

18 Weiss et al., 1997.

19 Camp et al. 1997

20 Robinson and Kolb, 1997.

21 Wren, 1996.

22 Melega al., 1997b; Schmued and Bowyer, 1997; Sheng et al., 1996; Sonsalla et al.,
    1997; Wagner et al., 1980; Zaczek et al., 1989; Battaglia et al., 1987.
    Methamphetamine causes destructive changes in all three of the neurotransmitter
    systems that are stimulated by the drug (also see Zaczek et al., 1989). I have
    reviewed these studies in Breggin, 1999b&c.

23 Melega used 2 doses of 2 mg/kg 4 hours apart.

24 Battaglia et al, 1987. Also see Psychiatric Times, 1995, and Psychiatric News,
    1997c.

25 Jaffe, 1995.

26 Wilson et al., 1996.

27 Harvey, 1996a.

28 See chapter for a detailed comparison.

29 Barnett and Kuczensk, 1986.

30 Mathieu et al., 1989.

31 Lacroix and Ferron, 1988.

32 National Toxicology Program, 1995.

33 Mathieu et al., 1989; Lacroix and Ferron, 1988; Juan et al., 1997.

34 Wagner et al., 1980; Yuan et al., 1997; Zaczek et al., 1989.

35 P. 14.

36 P. 796. A word was left out in the original text.

37 Bell et al., 1982.

38 Wang et al., 1994. The dose was 0.5 mg/kg intravenously.

39 Porrino and Lucignani, 1987. The doses were 1.25 to 15 mg/kg.

40 Antelman et al., 1995.

41 For stimulants, see Kosten 1990. For Prozac-like drugs, see Breggin and Breggin (1994).

42 Associated Press, 1997c. The quotes from the article are paraphrases of what the researchers said.

43 Connolly et al., 1997.

44 McCann et al., 1997.

45 P. 1211

46 Teicher et al. (1997) review brain development.

47 Perry, 1994; Perry et al., 1995; Schwartz and Perry, 1994.

Chapter 4: How Stimulants Really Work

1 Dulcan, 1994; Dulcan and Popper, 1991; Rapoport et al., 1978; Sroufe and Stewart, 1973; Swanson et al., 1992; Taylor, 1994.

2 Dulcan, 1994; Dulcan and Popper, 1991; Porrino and Lucignani, 1987; Rapoport et al., 1980; Rapoport et al., 1978; Taylor, 1994.

3 See chapters 5 and 6 for further discussion.

4 Early research into new treatments often tends to be more honest than later efforts in which ardent advocates try to improve the image of the treatment. This principle has been consistently reconfirmed throughout my research in psychiatry. The older, pioneering literature presents a truer picture of the treatment effects on the human brain and mind. Early research on stimulant drugs is no exception.

5 Rie et al., 1976a; also see Rie et al., 1976b.

6 Granger et al., 1993, p. 535.

7 Cotton and Rothberg, 1988.

8 Cunningham and Barkley, 1978.

9 Barkley and Cunningham, 1979.

10 Barkley et al., 1985.

11 Arakawa, 1994; Bhattacharyya et al., 1980; Hughes, 1972; Mueller, 1993; Randrup and Munkvad, 1970; Sams-Dodd and Newman, 1997; Schiørring, 1979, 1981.

12 Battacharyya et al., 1980; Hughes, 1972; Melega et al. 1997a; Randrup and Munkvad, 1970; Sams-Dodd and Newman, 1997; Schiørring, 1979, 1981.

13 See endnotes 11 and 12 in this chapter for a selection of these citations.

14 In Kramer, Lipton, Ellinwood, and Sulser, 1970.

15 Barnett and Kuczenski, 1986; Kuczenski and Segal, 1997.

16 For the anatomy, see Alheid et al., 1990. Also see explanations and diagrams in chapter 3 of this book. I discuss drug-induced loss of autonomy and willpower (zombie-like behavior) in more technical detail in Breggin, 1993 and 1997a.

17 Shih et al., 1975.

18 Bell et al., 1982.

19 See definition of perseveration in *Dorland's*, 1994.

20 My determination to stop these practices led to a largely successful campaign to prevent the resurgence of lobotomy and psychosurgery in the 1970s (Breggin and Breggin, 1998).

21 These syndromes are reviewed with many citations to the literature in Breggin 1991, 1997a. Also, see the annual *Physicians' Desk Reference* for warnings about these disorders.

22 Breggin, 1997a, describes the brain-disabling effects of the complete range of drugs routinely used in psychiatry. Writing in *USA Today*, journalist Tim Friend, 1995, criticizes some of the fad drugs used to treat ADHD.

23 P. 141.

24 P. 184.

Chapter 5: Vitamin R: The Road to Addiction and Abuse

1 Quoted by reporter Diane Struzzi, 1995.

2 Quoted in Thomas, 1995.

3 Pediatrician Patricia Quinn (1997) discusses some adverse effects at length in *Attention Deficit Disorder*, but fails to mention anything about Ritalin or Dexedrine abuse and addiction. Barbara Ingersoll (1988), a psychologist and active member of the ADHD/Ritalin advocacy community, specifically denies in *Your Hyperactive Child* that Ritalin or amphetamine can cause addiction or abuse in children being treated for ADHD. Sam Goldstein, a child psychologist, and Michael Goldstein (1992), a child neurologist, at least acquaint the parent with the fact that Ritalin and amphetamine are addictive drugs that are carefully controlled by the DEA. Typical of advocates, they conclude there's no significant danger.

4 Dialogue, 1997.

5 In general, if an addictive drug can be absorbed into the body by a particular route—such as orally, nasally, or intravenously—it can become addictive through that route. Often the intravenous use will produce particularly severe addictions and other health risks because it initially bypasses degradation by the liver and because it has a more immediate impact. Also, the intravenous injection of crushed pills poses additional risks due to the fragments of the pill and any filler substances.

6 P. 94.

7 P. 1221.

8 Pp. 204–205.

9 Pp. 19–20, 56.

10 Hammack, 1996; Turner, 1996.

11 Welsh, 1995.

12 St. Dennis and Synoground, 1996.

13 Wiley, 1971.

14 Subcommittee, 1970.

15 United Nations Information Service, p. 1997a.

16 P. 60.

17 Kennedy, 1972.

18 Martin et al., 1971, p. 255. Also see Ellinwood and Cohen, 1972, and Spotts and Spotts, 1980.

19 Pp. 58–59.

20 Spotts and Spotts, 1980.

21 See review by Lake and Quirk, 1984.

22 Haglund and Howerton, 1982.

23 Fulton and Yates, 1988.

24 P. 29

25 P. 14.

26 Drug Enforcement Administration, 1995c, p. 26; Greene, 1995.

27 Dackis and Gold, 1990.

28 Dackis and Gold, 1990, p. 18.

29 Dackis and Gold, 1990, p. 21.

30 Haglund and Howerton, 1982; Medical News, 1979.

31 Cahill et al, 1981.

32 Ellinwood and Cohen, 192; Spotts and Spotts, 1980.

33 P. 53.

34 Suro, 1997.

35 Baberg et al., 1996 (Germany); Williamson et al., 1997 (Great Britain); Hall et al., 1996 (Australia).

36 The more recent *DSM-IV* is more abbreviated and less informative.

37 Pp. 74–75. Citations omitted from the quote.

38 International Narcotics Control Board, 1996a.

39 International Narcotics Control Board, 1996a.

Chapter 6: "They Never Like the Medication"

1 Unsolicited remark from A.G., an adult, talking about when he was a child.

2 Sleator, Ullmann, and von Neumann, 1982. The average age was almost 12.

3 Jensen et al., 1989.

4 Bauer, 1989.

5 The children ranged in age from 8 to 14, with 16 boys and 4 girls. They were fairly evenly divided between children who had taken the drug for less than a year, for 1–3 years, and for more than 3 years.

6 Ellipses in original, p. 60.

7 Emonson and Vanderbeek, 1995.
8 P. 1218.
9 The phrase is from the title of psychiatrist Nancy Andreasen's 1984 book.
10 Discussed in chapter 10.
11 Chapter 10.
12 Chapter 14.

Chapter 7: Do Stimulants Help Children and Will Doctors Tell You the Truth?

1 Mannuzza et al., 1991; also see Gittelman et al., 1985.
2 Popper and Steingard, 1994
3 Richters et al., 1995.
4 Chapter 14.
5 Swanson et al., 1995.
6 Drug Enforcement Administration, 1993 and 1995a,b&c.
7 International Narcotics Control Board, 1995, 1996a&b, 1997.
8 Neurological Drugs Advisory Committee, 1977, p. 70. There has been no improvement in that estimate in the years since then.
9 Chapters 2 and 5.
10 Regier and Leshner, 1992.
11 Richters et al., 1995.
12 Italics in original, p. 991. With the caveat that the studies are flawed, Dulcan and Popper, 1991, also conclude "Stimulants have not been demonstrated to have long-term therapeutic effects" (p. 189). But investigator bias tends to make flawed studies come out too positive, not too negative. Whatever inadequacies there are in the stimulant literature, they would tend to exaggerate the drug's benefits, not its liabilities.
13 Bold type in original, p. 20.
14 Brown et al., 1986, p. 493.
15 Barkley and Cunningham, 1978; See discussion in Schrag and Divoky, 1975.
16 P. 2404.
17 Richters et al., 1995.
18 Whalen and Henker, 1997.
19 Breggin, 1997a.
20 These adverse drug effects are discussed in detail in earlier chapters.
21 P. 2304.
22 See Valentine, 1987 & 1988, for methods of effective communication with children.
23 Associated Press, 1997a.
24 Dulcan, 1994.
25 Kauffman et al., 1981.
26 When a child takes stimulants, the obvious side effects—such as a racing heart, insomnia, or loss of appetite—are likely to convince child and parent alike that

the child is taking "strong medication." This is the "snake oil" phenomenon in which a very bad tasting medicine seems like especially "strong medicine," enhancing its subjective effects. This has been confirmed by recent studies of research on depression which show that patients recover as well from placebo as from antidepressants if the placebo has noticeable side effects (Fisher and Greenberg, 1989, 1995. Reviewed in Breggin, 1997a).

27 Kauffman et al., 1981.

28 Richters et al., 1995.

29 P. 3.

30 P. 94.

31 P. 95.

32 P. 253.

33 P. 169.

34 P. 249.

35 IMS Canada, 1996; Harvey, 1996b.

36 Zametkin stated in the deposition that his fee was $500 per hour and that he had already been paid for "somewhere between 15 and 25 hours" as of one year earlier.

37 The case was eventually withdrawn by the plaintiff.

38 P. 74.

39 P. 82.

40 See chapter 10 for analysis of Zametkin's studies.

41 Gilbert, 1997. Also see B.B., 1997.

42 Gilbert, 1997.

43 Ten of the 62 children who remained after the first month of the study had mental retardation, seven had numerous signs of autism, and many others had a variety of diagnoses in addition to ADHD.

44 Gilbert, 1997.

45 Breggin, 1991 and 1997a; Breggin and Breggin, 1994.

46 Breggin, 1992a, 1997b&c.

47 I have devoted a book, *The Heart of Being Helpful*, 1997b, to self-transformation as the key to becoming a healing presence. Also see Breggin, 1997c.

48 How to help children is the subject of the final chapters of the book.

Chapter 8: Definitive Study or Scientific Hoax?

1 National Institute of Mental Health (undated).

2 MTA Cooperative Group (1999a&b).

3 Nies and Spielberg (1996, p. 45); also see Fisher and Greenberg (1989, 1997).

4 The principal investigators in the NIMH Ritalin study have claimed that it would have been unethical to use a placebo group because stimulants have been proven effective as a treatment for ADHD. In reality, placebo groups are commonly used in ADHD and stimulant research. For example, I recently reviewed eight double-blind placebo controlled studies of stimulants for ADHD that were

conducted from 1990–98 (Breggin, 1999a&b; also see chapter 2 of this book). Furthermore, placebo-controlled trials are routinely carried out in psychiatry for far more dangerous "disorders" than ADHD, including "major depression" and "schizophrenia." Also, a number of the children in the NIMH study went without medication while they were in the community and behavior treatment groups. It would have been no more "unethical" to add an actual placebo group. In addition, since this study exposes children to drugs for many weeks and even months, it has entered uncharted territory requiring a scientifically valid evaluation of safety and efficacy. Finally, there can be no ethical problem surrounding the use of double-blind procedures. It was unethical not to use them. Yet this basic methodology was also omitted.

5   MTA Cooperative Group (1999a, p. 1079) shows that of 144 medication management subjects, 46 (32%) were on medication for ADHD at the start of the selection process.

6   Borcherding et al. (1990) discuss how no one notices adverse drug effects such as drug-induced obsessions and compulsions unless they are trained to do so and unless the study focuses on them.

7   NIMH MTA Study (undated, b).

8   NIMH MTA Study (undated, a).

9   MTA Cooperative Group, 1999a, p. 1074). The data from these raters are produced in Table 5 (pp. 1082–3) of the study.

10 The children rated themselves on the MASC anxiety scale (results on Table 5 in the study).

11 New York State Psychiatric Institute and Columbia University Division of Child & Adolescent Psychiatry (1994). It was handed out at a conference held in New York City.

12 MTA Cooperative Group (1999a, bottom of p. 1075).

13 MTA Cooperative Group (1999a, table 4).

14 In a personal communication to me dated January 24, 2000, Dr. Karon explained that the Bonferroni correction of six was too small.

15 MTA Cooperative Group (1999a, p. 1077).

16 NYSPI Sponsored Research (1998).

17 The italicizing of "not" is added.

Chapter 9: The "Science" behind Making an ADHD Diagnosis

1   Dulcan and Popper, 1991.

2   International Narcotics Control Board, 1996b.

3   See Chapter 2.

4   United Nations Information Service, 1997a.

5   Rappley et al., 1995.

6   Breggin and Breggin, 1998. There were also a number of local malpractice suits involving Ritalin that also generated some publicity critical of Ritalin (Granat, 1997).

7   For a humorous critique of the widely shifting positions held by various states in regard to rates of prescribing Ritalin, see Parry, 1997. The DEA publishes a list each year of Ritalin usage state by state.

8   Caplan, 1995; Kirk and Kutchins, 1992.

9   P. 221, italics added.

10 Chapters 1, 3, and 10.

11 P. 20.

12 P. 40.

13 P. 140.

14 Drug Enforcement Administration, 1996, p. 12.

15 Rosenthal and Jacobson, 1968, studied teachers in three different classes who were told that a group representing 20% of their incoming students from a lower-class neighborhood were "intellectual bloomers" who would make substantial gains in the coming year. Probably due to the teachers' improved attitude toward the children, the IQ's of these supposed "bloomers" did increase over the year in comparison to the controls. Langer and Abelson, 1974, looked at how clinical psychologists tend to evaluate a videotaped job applicant. The psychologists perceived more mental disorder if they were told the person was a "patient" rather than a "job applicant."

16 Goldman, 1995.

17 P. 79.

18 See later chapters for further discussions of childhood.

19 Goldman, 1995.

20 Chapter 4.

21 Wender, 1973, p. 9.

22 Zachary, 1997.

23 Sexton and Swarns, 1997.

24 Chapters 6 and 9.

25 Pp. 25–25, italics in original.

26 Quoted in Azepeitia and Rocamora, 1997.

27 P. 2.

28 Pp. 21 and 22.

29 Chapter 6.

30 P. 13.

31 P. 4.

32 *Dorland's Illustrated Medical Dictionary*, 1994.

33 *Dorland's Illustrated Medical Dictionary*, 1994, p. 1627.

34 P. 11.

35 Teicher et al., 1997.

36 Goldman, 1995.

37 For a similar criticism, see Coles, 1987, p. 203

38 Coles, 1987, p. xii.

39 I have dealt with learning disabilities in more detail in *Toxic Psychiatry*, 1991.

40 P. 162.
41 Athans, 1997.
42 Applebome, 1996.
43 Discussed in chapters 12 and 21.
44 Speech et al., 1993.
45 Morrow, 1997. The estimate is from IMSAmerica which collects marketing data for industry.
46 Chapters 2 and 3.
47 See chapter 2 for McGinnis's description of a Ritalin-induced toxic psychosis.

Chapter 10: Scientific Evidence for a Biological Cause of ADHD

1 Zametkin et al., 1990.
2 The timing is discussed in Counterpoint, 1990.
3 Popper and Steingard, 1994, p. 739.
4 Granat, 1995.
5 Zametkin et al., 1993.
6 The same observation is made by Ernst, 1996.
7 Breggin and Breggin, 1998.
8 Morton, 1996.
9 P. 73.
10 E.g., Barkley, 1995; Ingersoll, 1988; Quinn, 1997.
11 Teicher et al., 1997, p. 908.
12 Breggin, 1991, 1997a; Breggin and Breggin, 1998; Gould, 1981; Hubbard, 1994; Hubbard and Wald, 1993; Lewontin, 1992; Lewontin, Rose, and Kamin, 1984; Mosher and Burti, 1994.
13 Twin studies..., 1992.
14 Wender, 1995. Quoted at length at end of chapter 6.
15 Leutwyler, 1996.
16 The disorder is characterized by mutant receptors for thyroid hormone (Hauser, 1993).
17 Psychiatric Times, 1993.
18 Chapter 13.
19 Haney, 1993.
20 The authors also compare it to other variables such as intellectual disability, but this is inaccurate. Intellectual disability, such as developmental retardation, is not merely a variation from the normal. It can be a genetic and physiological disorder.

Chapter 11: Back to the Future

1 Summarized in Ernst 1996.
2 See Bhandary, 1997, for history.
3 Conners and Eisenberg, 1963.
4 Conners, 1969.

5   Rapoport et al., 1970.
6   See chapter 7 about Rapoport and the holy grail. Rapoport's work is further reviewed in Breggin, 1991, and Breggin and Breggin, 1998.
7   Reviewed in Lambert et al., 1976.
8   Now deceased.
9   Chapters 14–16.
10 P. 26.
11 P. 27.
12 P. 1.
13 P. 33.
14 P. 45.
15 Chapter 9 discusses the concept of syndrome.
16 Schmidt, 1987.
17 Williams, 1988.
18 Henig, 1988.
19 Treadwell, 1987.
20 Blum, 1987; Hausman, 1987.
21 Examples of newspaper articles include, Kolata, 1996, McGinnis, 1997, Vatz, 1994, Vatz and Weinberg, 1995, and Zachary, 1997.
22 For the controversy, also see Kolata, 1996.
23 Also Crossette, 1996; Ladika, 1996.
24 Ladika, 1996.
25 United Nations Information Service, 1995.
26 *Psychiatric News*, 1992.
27 Safer and Krager, 1992.
28 Welke, 1990.
29 Described in Breggin and Breggin, 1998.
30 Data in Safer, Zito, and Fine, 1996.

Chapter 12: Parents, Caregivers, and Teachers Make the Difference

1   Pp. 83 and 134.
2   Nidecker, 1997.
3   Perry, 1994.
4   The studies cited are McLeer et al., 1994, and Glod and Teicher, 1996.
5   Azar, 1997a.
6   Baldwin et al., 1995. The primary caregivers included two fathers, 24 mothers, three grandmothers, and an aunt.
7   P. 83.
8   Schwarz and Perry, 1994. Also, Perry 1994.
9   Schwarz and Perry, 1994.
10 Reviewed in Breggin, 1992a.
11 DeAngelis, 1997.
12 Leff and Berkowitz, 1996.

13 Koslow, 1995, p. 173. Also see Greenough and Black, 1992.

14 Reviewed in Ounce of Prevention Fund, 1996.

15 Weiler et al., 1995.

16 Vobejda, 1997.

17 I initially found out about it from a short article in USA Today (Henry, 1997). The study is Nord et al., 1997. It was based on survey interviews with parents and guardians of almost 17,000 students spanning kindergarten through high school.

18 A parent who participated in three out of the four activities was considered "highly involved."

19 Discussed by Azar, 1997a. The research drew on 1,300 families and their children up to three years of age.

20 Burchinal et al., 1996.

21 Azar, 1997b.

22 Also see Kuhl, 1994.

23 Quoted in Azar, 1997a.

24 Estrada and Pinsof, 1995, reviewed the literature on parent management training (PMT). Also see Greenfield and Senecal, 1995, for an interesting approach involving teaching parents to play with their children. A parent-training group based on Barkley's methods was effective for children most of whom were not taking any medication (Anastopoulos et al., 1993).

25 Seppa, 1997.

26 For books on parenting, see chapter 17.

27 Breggin, 1997b.

Chapter 13: Physical Causes of ADHD-like Symptoms

1 As examples of sources that fail to review a wide range of possible medical causes for ADHD-like symptoms, see Barkley, 1995; Ingersoll, 1988; Quinn, 1997; Wender, 1973, 1987, 1995.

2 Wolraich, 1996.

3 Chapters 2–4.

4 Ojito, 1997. A study in New York is exploring the possibility of widespread mercury poisoning in apartments due to its use in religious rituals. Sprinkled or spread on floors, it can remain undetected for years causing irritability and insomnia, and physical symptoms such as skin problems, leg cramps, and excessive salivation.

5 Wolraich, 1996.

6 The experiment began with a 3-week baseline, followed by a 3-week placebo period, and then a 4-week experimental diet. Ten of their 24 hyperactive children showed an approximately 50% improvement by parental ratings. Another four showed some improvement. The remaining 10 showed none.

7 Egger et al., 1992. Out of a group of 185 children, they selected 40 children whose behavior improved on special diets low in antigens. These children were then placed in a double-blind study in which they were treated with injections of an

enzyme (beta-glucuronidase) thought to reduce food allergies, although its mechanism is unknown. Sixteen of twenty children who received the active treatment no longer responded with so much hyperactivity to their food intolerance.

8 Rowe and Rowe, 1994.
9 Pp. 73–74 and p. 79.

Chapter 14: Who's Behind All This? Part I

1 Breggin, 1991, 1997a.
2 Kirk and Kutchins, 1992; Breggin, 1991.
3 Chapter 3.
4 Breggin, 1992b.
5 Jonas, 1992.
6 Benedek, 1993.
7 Italics added.
8 Thomson, 1997. Reproduced on web site www.breggin.com.
9 Breggin and Breggin, 1994; Breggin and Breggin, 1998.
10 Novartis, 1996.
11 Moore, 1997.
12 Chapter 2.
13 Stout, 1996.
14 Moore, 1997.
15 Office of the Inspector General, 1992.
16 Jacoby and Small, 1975; Millstein, 1983.
17 Leber, 1994. Discussed in chapter 11.
18 Silver, 1990.
19 Office of the Inspector General, 1992.
20 P. 89.
21 Cody, 1992.
22 Ciba, 1976.
23 For Prozac, see Breggin and Breggin, 1994, and for the FDA, see Breggin, 1991, 1997a, and 1998a.
24 *Medical News Letter*, 1969.
25 Scoville, 1970.
26 Methyl-testosterone and ethinyl estradiol.
27 Scoville, 1970.
28 Associated Press, 1996b.
29 Reviewed in Breggin and Breggin, 1994, and Breggin, 1991, 1997a.
30 Nemeroff, 1996.
31 Stecklow and Johannes, 1997a.
32 Stecklow and Johannes, 1997b.
33 *PT* staff, 1997.
34 Ciba, 1991; also see Anafranil section of the *Physicians' Desk Reference*, 1997.
35 CHADD, 1996a.

36 See chapter 16.

37 Southam News Media, 1996.

38 P. 2.

39 Kaplan, 1997.

40 Food and Drug Administration, 1995, 1996; reviewed in Breggin, 1997a and 1998a. See ahead this chapter.

41 CHADD, 1995b, 1996b.

42 Euren, 1993. The Quinn and Stern book is discussed in chapter 6.

43 Excerpted statements from *Pay Attention!!!* by Craig B. Liden (a physician), Jane Zalenski, and Roberta Newman, circa 1989.

44 CHADD, 1994; Riordan and Matyas, 1994.

45 21 CFR Ch. II, Paragraph 1308.12.

46 Riordan and Matyas, 1994.

47 United Nations Information Service, 1997a.

48 1-800-742-2422.

49 Leary, 1993.

50 Drug Enforcement Administration, 1995.

51 See Morales, 1995.

52 Thomas, 1995.

53 1995, p. 29; 1996a, p. 13.

54 Schaepe, 1995.

55 Drug Enforcement Administration, 1995c, p. 62.

56 P. 12.

57 Breggin, 1991.

58 Lilly, 1997a.

59 Breggin, 1991.

60 Armstrong, 1993; Howe, 1994.

61 Howe, 1994.

62 Hoss and Bartlett, 1994.

63 Pp. 166–167. I use the term "complex" rather than "combine."

Chapter 15: Who's Behind All This? Part II

1 Livingston, 1997.

2 Lang, 1997.

3 Power et al.,1995.

4 Lucker and Molloy, 1995.

5 Schwiebert et al., 1995.

6 Athans, 1997.

7 The conduit for support of ADHD/Ritalin comes mainly through The Office of Special Education Programs (OSEP), a component of the Office of Special Education and Rehabilitative Services (OSERS).

8 Dialog, 1997.

9 U. S. Department of Education, circa 1993.

10 Axelrod and Bailey, 1979; Divoky, 1989; George, 1993a&b; Maag and Reid, 1994. Also see chapter 21.

11 U. S. Department of Education, undated.

12 The government Office of Special Education and Rehabilitative Services (1997) describes NICHCY as one of five "key federally supported clearinghouses on disability."

13 A number of professional educators read this manuscript.

14 From the Office of Special Education Programs (OSEP).

15 The reauthorization of the Education of the Handicapped Act which was renamed the Individuals with Disabilities in Education Act (IDEA),

16 Summarized in OSHERS, 1992.

17 Shapiro, 1996.

18 Schiller and Hauster, 1992a&b.

19 Moss, 1996 & 1997.

20 Lewis, 1997; Ansorge, 1997.

21 See Zito et al., 1997.

22 Republished with an update as *The War Against Children of Color* (1998).

23 Chandler, 1997.

24 E.g., Lewis, 1997.

25 Perkins, 1994.

26 Chapters 2-4.

27 In February 1990 the U. S. Supreme court mandated in Sullivan v. Zebley that the Social Security Administration broaden its concept of disability to include children whose impairments limit their ability to act and to behave in an age appropriate manner. Regulations were then written to make it possible for children with ADHD to qualify for disability payments under Supplemental Security Income (SSI) (General Accounting Office, 1994; Woodward and Weiser, 1994).

28 Bello and Latty, 1997.

29 National Center, 1996–1997.

30 Woodward and Weiser, 1994. The number of children receiving benefits leaped from 300,000 in 1989 to more than 770,000 in 1993. Under the broadened category of mental impairment, 61% of the awards went to children diagnosed with "mental retardation," followed by 10% diagnosed with ADHD (General Accounting Office, 1994). These numbers may begin to reverse during the welfare cutbacks.

31 Chapter 21.

32 National Institute of Mental Health and Food and Drug Administration, 1995.

33 The conference is discussed in chapter 16.

34 Herbert, 1997.

35 Breggin and Breggin, 1998, discuss recent NIMH policies in detail.

36 National Institute of Mental Health, 1993.

37 Dialog, 1997.

38 Mackie, 1997.

39 Chapter 5.

40 Discussed in chapter 14.

41 Schrag and Divoky, 1975.

42 Regier and Leshner, 1992; Richters et al., 1995. See chapter 8 for a critical analysis of the funded studies.

43 See critique in chapter 10.

44 Breggin and Breggin, 1998.

45 Silver, 1989.

46 Ross and Pam, 1995. Also see Breggin, 1991.

47 Breggin, 1991, 1997a, and 1998a.

48 Chapter 14.

49 Skrzycki, 1996.

50 Kuttner, 1997.

51 Food and Drug Administration, 1997.

52 Chapter 14.

53 Schwartz, 1997; Stout, 1997.

54 Finkel, 1982.

55 Food and Drug Administration, circa 1981.

56 Cinque, 1978.

57 Schary, 1980.

58 Leber, 1985.

59 Breggin, 1991, 1997a, 1998a; Breggin and Breggin, 1994.

60 I attempted to find them through the Freedom of Information Act and was informed by the FDA that they were too old to be located.

61 Lee, 1981.

62 Breggin, 1991, 1997a; Breggin and Breggin, 1994, and 1998.

63 Breggin, 1991, 1997a; Breggin and Breggin, 1994, and 1998.

64 Food and Drug Administration, 1985; discussed in Breggin and Breggin, 1998.

65 American Medical Association et al., 1997.

66 Kealey, 1997.

67 Chapter 3.

68 Chapter 2.

69 Receptor loss, causing reduced sensitivity of the receptor system (subsensitivity), is discussed in regard to Prozac in Breggin and Breggin, 1994, and in Breggin, 1997a, as well as in chapter 3.

70 Kolata, 1997.

71 McCann et al., 1997.

72 Wyeth-Ayerst, 1997.

73 Sackeim et al., 1993.

74 Chapters 14 to 16 for the politics of psychiatry.

Chapter 16: Brave New World of Childhood

1   IMS Canada, 1996; Harvey, 1996.

2   International Narcotics Control Board, 1996b.

3   PR Newswire, 1997.

4   Seattle Clinical Research Center, Inc., 1997.

5   Data from IMS America reported by Leonard, 1997; Tanouye, 1997.

6   IMS America, 1997.

7   Reuters, 1997c.

8   Reuters, 1997b.

9   Reuters, 1997d.

10 Price, 1997; Strauch, 1997.

11 Crowley, 1997.

12 See ahead in this chapter.

13 National Advisory Mental Health Council, 1988.

14 Crowley, 1997.

15 Leonard, 1997.

16 Schrag and Divoky, 1975, p. 79.

17 Knapp et al., 1995.

18 Knapp et al., 1995.

19 Fisher and Fisher, 1996; Hazell et al.,1995.

20 Fisher and Fisher, 1996; Pelliegrino, 1996.

21 Baker, 1995. I have reviewed both the lack of efficacy and the dangers of using these newer drugs in children (Breggin and Breggin, 1994; Breggin, 1997a).

22 Chapter 3.

23 The study (Emslie et al., 1997) was reported in a psychiatric newspaper (Sherman, 1995) prior to publication. My analysis, published in a letter to the paper, indicated a rate of Prozac-induced mania of 6% (Breggin, 1995). The newspaper reported that Emslie, the senior author of the study, refused to respond to my observations.

24 Susman, 1996.

25 Grinfeld, 1997.

26 Reuters, 1997d.

27 Pear, 1997.

28 Pear, 1997.

29 Breggin and Breggin, 1994; Breggin, 1997a.

30 Breggin and Breggin, 1994; Breggin, 1997a.

31 Breggin and Breggin, 1998.

32 Gostin et al., 1997.

33 Chapter 2.

34 Maurer, 1996.

35 Breggin and Breggin, 1998.

36 Reviewed in Breggin and Breggin, 1998.

37 E.g., Mason, Jr., 1994a&b.

38 Mason, Jr., 1994b.

39 McKinney et al., circa 1993.

40 The brain-disabling principle of drug treatment is most recently and thoroughly discussed in Breggin, 1997a.

41 Pp. 65–66.

42 Dialog, 1997.

43 For information on the upsurge of electroshock, see Breggin 1991 and 1997a, and for efforts to revive psychosurgery, see Breggin and Breggin, 1998.

Chapter 18: The Environmental Stressor Checklist

1 Pedism was coined by Breggin and Breggin, 1998.

Chapter 19: Making Ourselves Ready to Help Our Children

1 Research on the importance of love and relationship is reviewed in chapter 12.

2 See especially my book, *The Heart of Being Helpful*. Also Breggin, 1992a and 1997c.

3 Breggin, 1991 pp. 287 ff.

4 Breggin, 1991; Breggin and Stern, 1996; Karon and Vandenbos, 1981; Mosher and Burti, 1994.

5 Kuehnel and Slama, 1984.

Chapter 20: When Adults Are in Conflict with the Children They Love

1 Seppa, 1997.

2 Fowler, 1992. See chapter 14 for entire quote.

3 Discussed in chapter 9, and Coles. (1987)

Chapter 21: What to Do When the Teacher Says Your Child Has ADHD

1 Psychologist Brian Kean, 1997, has written to me from Australia: "Gaining a special education label or being classified into a category virtually guarantees failure.... In fact, what occurs in many cases is all the failing kids and kids with behaviour and emotional problems are grouped together which in itself creates a significant educational disadvantage. The current push in special education internationally is for 'full inclusion' with no labeling. The traditional special education model is outmoded and is seen in enlightened practice as detrimental to basic human rights."

2 Chapter 15.

3 For a critique of learning disorders, see chapter 9, and coles (1987).

4 Calahan, 1995.

5 p. 38

6 U.S. Department of Education, undated, Attention deficit disorder: Beyond the myths. Discussed in chapter 15.

7 Chapter 12.

8 Murray, 1996, for home schooling data.

9 Murray, 1996.

BIBLIOGRAPHY

Aarskog, D., Fevang, F., Kløve, H., Støa, K., and Thorsen, T. (1977). The effect of stimulant drugs, dextroamphetamine and methylphenidate, on secretion of growth hormone in hyperactive children. *Journal of Pediatrics, 90,* 136–139.

Abbott Laboratories. (1996, December). Dear Doctor letter [warning about hepatotoxicity from Cylert (pemoline)]. Abbott Park, Illinois: Author.

Accardo v. Cenac. (1997). 19th Judicial District Court. Parish of East Baton Rouge, State of Louisiana, Docket No. 350.125. Div. "F." Civil Action.

Alheid, F., Heimer, L., and Switzer, R. (1990). Basal ganglia. In G. Paxinos (Ed.), *The Human Nervous System,* pp. 483–582. New York: Academic Press.

Alcohol, Drug Abuse, and Mental Health Administration. (ADAMHA) (1984). *Cocaine and stimulants.* Washington, DC: Department of Health and Human Services, Public Health Service, ADAMHA. DHHS Publication No. (ADM) 84–1306.

Allen, A. (1997, July). readin', ritin' and ritlin. A Salon special on legal drugs. http://www.salonmagazine.com/

Amen, D. (1997, fall). Advances in the treatment of attention deficit disorder in children and adults (workshop brochure). Minneapolis, Minnesota: Institute for Behavioral Healthcare.

American Academy of Pediatrics. (2000a). Practice guideline: Diagnosis and evaluation of a child with attention-deficit/hyperactivity disorder. *Pediatrics, 105,* 1158–70. Also available at http://www.aap.org/policy/ac0002.html

American Academy of Pediatrics. (2000b, May 1). Press Release: AAP releases new guidelines for diagnosis of ADHD. http://www.aap.org/advocacy/releases/mayadhd.htm.

American Medical Association, Association of American Medical Colleges, National Medical Association, and PhARMA. (1997, June 25). Restore FDA Funding. (advertisement). *Washington Post,* p. A16.

American Psychiatric Association. (1987). *Diagnostic and statistical manual of mental disorders, Third Edition, Revised (DSM-III-R).* Washington, DC: author.

American Psychiatric Association (1989). *Treatments of psychiatric disorders: A task force report of the American Psychiatric Association.* Washington, D.C.: author.

American Psychiatric Association. (1994). *Diagnostic and statistical manual of mental disorders, Fourth Edition (DSM-IV).* Washington, D.C.: author.

America's Pharmaceutical Research Companies. (1996, September 2). Advertisement for booklet, *New Hope For Depression and Other Mental Illnesses. Time,* unnumbered page.

American Psychiatric Association. (1992). *Tardive dyskinesia: A task force report.* Washington, DC: Author.

Anastopoulos, A, Shelton, T., DuPaul, G., and Guevremont, D. (1993). Parent training for attention-deficit hyperactivity disorder: Its impact on parent functioning. *Journal of Abnormal Child Psychology, 21,* 581–5966.

Andreasen, N. (1984). *The broken brain: The biological revolution in psychiatry.* New York: Harper & Row.

Ansorge, R. (1997, February 2). Drug gets results, but parents worry: is it safe for kids. *The Sun News* (Myrtle Beach, S.C.) (Reprinted from the Colorado Springs *Gazette Telegraph*), p. 1E.

Antelman, S.M., Caggiula, A.R., Kiss, S., Edwards, D.J., Kocan, D., and Stiller, R. (1995). Neurochemical and physiological effects of cocaine oscillate with sequential drug treatment: Possibly a major factor in drug variability. *Neuropsychopharmacology, 12,* 297–306.

Applebome, P. (1996, November 21). Americans straddle the "average" mark in math and science. *New York Times,* p. B14.

Arakawa, O. (1994). Effects of methamphetamine and methyl-phenidate on single and paired rat open-field behaviors. *Physiology & Behavior, 55,* 441–446.

Archives of General Psychiatry. (1995, June). Editorial. *52,* 422–423.

Armstrong, L. (1993). *And they call it help: The psychiatric policing of America's Children.* New York: Addison-Wesley Publishing Co.

Armstrong, T. (1995). *The myth of the A.D.D. child.* New York: Dutton.

Arnold, L. E., and Jensen, P. S. (1995). Attention-deficit disorders. In H. I. Kaplan and Sadock, B. (Eds.). *Comprehensive Textbook of Psychiatry, VI,* pp. 2295–2310. Baltimore: Williams & Wilkins.

Ascoli, M., and Segaloff, M. L. (1996). Adrenohypophyseal hormones and their hypothalamic releasing factors.

In J. G. Harman and Limbird, L. E. (Eds.). *The pharmacological basis of therapeutics, 9th edition,* pp. 1363–1382. New York: McGraw-Hill.

Associated Press. (1996a, January 13). Federal agency issues a mild caution on a hyperactivity drug. *New York Times.*

Associated Press. (1996b, March 27). Maker of Ritalin warns against misuse. *Huntington Herald-Express* (Indiana), p. 5A.

Associated Press. (1997a, April 16). Study: Placebo effect can last. Press release.

Associated Press. (1997b, July 7). Study: High blood pressure speeds brain shrinkage. *USA Today Health.*

Associated Press. (1997c, September 26). Precise cocaine effects are seen in brain scans. *New York Times,* p. A18.

Associated Press. (2000, April 16). Doc: Ritalin led to boy's death. Press release.

Athans, M. (1997, November 2). Young readers left to struggle. *Baltimore Sun,* p. 1.

Axelrod, S. and Bailey, S. (1979, April). Drug treatment for hyperactivity: Controversies, alternatives, and guidelines. *Exceptional Children,* 544–550.

Azar, B. (1997a, June). It may cause anxiety, but day care can benefit kids. *Monitor,* p. 13.

Azar, B. (1997b, June). Consistent parenting helps children regulate emotions. *Monitor,* p. 17.

Azepeitia, L. and Rocamora, M. (1997, February) cited in *Attention Deficit (/Hyperactivity) Disorder, Giftedness, and Ritalin. nafi, second quarter* [newsletter of the National Association for the Fostering of Intelligence], p. 2.

Baberg, HT, Nelesen, R.A., and Dimsdale, J.E. (1996). Amphetamine use: Return of an old scourge in a consultation psychiatric setting. *American Journal of Psychiatry, 153,* 789–793.

Bailey, W. J. (1995). Factline on nonmedical use of Ritalin (methylphenidate). Indiana Prevention and Resource Center at Indiana University. http://www.drugs.indiana.edu/pubs/factline/ritalin.

Baker, B. (1995, March). Though data lacking, antidepressants used widely in children. *Clinical Psychiatry News,* p. 16.

Baldwin, J. (1997, April). Military policy on Ritalin use under examination. *Psychiatric Times,* p. 30.

Baldwin, K., Brown, R.T., and Milan, M.A. (1995). Predictors of stress in caregivers of attention deficit hyperactivity disordered children. *The American Journal of Family Therapy, 23,* 149–159.

Barker, R. (1997). *And the waters turned to blood.* New York: Simon & Schuster.

Barkley, R. A. (1977). A review of stimulant drug research with hyperactive children. *Journal of Child Psychology and Psychiatry, 18,* 137–165.

Barkley, R. A. (1981). *Hyperactive children: A handbook for diagnosis and treatment.* New York: Guilford Press.

Barkley, R. A. (1990). *Attention deficit hyperactivity disorder: A handbook for diagnosis and treatment.* New York: Guilford Press.

Barkley, R. A. (1991). *Attention-deficit hyperactivity disorder: A clinical workbook.* New York: Guilford Press.

Barkley, R. A. (Ed.) (1995). *Taking charge of ADHD: The complete, authoritative guide for parents.* New York: Guilford Press.

Barkley, R.A. (1996). ADD research: A look at today and tomorrow (interview). CHADD: http://www.chadd.org/barkley.htm.

Barkley, R. A. and Cunningham, C. E. (1978). Do stimulant drugs improve the academic performance of hyperkinetic children? A review of outcome studies. *Clinical Pediatrics, 8,* 137–146.

Barkley, R.A., and Cunningham, C.E. (1979). The effects of methylphenidate on the mother-child interactions of hyperactive children. *Archives of General Psychiatry, 36,* 201–208.

Barkley, R. A., Karlsson, J., Pollard, S., and Murphy, J.V. (1985). Developmental changes in the mother-child interactions of hyperactive boys: Effects of two dose levels of Ritalin. *Journal of Child Psychology, 26,* 705–715.

Barkley, R.A., McMurray, M.B., Edelbrock, C.S., and Robbins, K. (1989). The response of aggressive and nonaggressive ADHD children to two doses of methylphenidate. *Journal of the American Academy of Child and Adolescent Psychiatry, 28,* 873–871.

Barkley, R.A., McMurray, M.B., Edelbrock, C.S., & Robbins, K. (1990). Side effects of methylphenidate in children with attention deficit disorder: A systemic, placebo-controlled evaluation. *Pediatrics, 86,* 184–192.

Barnett, J.V., and Kuczenski, R. (1986). Desensitization of rat striatal dopamine-stimulated adenylate cyclase after acute amphetamine administration. *Journal of Pharmacology and Experimental Therapeutics, 237,* 820–825.

Bates, G. (1997, September 5). Personal communication from the publisher at

Common Courage Press to Peter R. Breggin.

Battaglia, G., Yeh, S.Y., O'Hearn, E., Molliver, M.E., Kuhar, M.J. and DeSouza, E.B. (1987). 3,4-methylenedioxymethamphetamine and 3,4-methylenedioxyamphetamine destroy serotonin terminals in rat brain. *Journal of Pharmacology and Experimental Therapeutics, 142,* 911–916.

Baughman, C. (1997, March 15). BR jury awards $1.3 million to injured woman. *Advocate* (Baton Rouge, LA)., p. 7c.

Baughman, Jr., F.A. (1992, October). Says drug companies too powerful. (letter). *Clinical Psychiatry News,* p. 5.

Baughman, Jr., F.A. (1993). Treatment of attention-deficit hyperactivity disorder. (letter). *Journal of the American Medical Association, 269,* 2368–2369.

Baughman, Jr., F.A., (1996, January). Fundamentally flawed. (letter). *Clinical Psychiatry News,* p. 8.

B.B. (B. Bauer) (1997, September 27). Meds may give attention a lasting boost. *Science News, 152,* 204.

Begley. S. (1993, June 28). The puzzle of genius. *Newsweek,* p. 46.

Begley, S. (2000, February 28). Getting inside a teen brain. *Newsweek,* p. 58.

Bell, R.D., Alexander, G.M., Schwartzman, R.J., and Yu, J. (1982). The methylphenidate-induced stereotypy in the awake rat: Local cerebral metabolism. *Neurology, 32,* 377–381.

Bello, M., and Latty, Y. (1997, June 23). Mental clinics under fire: Agencies believed ripping off SSI and overmedicating poor kids for big profits. *Philadelphia Daily News,* p. 5.

Benedek, E. (1993, February 8). Letter to Peter Roger Breggin, M.D., as a part of a mass mailing soliciting funds for the American Psychiatric Foundation.

Bhandary, A. N. (1997). The chronic attention deficit syndrome. *Psychiatric Annals, 27,* 543–544.

Bhattacharyya, A.K., Ghosh, B., Aulakh, C.S. and Pradhan, S.N. (1980). Correlation of behavioral and neurochemical effects of acute administration of methylphenidate in rats. *Progress in Neuro-Psychopharmacology, 4,* 129–136.

Bielski, V. (1990, July 4). The assault on patients' rights. *The San Francisco Bay Guardian,* p. 17.

Billing, L., Eriksson, M., Jonsson, B., Steneroth, G., and Zetterstrom, R. (1994). The influence of environmental factors on behavioural problems in 8-year-old children exposed to amphetamine during fetal life. *Child Abuse & Neglect, 18,* 3–9.

Blair, J. (1997, May 26). School survey prompts lawsuit. Associated Press wire service release.

"Mrs. Blair." (1997). Anonymous communication from a parent provided by psychologist Peter Oas, Niceville, Florida.

Blakeslee, S. (1997, April 17). Studies show talking with infants shapes basis of ability to think. *New York Times,* p. A22.

Blanton, S. (1956). *Love or perish.* New York: Simon & Schuster.

Block, M. A. (1996). *No more Ritalin: Treating ADHD without drugs.* New York: Kensington Books.

Bloom, A.S., Russell, L.J., Weisskopf, B., and Blackerby, J. L. (1988). Methylphenidate-induced delusional disorder in a child with attention deficit disorder with hyperactivity. *Journal of the American Academy of*

Child and Adolescent Psychiatry, 27, 88–89.

Blum, A. (1987, November 23). Legal attack on Ritalin expands. *National Law Journal, 10* (11).

Blum, N.J., Mauk, J.E, McComas, J.J., and Mace, F.C. (1996). Separate and combined effects of methylphenidate and a behavior intervention on disruptive behavior in children with mental retardation. *Journal of Applied Behavioral Analysis, 29,* 305–319.

Blume, E. S. (1990). *Secret survivors: Uncovering incest and its aftereffects in women.* New York: John Wiley.

Bodenheimer, T. (2000, May 18). Uneasy alliance: Clinical investigators and the pharmaceutical industry. *New England Journal of Medicine, 342,* 1539–1544.

Boneau, C.A. (1992). Observations on psychology's past and future. *American Psychologist, 47,*1586–1596.

Boris, M., and Mandel, F.S. (1994). Foods and additives are common causes of the attention deficit hyperactive disorder in children. *Annals of Allergy, 72,* 462–468.

Borcherding, B.V., Keysor, C.S., Rapoport, J.L., Elia, J., & Amass, J. (1990). Motor/vocal tics and compulsive behaviors on stimulant drugs: Is there a common vulnerability. *Psychiatric Research, 33,* 83–94.

Boutros, N. N., and Bowers, M.B. (1996). Chronic substance-induced psychotic disorders: State of the literature. *Journal of Neuropsychiatry and Clinical Neurosciences, 8,* 262–269.

Bower, B. (1988). Hyperactivity: The family factor. *Science News, 134,* p. 399.

Bower, B. (1989). Kids talk about the 'good pill.' *Science News, 135,* p. 332.

Bradley, C. (1937). The behavior of children receiving benzedrine. *American Journal of Psychiatry, 94,* 577–585.

Bradshaw, J. (1988). *Healing the shame that binds you.* Deerfield Beach, Florida: Health Communications.

Breedlove, S. M. (1997, August 13). Disregard anecdotes. *New York Times,* p. A28.

Breggin, P. (1990). Brain damage, dementia and persistent cognitive dysfunction associated with neuroleptic drugs: Evidence, etiology, implications. *Journal of Mind and Behavior 11,* 425–464.

Breggin, P. (1991). *Toxic psychiatry: Why therapy, empathy and love must replace the drugs, electroshock and biochemical theories of the 'new psychiatry'.* New York: St. Martin's Press.

Breggin, P. (1992a) *Beyond conflict: From self-help and psychotherapy to peacemaking.* New York: St. Martin's Press.

Breggin, P. (1992b, February 11). The president's sleeping pill and its makers (letter). *New York Times,* p. A. 18.

Breggin, P. (1993). Parallels between neuroleptic effects and lethargic encephalitis: The production of dyskinesias and cognitive disorders. *Brain and Cognition 23,* 8–27.

Breggin, P. (1995, September). Prozac "hazardous" to children (letter). *Clinical Psychiatry News,* p. 10.

Breggin, P. (1997a). *Brain-disabling treatments in psychiatry: Drugs, electroshock and the role of the FDA.* New York: Springer Publishing Company.

Breggin, P. (1997b). *The heart of being helpful: Empathy and the creation of a healing presence.* New York: Springer Publishing Company.

Breggin, P. (1997c). Psychotherapy in emotional crises without resort to psychiatric medication. *Humanistic Psychologist, 25,* 2–14.

Breggin, P. (1998a). Analysis of adverse behavioral effects of benzodiazepines with a discussion on drawing scientific conclusions from the FDA's spontaneous reporting system. *Journal of Mind and Behavior, 19,* 21–50, 1998.

Breggin, P. (1998b). Risks and mechanism of action of stimulants. *Program and Abstracts,* pp. 105–120. NIH Consensus Development Conference on the Diagnosis and Treatment of Attention Deficit Hyperactivity Disorder. November 16–18, 1998. William H. Natcher Conference Center. National Institutes of Health. Bethesda, Maryland.

Breggin, P. (1998c). *Talking back to Ritalin: What doctors aren't telling you about stimulants for children.* Monroe, Maine: Common Courage Press.

Breggin, P. (1998d), December). Psychostimulant effects on chldren: A primer for school psychologists and counselors. *Communique; pp. 8–9. (Newspaper of the National Association of School Psychologists.)*

Breggin, P. (1999a). Psychostimulants in the treatment of children diagnosed with ADHD: Part I: Acute risks and psychological effects. *Ethical Human Sciences and Services, 1,* 13–33.

Breggin, P. (1999b). Psychostimulants in the treatment of children diagnosed with ADHD: Part II: Adverse effects on brain and behavior. *Ethical Human Sciences and Services, 1,* 213–241.

Breggin, P. (1999c). Psychostimulants in the treatment of children diagnosed with ADHD: Risks and mechanism of action. *International Journal of Risk and Safety in Medicine, 12,* 3–35. By special arrangement, this report was orig-

inally published in two parts by Springer Publishing Company in *Ethical Human Sciences and Services* (Breggin 1999a&b).

Breggin, P. (2000a). *Reclaiming our children: A healing solution for a nation in crisis.* Cambridge, Massachusetts: Perseus Books.

Breggin, P. (2000b, February 28). Don't let "experts" parent your children. *USA Today,* p. 19A.

Breggin, P. (2000c, Spring). "What psychologists and psychotherapists need to know about ADHD and stimulants." *Changes: An International Journal of Psychology and Psychotherapy* 18:13–23.

Breggin, P. (2000d, September 29). Testimony concerning behavioral drug use in the schools before the U.S. House of Representatives Committee on Education and the Workforce, Subcommittee on Oversight and Investigations, Washington, DC. Text of Breggin's formal submission to the committee available at www.breggin.com. See U.S. House of Representatives, 2000, for how to purchase C-Span film of entire hearing.

Breggin, P. (2001). *The antidepressant fact book: What doctors won't tell you about Prozac, Zoloft, Paxil, Celexa, and Luvox.* Cambridge, Massachusetts: Perseus Books.

Breggin, P. and Breggin, G. (1994). *Talking back to Prozac.* New York: St. Martin's Press.

Breggin, P. and Breggin, G. (1998). *The war against children of color.* Monroe, Maine: Common Courage Press.

Breggin, P. and Cohen, D. (1999). *Your drug may be your problem: How and why to stop taking psychiatric medications.* Cambridge, Massachusetts: Perseus Books.

Breggin, P. and Stern, E.M. (Eds.). (1996). *Psychosocial approaches to deeply disturbed persons*. New York: Haworth Press.

Brenna, S. (1997, November 12). This is your child. This is your child on drugs. *New York*, p. 46.

Brody, D. (1997, August 15). Drug company support. *Psychiatric News*, p. 24.

Brody, J. (1997, February 4). Quirks, oddities may be illnesses. *New York Times*, p. C1.

Brown, J. L., and Bing, S.R. (1976). Drugging children: Child abuse by professionals. In G. P. Koocher (Ed.): *Children's rights and the mental health professions*. New York: John Wiley.

Brown, R. T., Borden, K.A., Wynne, M.E., Schleser, R., and Clingerman, S.R. (1986). Methylphenidate and cognitive therapy with ADD children: A methodological reconsideration. *Journal of Abnormal Child Psychology*, 14, 481–497.

Brown, R.T., and Sexson, S.B. (1988). A controlled trial of methylphenidate in black adolescents. *Clinical Pediatrics*, 27, 74–81.

Brown, R.T., and Sexson, S.B. (1989). Effects of methylphenidate on cardiovascular responses in attention deficit hyperactivity disordered adolescents. *Journal of Adolescent Health Care*, 1989, 179–183.

Brown, W.A. and Williams, B.W. (1976). Methylphenidate increases serum growth hormone concentrations. *Journal of Clinical Endocrinology and Metabolism*, 43, 937–938.

Burchinal, MR, Roberts, J.E., Nabors LA, and Bryant, D.M. (1996). Quality of center child care and infant cognitive and language development. *Child Development*, 67, 606–620.

Burgess, K. (1985, July). Nursing alert: Understanding the spectrum of cerebral stimulants. *Nursing85*, pp. 50–56.

Cahill, D.W., Knipp, H., and Mosser, J. (1981) (letter). Intracranial hemorrhage with amphetamine abuse. *Neurology*, 31, 1058–1059.

Cahill, Jr., G.F. (1970). And pep in America. *New England Journal of Medicine*, 282, 761–762.

Calahan, C. A. (1995). Temperament of primary caregivers and development of literacy. *Perceptual and Motor Skills*, 81, 828–830.

Calhoun, Jr., G., Fees, C., and Bolton, J. (1994). Attention-deficit hyperactivity disorder: Alternatives for psychotherapy? *Perceptual and Motor Skills*, 79, 657–658.

Camp, D.M., DeJonghe, D.K., & Robinson, T.E. (1997). Time-dependent effects of repeated amphetamine treatment on norepinephrine in the hypothalamus and hippocampus assessed with in vivo microdialysis. *Neuropsychopharmacology*, 17, 130–40.

Campbell, M. (1997, August 9). A pill before lunch at Camp Ritalin. *The Globe and Mail* (Toronto).

Cantwell, D. P. (1972). Psychiatric illness in families with hyperactive children. *Archives of General Psychiatry*, 27, 414–417.

Cantwell, D. P. (1996). Attention deficit disorder: A review of the past 10 years. *Journal of the American Academy of Child and Adolescent Psychiatry*, 35, 978–987.

Caplan, P. (1995). *They say you're crazy: How the world's most powerful psychiatrists decide who's normal*. New York: Addison-Wesley.

Carey, W.B. (1998). Is attention deficit hyperactivity a valid disorder? *NIH consensus development conference program and abstracts: Diagnosis and treatment of attention deficit hyperactivity disorder*, pp. 33–6. Rockville, Maryland: National Institutes of Health.

Carnegie Council on Adolescent Development. (1989). *Turning Points:Preparing American youth for the 21st century.* New York:Carnegie Corporation.

Carrey, N. J., Wiggins, D.M., and Milin, R. P. (1996, May). Pharmacological treatment of psychiatric disorders in children and adolescents: Focus on guidelines for the primary care physician. *Drugs 1996, 51,* 750–759.

Carrns, A. (1997, November 12). Schools aren't brick boxes anymore. *Wall Street Journal,* p. B1.

Castellano, M. (1995, May 15). Kentucky fried verdict up for grabs. *New Jersey Law Journal,* p. 39.

Castellanos, F.X., Giedd, J.N., Marsh, W.L., Hamburger, S.D., Vaituzis, A.C., Dickstein, D.P., Sarfatti, S.E., Vauss, Y.C., Snell, J.W., Lange, N., Kaysen, D., Krain, A.L., Ritchie, G.F., Rajapakse, J.C., & Rapoport, J.L. (1996). Quantitative brain magnetic resonance imaging in attention-deficit hyperactivity disorder. *Archives of General Psychiatry,* 53, 607–616.

Castellanos, F.X., Giedd, J.N., Elia, J., Marsh, W.L., Ritchie, G.F., Hamburger, S.D., & Rapoport, J.L. (1997). controlled stimulant treatment of ADHD and Comorbid Tourette's syndrome: Effects of stimulant and dose. *Journal of the American Academy of Child and Adolescent Psychiatry, 36,* 589–596.

Cernerud, L., Eriksson, M., Jonsson, B., Steneroth, G., and Zetterstrom, R. (1996). Amphetamine addiction during pregnancy: 14-year follow-up of growth and school performance. *Acta Paediatrica* (Oslo), 85, 204–208.

CHADD (undated). *CHADD: Children with attention deficit disorders: Hyperactive? inattentive? impulsive?* A mailing membership brochure. Plantation, Florida: CHADD.

CHADD (circa 1989). Facts about Ritalin. Plantation, Florida: CHADD.

CHADD (1992, October 15–17). Program for the Fourth Annual Conference: Pathways to Progress. Hyatt Regency Chicago in Illinois Center, Chicago, Illinois.

CHADD (1993a). CHADD Facts, 1: The disability named ADD. Plantation, Florida: CHADD.

CHADD (1993b). CHADD Facts, 2: Parenting a child with Attention Deficit Disorder. Plantation, Florida: CHADD.

CHADD (1994, October 11, date on cover letter). Petition for rulemaking to reclassify methylphenidate from Schedule II to Schedule III. Attachment B to Riordan and Matyas (1994).

CHADD (1995a, October 13). PBS's Merrow Report inaccurate on ADD says national parent support group. Plantation, Florida: Author.

CHADD (1995b, November 14). C. Keith Conners, Ph.D., Duke University, inducted into Attention Deficit Disorder Hall of Fame. Plantation, Florida: Author. http://www.chadd.org/press6.htm.

CHADD (1996a). CHADD events. http://www.chadd.org/events.htm.

CHADD (1996b). Annual Report. http://www.chadd.org/ann96.htm.

Chandler, T. (1997, June 25). Memo to elementary principals: Information

[On Ritalin referrals] to be included in teacher handbook. Horry County Schools, South Carolina.

Charles, G. (1997, May 15). Silence sur le Prozac! *L'Express* [France], p. 68.

Chira, S. (1993, July 14). Is small better? Educators now say yes for high school. *New York Times*, p. 1.

Chronicle of Higher Education. (1998, January 9). Ex-professor admits he diverted funds, p. A12.

Chronis, P. G. (1999, November 10). Drugs for unruly children attacked: State legislators told of school-violence ties. *Denver Post*, p. 1.

Ciba Pharmaceutical Company. (1969). Ritalin and Ritonic. *Physicians' desk reference*, pp. 653–655. Oradell, New Jersey: Medical Economics.

Ciba Pharmaceutical Company. (1970). Ritalin and Ritonic. *Physicians' desk reference*, pp. 654–655. Oradell, New Jersey: Medical Economics.

Ciba Pharmaceutical Company. (1976, May). Advertisement: Tested by time and experience in the treatment of MBD. *American Journal of Psychiatry*, *133*, A66–A68.

Ciba Pharmaceutical Company. (1986, October). Advertisement: Now... The standard ADD medication in once-a-day dosage. *American Journal of Psychiatry*, *143*, A21–22.

Ciba-Geigy Corporation. (1991). OCD: When a habit isn't just a habit. Pine Brook, NJ: author.

Ciba-Geigy Corporation. (1997). Ritalin. *Physicians' desk reference*, pp. 866–867. Montvale, New Jersey: Medical Economics.

Cinque, J. (1978, January 8). Clinical review for Ritalin-SR tablets, NDA # 18-029, Ciba-Geigy Corporation. Rockville, Maryland: Food and Drug Administration. Obtained through Freedom of Information Act (FOIA).

Clark, C. G. (1997). Attention Deficit Disorder—OCD and/or Tourette Syndrome evaluation/treatment fun package. Las Vegas: A.D.D. Clinic. Web site http://www.addclinic.com/fun-pack.html

Clarke, C. (1997a). *An exploratory study of the meaning of prescription medication to children diagnosed with Attention Deficit Hyperactivity Disorder*. Unpublished doctoral dissertation, Loyola University, Chicago, School of Social Work.

Clarke, C. (1997b, June 26). Personal letter to Peter R. Breggin.

Clinical Psychiatry News (1997, January). ADHD children have smaller, less active brains, p. 12.

Clinton, B. (1997, August 12). Remarks by the president at the DNC democratic mayors dinner. Washington, DC: The White House, Office of the Press Secretary.

Cocciarella, A., Wood, R., and Low K. (1995). Brief behavioral treatment for attention-deficit hyperactivity disorder. *Perceptual and Motor Skills, 81*, 225–226.

Cody, P. (1992, August 21). Numerous drug ads in journals judged misleading, inaccurate. *Psychiatric News*, p. 1.

Cohen, H.A., Ashkenazi, A., Nussinovitch, M., Gross, S., and Frydman, M. (1992). Fixed drug eruption of the scrotum due to methylphenidate. *Annals of Pharmacology, 26*, 1378–1379.

Colbert, T. C. (1997, June 15). Personal communication to Peter and Ginger Breggin from the psychologist who practices in Santa Ana, California.

Coles, G. (1987). *The learning mystique: A critical look at 'learning disabilities.'*

New York: Pantheon Books.

Collins, S. (1997, February 18). Is attention deficit-hyperactivity disorder over-diagnosed? Yes. *Washington Post Health*, p. 19.

Connell, P.H. (1961). Clinical manifestations and treatment of amphetamine type of dependence. *Journal of the American Medical Association, 196*, 718–723.

Conners, C.K. (1969). A teacher rating scale for use in drug studies with children. *American Journal of Psychiatry, 126*, 152–156.

Conners, C.K. (1972). Psychological effects of stimulant drugs in children with minimal brain dysfunction. *Pediatrics, 49*, 702–708.

Conners, C.K., and Eisenberg, L. (1963). The effects of methylphenidate on symptomatology and learning in disturbed children. *American Journal of Psychiatry, 120*, 458–464.

Connolly, H.M., Crary, J.L., McGoon, M.D., Hensrud, D.D., Edward, B.S., Edwards, W.D., and Schaff, H.V. (1997). Valvular heart disease associated with fenfluramine-phentermine. *New England Journal of Medicine, 337*, 581–588.

Cotton, M.F., and Rothberg, A.D. (1988). Methylphenidate v. placebo: A randomized double-blind crossover study in children with attention deficit disorder. *South African Medical Journal, 74*, 268–271.

Counterpoint. (1990, Winter). Researchers find brain link in attention deficit disorder, pp. 4–5.

Covey, S. R. (1997). *The 7 habits of highly effective families*. New York: Golden Books.

Cowart, V.S. (1988, May 6). The Ritalin controversy: What's made this drug's opponents hyperactive? *Journal of the American Medical Association, 259*, 252–253.

Coyle, J. T. (2000). Psychotropic drug use in very young children. *Journal of the American Medical Association, 283*, 1059–60.

Crossette, B. (1996, February 28). Agency sees risk in drug to temper child behavior: Worldwide survey cites overuse of Ritalin. *New York Times*, p. A14.

Crowley, M. (1997, October 20). Do kids need Prozac? *Newsweek*, pp. 73–74.

Cunningham, C.E. and Barkley, R.A. (1978). The effects of methylphenidate on the mother-child interactions of hyperactive identical twins. *Developmental Medicine And Child Neurology, 20*, 634–642.

Dackis, C. A., and Gold, M.S. (1990). Addictiveness to central stimulants. *Advances in Alcohol and Substance Abuse, 9*, 9–26.

David, R. (1997). Personal communication from the chief medical officer of D. C. General to Peter Breggin.

Davies, J. C. (1988). The existence of human needs. In R. A. Coat and Rosati, J.A. (Eds.). *The power of human needs in world society*. New York: Lynne Rienner.

Davy, T., and Rodgers, C.L. (1989). Stimulant medication and short attention span: A clinical approach. *Journal of Developmental and Behavioral Pediatrics, 10*, 313–318.

DeAngelis, T. (1997, June). Trauma at an early age inhibits ability to bond. *Monitor*, p. 11

de Girolamo, G. (1996). WHO studies on schizophrenia: An overview of the results and their implications for understanding the disorder. In P. Breggin, and Stern, E.M. (Eds.). *Psychosocial approaches to deeply disturbed persons*, pp. 213–231. New York: Haworth Press. Also published in (1996) a single volume of *The Psychotherapy Patient*, 9, 213–231.

Dew, J. C. (1997, May 17). Letter from J. Chappell Dew, Horry County Board of Education, District One, South Carolina, to Peter and Ginger Breggin, with accompanying tables on Ritalin daily doses administered in school.

Dialog. (1997, June 11). Generation Rx/Millions of U.S. kids on Ritalin. Busy parents, teachers like effect of 'smart pill.' *Microsoft Daily News*. http://pnp.individual.comm/cgi-bin/pnp.

Diller, L. H. (1996, March–April). The run on Ritalin: Attention deficit disorder and stimulant treatment in the 1990s. *Hastings Center Report 26 (2)*, 12–18.

Dinkmeyer, Sr., D., McKay, G.D., and Dinkmeyer, Jr., D. (1997). *The parent's handbook*. Circle Pines, Minnesota: AGS.

Divoky, D. (1989, April). Ritalin: Education's fix-it drug? *Phi Delta Kappan*, 70, 599–605.

Donovan, D. (1997, September 15). Personal communication to Peter R. Breggin.

Dorland's illustrated medical dictionary. (1994). Philadelphia: W.B. Saunders.

Drug Enforcement Administration (DEA). (1993, October 7). Public Affairs press release concerning Aggregate Production Quota for methylphenidate. Washington, DC: Public Affairs Section, DEA, U.S. Department of Justice.

Drug Enforcement Administration (DEA). (1995a, October 20). Methylphenidate: DEA press release [attached to DEA, 1995b]. Washington, DC: Drug and Chemical Evaluation Section, Office of Diversion Control, DEA, U.S. Department of Justice.

Drug Enforcement Administration (DEA). (1995b, October). *Methylphenidate (A background paper)*. Washington, DC: Drug and Chemical Evaluation Section, Office of Diversion Control, DEA, U.S. Department of Justice.

Drug Enforcement Administration (DEA). (1995c, August 7). Response to CHADD petition concerning Ritalin. See cover letter by Greene (1995). Washington, DC: DEA, U. S. Department of Justice.

Drug Enforcement Administration (DEA). (1996, December 10–12)). *Conference report: Stimulant use in the treatment of ADHD*. Washington, DC: DEA, U. S. Department of Justice.

Drug Facts and Comparisons (1997). St. Louis: Facts and Comparisons.

Drug Facts and Comparisons (2000). St. Louis: Facts and Comparisons.

Dulcan, M. (1994). Treatment of Children and Adolescents. In R. Hales, Yudofsky, S. and Talbott, J. (Eds.), *The American Psychiatric Press textbook of psychiatry*, (Second Edition) (pp. 1209–1250). Washington, D.C.: American Psychiatric Press.

Dulcan, M. and Popper, C. (1991). *Concise guide to child and adolescent psychiatry*. Washington, DC: American Psychiatric Press.

Dumont, M. P. (1990). In bed together at the market: Psychiatry and the pharmaceutical industry. *American Journal of Orthopsychiatry, 60,* 484–485.

Dunnick, J. K. and Hailey, J.R. (1995). Experimental studies on the long-term effects of methylphenidate hydrochloride. *Toxicology, 103,* 77–84.

DuPaul, G., and Costello, A. (1995). The stimulants. In R. Barkley (Ed.), *Taking charge of ADHD* (pp. 249–262). New York: Guilford Press.

During, M.J., Bean, A.J., and Roth, R.H. (1992). Effects of CNS stimulants on the in vivo release of colocalized transmitters, dopamine and neurotensin, from rat prefrontal cortex. *Neuroscience Letters, 140,* 129–133.

Dykman, R. A., Ackerman, P.T., and Raney, T. J. (circa 1993). Research synthesis on assessment and characteristics of children with attention deficit disorder. Executive Summary prepared for Division of Innovation and Development, Office of Special Education Programs, Office of Special Education and Rehabilitation Services, U.S. Department of Education, Washington, DC. Prepared by the Chesapeake Institute.

Dyme, I.Z., Sahakian, B.J., Golinko, B.E., and Rabe, E.F. (1982). Perseveration induced by methylphenidate in children: Preliminary findings. *Progress in Neuro-Psychopharmacology and Biological Psychiatry, 6,* 269–273.

Egeland, B. and Erickson, M.F. (1990). Rising above the past: Strategies for helping new mothers break the cycle of abuse and neglect. *Zero to Three, 11,* (2).

Egger, J., Stolla, A., and McEwen, L.M., (1992). Controlled trial of hyposensitisation in children with food-induced hyperkinetic syndrome. *Lancet, 339,* 1150–1153.

Eichlseder, W. (1985). Ten years of experience with 1,000 hyperactive children in private practice. *Pediatrics, 76,* 176–184.

Ellinwood, E. H., and Cohen, S. (1972). *Current concepts of amphetamine abuse.* Rockville, Maryland: National Institute of Mental Health. DHEW Publication No. (HSM) 72–9085.

Ellinwood, E.H., & Kilbey, M.M. (Eds.). (1977). *Cocaine and other stimulants.* New York: Plenum.

Emmett, A. J. (1993, October 1). "Dear doctor" letter from Senior Vice President, Medical & Public Affairs, Ciba-Geigy, to physicians throughout America. Summit, New Jersey: Ciba-Geigy Corporation.

Emonson, D.L, and Vanderbeek, R.D. (1995). The use of amphetamines in the U.S. Air Force tactical operations during Desert Shield and Storm. *Aviation, Space, and Environmental Medicine,* pp. 260–263

Emslie, G.J., Rush, A.J., Weinberg, W.A., Kowatch, R.A., Hughes, C.W., Carmody, T., & Rintelmann, J. (1997). A double-blind, randomized, placebo-controlled trial of fluoxetine in children and adolescents with depression. *Archives of General Psychiatry, 54,* 1031–1037.

Engelman, R. (1990, November 15). Study ties hyperactivity to disorder of the brain. *San Jose Mercury News.*

Ernst, M. (1996). Neuroimaging in attention-deficit hyperactivity disorder. In G. R. Lyon, and Rumsey, J. M. (Eds.). *Neuroimaging: A window to the neurological foundations of learning and behavior in children,* pp. 95–117. Baltimore: Paul H. Brookes Publishing Company.

Estrada, A. U., and Pinsof, W. (1995). The effectiveness of family therapies for selected behavioral disorders of childhood. *Journal of Marital and Family Therapy, 21,* 403–440.

Euren, S. (1993, May). Attention-Deficit Hyperactivity Disorder: A recommended reading list. Distributed by CHADD, Plantation, Florida.

Faber, A., and Mazlish, E. (1980). *How to talk so kids will listen & listen so kids will talk.* New York: Avon.

Fasnacht, B. (1993, September 3). Child and adolescent disorders get fine-tuning in DSM-IV. *Psychiatric News* p. 8.

Feingold, B. F. (1975). *Why is your child hyperactive.* New York: Random House.

Fiedler, N. L. and Ullman, D.G. (1983). The effects of stimulant drugs on curiosity behaviors of hyperactive boys. *Journal of Abnormal Child Psychology, 11,* 193–206.

Feussner, G. (1998). Diversion, trafficking, and abuse of methylphenidate. *NIH consensus development conference program and abstracts: Diagnosis and treatment of attention deficit hyperactivity disorder,* pp. 201–4. Rockville, Maryland: National Institutes of Health.

Finkel, M. J. (1982, March 30). Letter from the Associate Director for New Drug Evaluation, Bureau of Drugs, to Ciba Pharmaceutical Company, attention Ronald Gauch, for NDA 18-029. Rockville, Maryland: Food and Drug Administration. Obtained through Freedom of Information Act (FOIA).

Firestone, P., Musten, L. M., Pisterman, S., Mercer, J., & Bennett, S. (1998). Short-term side effects of stimulant medications in preschool children with attention-deficit/hyperactivity disorder: A double-blind placebo-controlled study. *Journal of Child and Adolescent Psychopharmacology, 8,* 13–25.

Fisher, R. and Fisher, S. (1996). Antidepressants for children: Is scientific support necessary? *Journal of Nervous and Mental Disease, 184,* 99–102.

Fisher, S., & Greenberg, R. (1989). *The limits of biological treatments for psychological distress: Comparisons with psychotherapy and placebo.* Hillsdale, New Jersey: Lawrence Erlbaum.

Fisher, S., & Greenberg, R. (1995 September/October). Prescriptions for Happiness. *Psychology Today,* pp. 32–37.

Flaum, M., and Schultz, S.K. (1996). When does amphetamine-induced psychosis become schizophrenia? *American Journal of Psychiatry, 153,* 812–815.

Food and Drug Administration. (circa 1981). Summary basis of approval, Ritalin S-R Tablets, NDA 18-029, Ciba-Geigy Corporation. Rockville, MD: Author. Obtained through Freedom of Information Act (FOIA).

Food and Drug Administration. (1985, January 31). Pharmacological advisory committee (workshop). Twenty-seventh meeting. Rockville, MD: Author. Obtained through Freedom of Information Act (FOIA).

Food and Drug Administration. (1995, June). *A MEDWatch continuing education article.* Rockville, Maryland: Staff College, Center for Drug Evaluation and Research, Food and Drug Administration.

Food and Drug Administration. (1996, January 12). Ritalin [cancer] studies. Rockville, MD: Author. Obtained through Freedom of Information Act (FOIA).

Food and Drug Administration. (1996, October). *A MEDWatch continuing ed-*

ucation article: The clinical impact of adverse event reporting. Rockville, Maryland: Staff College, Center for Drug Evaluation and Research, Food and Drug Administration.

Food and Drug Administration. (1997a, March). FDA proposes to withdraw Seldane approval. *FDA Medical Bulletin, 27,* p. 3. Rockville, Maryland: Food and Drug Administration.

Food and Drug Administration. (1997b, summer). FDA public health advisory: Reports of valvular heart disease in patients receiving concomitant fenfluramine and phentermine. *FDA Medical Bulletin, 27,* p. 2.

Food and Drug Administration. (1997c, March 10). Cylert adverse reaction report summary from the FDA's Spontaneous Reporting System (SRS). Division of Epidemiology and Surveillance. Rockville, Maryland: Food and Drug Administration. Obtained through Freedom of Information Act (FOIA).

Food and Drug Administration. (1997d, August). *Guidance for industry: Postmarketing adverse experience reporting for human drug and licensed biological products: Clarification of what to report.* Rockville, Maryland: Food and Drug Administration. Obtained through Freedom of Information Act (FOIA).

Food and Drug Administration. (1997e, March). *Spontaneous Reporting Systems (SRS) Data for Methylphenidate: 1985–March 3, 1997.* Rockville, MD: Author.

Forness, S. R. (1992, winter). Attention deficit disorders, academic functioning and stimulant medication. *OSERS News In Print,* U.S. Department of Education, Washington, DC, pp. 32–36.

Forward, S. (1989). *Toxic Parents: Overcoming their hurtful legacy and reclaiming your life.* New York: Bantam.

Fouse, B. and Morrison, J.A. (1997, February). Using children's books as an intervention for attention-deficit disorder. *The Reading Teacher, 50,* 442–444.

Fowler, M. (1992). *Educators manual:* A project of the CHADD National Education Committee. Plantation, FL: CHADD

Fowler, M. (1994). Attention-Deficit/Hyperactivity Disorder: A NICHCY Briefing Paper. Washington, DC: National Information Center for Children with Disabilities.

Frank, E. (1997, January 17). Synapse elimination: For nerves it's all or nothing. *Science, 275,* 324–325.

Friedberg, J. (1997, November 5). Letter from the Berkeley, California neurologist to Peter R. Breggin, M.D.

Friend, T. (1995, September 10). Patients, doctors face 'the uncertainty of medicine.' *USA Today.*

Frost, J. (1997, August 18). Letter to the editor. *Globe and Mail* (Toronto).

Fulton, A. I., and Yates, W.R. (1988). Family abuse of methylphenidate. *American Family Physician, 38,* 144–145.

Gaines, D. (1992). *Teenage wasteland: Suburbia's dead end kids.* New York: Harper Perennial.

Garcia, L. M. (1990, December 21). A tragedy of gross incompetence: Judge slams two decades of bureaucratic inaction. *Sydney Morning Herald,* p. 7.

Gardner, F. (1994, July 27). Notes from the city. *Synapse UCSF* (University of California, San Francisco).

Gardner, F. (1995, February 8). Ritalanalysis. *Anderson Valley Advertiser,* p. 1.

Gavin, M. (1988). *Otto learns about his*

medicine: A story about medication for hyperactive children. New York: Brunner/Mazel.

Gay, C.T. and Ryan, S.G. (1994). Paroxysmal kinesigenic dystonia after methylphenidate administration. *Journal of Child Neurology, 9*, 45–46.

General Accounting Office (GAO) (1994, September). *Rapid rise in children on SSI disability rolls follows new regulations.* Washington, DC: United States General Accounting Office, GAO/HEHS-94-225.

George, J. (1993a, September 13). Some information left out on ADD. *Harrisburg Patriot* (letter).

George, J. (1993b, October 15). Existence of ADD theoretical. *Leadership News* (Harrisburg), p. 3.

Gibeaut, J. (1996, August). Mood-altering verdict. *American Bar Association Journal*, p. 18.

Giedd, J.N., Castellanos, F.X., Casey, B.J., Kozuch, P., King, A. C., Hamburger, S.D., and Rapoport, J.L. (1994). Quantitative morphology of the corpus callosum in attention deficit hyperactivity disorder. *American Journal of Psychiatry, 151*, 665–669.

Gilbert, S. (1997, September 16). Study supports use of stimulants for children with hyperactivity. *New York Times*, p. C10.

Gillberg, C., Melander, H., von Knorring A-L, Janois, L-O, Thernlund, G., Hagglof, B., Eidevall-Wallin, L., Gustafsson, P., and Kopp, S. (1997). Long-term stimulant treatment of children with attention-deficit hyperactivity disorder symptoms. *Archives of General Psychiatry, 54*, 857–864.

Ginott, H. (1969). *Between parent & child.* New York: Avon.

Gittelman, R., Mannuzza, S., Shenker, R., and Bonagura, N. (1985). Hyperactive boys almost grown up, II: Psychiatric status. *Archives of General Psychiatry, 42*, 937–947.

Gittelman-Klein, R., Klein, D.F., Abikoff, H., Katz, S., Gloisten, A., and Kates, W. (1976). Relative efficacy of methylphenidate and behavior modification in hyperkinetic children: An interim report. *Journal of Abnormal Child Psychology, 4*, 361–379.

Glick, D. (1997, spring/summer). Rooting for intelligence. *Newsweek Special Issue*, p. 32.

Glod, CA, and Teicher, M.H. (1996). Relationship between early abuse, post-traumatic stress disorder, and activity levels in prepubertal children. *Journal of the American Academy of Child and Adolescent Psychiatry, 35*, 1384–1393.

Goeders, N.E., and Kuhar, J.J. (1987). Chronic cocaine administration induces changes in dopamine receptors in the striatum nucleus accumbens. *Alcohol and Drug Research, 7*, 207–216.

Golden, G.S. (1974). Gilles de la Tourette's syndrome following methylphenidate administration. *Developmental Medicine and Child Neurology, 16*, 76–78.

Golden, G.S. (1991, March). Role of attention deficit hyperactivity disorder in learning disabilities. *Seminars in Neurology, 11*, 35–41.

Goldman, E. L. (1995, February). Subtypes, comorbidities make definitive ADHD diagnosis difficult. *Pediatric News*, p. 28.

Goldsmith, S. (1997a, March 31). Medicating foster care: Unmonitored stream of mood drugs imperils children entrusted to state. *Seattle Post-In-*

telligencer, p. 1.

Goldsmith, S. (1997b, April 1). A drug poisoning: 6-year-old died while in state's hands. *Seattle Post-Intelligencer*, p. 1.

Goldsmith, S. (1997c, April 2). Drugs and doubt in Wenatchee: Medications cloud investigation of sex cases. *Seattle Post-Intelligencer*, p. 1.

Goldsmith, S. (1997d, April 3). Boy's death spurs Oregon act. *Seattle Post-Intelligencer*, p. 1.

Goldstein, S. and Goldstein, M. (1992). *Hyperactivity: Why won't my child pay attention*. New York: John Wiley & Sons.

Goleman, D. (1995). *Emotional intelligence*. New York: Bantam.

Gong, Jr., E. J. (1997, July 8). Hypertension damages the brain. ABC News Commentary. http://www.abcnews.com.

Goodman, A.G., Rall, T.W., Nies, A.S., Taylor, P. (1991). *The pharmacological basis of therapeutics, 8th edition*. New York: Pergamon Press.

Goodnow, C. (1994, July 7). Experts say it's not a prescription for trouble. *Seattle Post-Intelligencer*, p. C3.

Gordon, J. S. (1996). *Manifesto for a new medicine*. Reading, Massachusetts: Addison-Wesley.

Gordon, T. (1970). *P.E.T.: Parent effectiveness training*. New York: Peter H. Wyden, Inc.

Gostin, L. O., Arno, P. S., and Brandt, A.M. (1997, March 13). Free-speech smokescreen. *Washington Post*, p. A23.

Gottlieb, F. (1985). Report of the Speaker. *American Journal of Psychiatry, 142*, 1246–1249.

Gould, S.J. (1981). *The mismeasure of man*. New York: W.W. Norton.

Government Accounting Office (GAO). (released 1990, April). *FDA drug review: Postapproval risks 1976–1985*. Report to the Chairman, Subcommittee on Human Resources and Intergovernmental Relations, Committee on Government Operations, U.S. House of Representatives.

Goyer, P.F., Davis, G.C., and Rapoport, J.L. (1979). Abuse of prescribed stimulant medication by a 13-year-old hyperactive boy. *Journal of the American Academy of Child Psychiatry, 18*, 170–175.

Grahame-Smith, D.G., and Aronson, J.K. (1992). *Oxford textbook of clinical pharmacology and drug therapy*. Oxford: Oxford University Press.

Granat, D. (1995, April). The young and the restless. *Washingtonian*, p. 60.

Granger, D.A., Whalen, C.K., and Henker, B. (1993). Perceptions of methylphenidate effects on hyperactive children's peer interactions. *Journal of Abnormal Child Psychology, 21*, 535–549.

Green, A. (1989). Physical and sexual abuse of children. In Kaplan, H. and Sadock, B. (Eds.) *Comprehensive textbook of psychiatry*, pp. 1962–1970. Baltimore: Williams and Wilkins.

Greene, S. H. (1995, August 7). Letter from Deputy Administrator, Drug Enforcement Administration (DEA), to Phillip R. Lee, M.D., Assistant Secretary for Health, Department of Health and Human Services. Cover letter, followed by untitled 111 page DEA response to Child and Adults with Attention Deficit Disorder (CHADD) petition to change Ritalin from Schedule II to Schedule II, plus other attachments. Washington, DC: Drug Enforcement Administration, U.S. Department of Justice. Obtained under Freedom of Information Act (FOIA).

Greenfield, B. J. and Senecal, J. (1995). Recreational multifamily therapy for troubled children. *American Journal of Orthopsychiatry, 65,* 434–439.

Greenhill, L. (1998, July 8). Full disclosure of speaker financial interests or relationships. A form provided by the National Institute of Mental Health to all potential scientific presenters at the NIH Consensus Development Conference on Diagnosis and Treatment of Attention Deficit Hyperactivity Disorder (November 1998). Obtained through the Freedom of Information Act (FOIA).

Greenough, WT, and Black J.E. (1992). Induction of brain structure by experience: Substrates for cognitive development. In M. Gunnar, and Nelson, C. (Eds.), *Developmental Behavioral Neuroscience, Volume 24: Minnesota symposia on child development,* pp. 155–200. Hillsdale, NJ: Lawrence Erlbaum.

Grinfeld, M.J. (1997, September). Ad campaign targets depression. *Psychiatric Times,* p. 1.

Grinfeld, M. J. (2000, May). More kids on drugs: Is the research worth the furor. *Psychiatric Times,* p. 1.

Grob, C. S., and Coyle, J.T. (1986). Suspected adverse methylphenidate-imipramine interactions in children. *Developmental and Behavioral Pediatrics, 7,* 265–267.

Grossman, L.K., and Grossman, N.J. (1985). Methylphenidate and idiopathic thrombocytopenic purpura—Is there an association. *Journal of Family Practice, 20,* 302–304.

Gualtieri, C.T., Kanoy, R., Hawk, B., Koriath, U., Schroeder, S., Young-

blood, W., Breese, G., and Prange, Jr., A. (1981). Growth hormone and prolactin secretion in adults and hyperactive children: Relation to methylphenidate serum levels. *Psychoneuroendocrinology, 6,* 331–339.

Haglund, R.M. and Howerton, L.L. (1982). Ritalin: Consequences of abuse in a clinical population. *The International Journal of Addictions, 17,* 349–356.

Haislip, G. R. (1995, October 25). Letter to Fred A. Baughman, Jr., from Gene R. Haislip, Deputy Assistant Administrator, Office of Diversion Control, Drug Enforcement Administration, Department of Justice, Washington, DC.

Hall, W, Hando, J., Darke, S., and Ross, J. (1996). Psychological morbidity and route of administration among amphetamine users in Sydney, Australia. *Addiction, 91,* 81–87.

Hallowell, E. (1997, May/June). What I've learned from A.D.D. *Psychology Today,* pp. 41 ff.

Hammack, L. (1996, June 4). Ritalin sharer scolded. *Roanoke Times,* p. A.

Handen, B.L., Feldman, H., Gosling, A., Breaux, A.M., and McAuliffe. B. S. (1991). Adverse side effects of methylphenidate among mentally retarded children with ADHD. *Journal of the American Academy of Child and Adolescent Psychiatry, 30,* 241–245.

Haney, D. Q. (1993, April 8). Scientists find gene defect tied to hyperactivity. *Pittsburgh Post-Gazette,* p. A2.

Harvey, R. (1996a, June 6). Study raises concerns about use of Ritalin. *Toronto Star.*

Harvey, R. (1996b, August 4). Use of drug for hyperactivity soaring, study finds. *Toronto Star,* p. A14.

Hauser, P., Zametkin, A.J., Martinez, P., Vitiello, B., Matochik, J.A., Mixson, A.J., and Weintraub, B.D. (1993). Attention deficit-hyperactivity disorder in people with generalized resistance to thyroid hormone. *New England Journal of Medicine, 328,* 997–1001.

Hausman, K. (1987, December 18). Woman sues APA for "fraudulent" ADHD diagnosis, "vague" criteria in *DSM-III. Psychiatric News,* p. 2.

Hazell, P., O'Connell, D., Heathcote, D., Robertson, J., and Henry, D. (1995). Efficacy of tricyclic drugs in treating child and adolescent depression:A meta-analysis. *British Medical Journal, 310,* 897–901.

Healy, D. (1994). The fluoxetine and suicide controversy. *CNS Drugs, 1(3),* 223–231.

Healy, J. M. (1991). *Endangered minds: Why our children don't think.* New York: Simon & Schuster.

Hellmich, N., and Sternberg, S. (1997, September 16). Critics say known side effects were enough to stop approval. *USA Today,* p. 1A.

Henig, R. M. (1988, March 15). Courts enter hyperactivity fray. *Washington Post.*

Henry, T. (1997, October 3–5). Kids do better in school when dad involved. *USA Today,* p. 1.

Henry, T. (2000, August 22). School rolls hit record. *USA Today,* p. 1.

Herbert, W. (1997, April 21). Politics of biology. *U.S. News & World Report,* pp. 72–80.

Hibbs, E.D., and Jensen, P.S. (1996). *Psychosocial treatments of child and adolescent disorders.* Washington, DC: American Psychological Association.

Hoeller, K. (1997, August 13). Against their will. *New York Times,* p. A28.

Hoss, J. and Bartlett, P. (1994, October). *Information, treatment and services for the mentally ill in California.* Sutter-Yuba Mental Health Services & The Alliance for the Mentally Ill of Yuba and Sutter Counties.

Howe, C. (1994). A history of NAMI CAN. *The Journal: Quarterly Publication of the California Alliance for the Mentally Ill, 5(4),* 67–69.

Huang, N.-K., Wan, F.-J., Tseng, C.-J., and Tung, C.-S. (1997). Amphetamine induces hydroxyl radical formation in the striatum of rats. *Life Sciences, 61,* 2219–2229.

Hubbard, R. (1994). *Profitable promises: Essays on women, science and health.* Monroe, Maine: Common Courage Press.

Hubbard, R. and Wald, E. (1993). *Exploding the gene myth.* Boston: Beacon Press.

Huffington, A. (1997a, July 21). Exit Joe Camel, but here comes Joe Prozac. *Los Angeles Times.*

Huffington, A. (1997b, August 26). Lilly markets Prozac for the family medicine chest. Obtained from web site of Creators Syndicate.

Huffington, A. (2000, March 22) (syndicated). Trading pacifiers for Ritalin. *Washington Times,* p. A15.

Huget, J. (2000, August 22). Readin' and writin' and Ritalin: New drug delivers a dose that lasts all day. *Washington Post Health,* p. 7.

Hughes, R. N. (1972). Methylphenidate induced inhibition of exploratory behavior in rats. *Life Sciences, 11,* 161–167.

Hyman, S.E., and Coyle, J.T. (1994). The neuroscientific foundations of psychiatry. In R. Hales, Yudofsky, S. and Talbott, J. (Eds.), *The American*

Psychiatric Press textbook of psychiatry, (Second Edition) (pp. 1–33). Washington, D.C.: American Psychiatric Press.

Hynd, G.W., Semrud-Clikeman, M., Lorys, A.R., Novey, E.S., Eliopulos, D., and Lyytinen, H. (1991). Corpus callosum morphology in attention deficit-hyperactivity disorder: Morphometric analysis on MRI. *Journal of Learning Disabilities, 24*, 141–145.

IMS America. (1997). Top 10 Uniform System of Classification—US. Moving annual totals. Total sales dollars. December, 1996. http://www.ims-america.com/html/today/top10usc.html.

IMS Canada. (1996, July 22). Now pay attention...ADD and the drug debate. *Health points: A compendium of health information by IMS Canada, 1 (1), 1.*

Ingersoll, B. (1988). *Your hyperactive child: A parent's guide to coping with attention deficit disorder*. New York: Doubleday.

International Narcotics Control Board. (INCB) (1995). Report for 1995. United Nations Publications: No. E.96.XI.1. http://www. undep.org/reports/incb95/incb95en.htm#IIB4.

International Narcotics Control Board. (INCB) (1996a). Report for 1996. Vienna, Austria: Author. United Nations Publications: No. E.97XI.3 http://www.undep.org/reports/incb96/e/index.htm

International Narcotics Control Board. (INCB). (1996b, November). *Control of use of methylphenidate in the treatment of ADD: Expert meeting on amphetamine-type stimulants, Shanghai, 25–29 November 1996.* Vienna, Austria: Author.

International Narcotics Control Board.

(INCB). (1997, March 4). INCB sees continuing risk in stimulant prescribed for children. INCB Annual report background note no. 4. Vienna, Austria: Author.

International Narcotics Control Board (INCB). (1999, February 23). Europeans taking "downers." Americans taking "uppers." *INCB annual report 1998: Release no. 4.* Vienna, Austria: Author.

Jacobovitz, D., Sroufe, L. A., Stewart, M., and Leffert, N. (1990). Treatment of attentional and hyperactivity problems in children with sympathomimetic drugs: A comprehensive review. *Journal of the American Academy of Child and Adolescent Psychiatry, 29,* 677–688.

Jacoby, J. and Small, C. (1975, October). The FDA approach to defining misleading advertising. *Journal of Marketing, 39,* 65–73.

Jaffe, J.H. (1995). Amphetamine (or amphetaminelike)-related disorders. In H.I. Kaplan and Sadock, B. (Eds.). *Comprehensive Textbook of Psychiatry, VI,* pp. 791–799. Baltimore:Williams &Wilkins.

Jain, K.K. (1996). *Drug-induced neurological disorders.* Seattle: Hogrefe & Huber.

Jain, J.; Birmaher, B.; Garcia, M.; Al-Shabbout, M.; and Ryan, N. (1992). Fluoxetine in children and adolescents with mood disorders: A chart review of efficacy and adverse reactions. *Journal of Child and Adolescent Psychopharmacology* 2:259–265

Janofsky, M. (1999, November 25). Colorado fuels U.S. debate over use of behavioral drugs. *New York Times,* p. A1.

Jensen, P.S. (1996, December). Letter from the chief of NIMH's Child and

Adolescent Disorders Research Branch to Michael F. Parry, a concerned parent.

Jensen, P. (2000). Commentary: the NIH ADHD Consensus Statement: Win, lose, or draw? *Journal of the American Academy of Child and Adolescent Psychiatry, 39,* 194–7.

Jensen, P. (2000, August 15). Child's well-being is priority. *USA Today.*

Jensen, P., Bain, M.W., and Josephson, A. M. (1989). Why Johnny can't sit still: Kids' ideas on why they take stimulants. Unpublished paper from the Division of Neuropsychiatry, Walter Reed Army Institute of Research, Washington, DC.

Johnston, C. (1996). Parent characteristics and parent-child interactions in families of nonproblem children and ADHD children with higher and lower levels of oppositional-defiant disorder. *Journal of Abnormal Child Psychology, 24,* 85–103.

Johannes, L. and Stecklow, S. (1997, September 16). Withdrawal of Redux spotlights predicament FDA faces on obesity. *Wall Street Journal,* p. 1.

Jonas, J.M. (1992, October). Dr. Jeffrey M. Jonas, director of CNS clinical development at Upjohn, replies [to neurologist, Fred Baughman, Jr. (1992)]. *Clinical Psychiatry News,* p. 5.

Jones, T., Borg, W.P., Boulware, S.D., McCarthy, G., Sherwin, R.S., and Tamborlane, W.V. (1995). Enhanced adrenomedullary response and increased susceptibility to neuroglycopenia: Mechanisms underlying the adverse effects of sugar ingestion in healthy children. *Journal of Pediatrics, 126,* 171–177.

Joyce, P.R., Donald, R.A., Nicholls, M.G., Livesey, J.H., and Abbott, R.M. (1986). Endocrine and behavior responses to methylphenidate in normal subjects. *Biological Psychiatry, 21,* 1015–1023.

Joyce, P.R., Nicholls, M.G., and Donald, R.A. (1984). Methylphenidate increases heart rate, blood pressure and plasma epinephrine in normal subjects. *Life Sciences, 34,* 1701–1711.

Juan, J., McCann, U., and Ricaurte, G. (1997). Methylphenidate and brain dopamine neurotoxicity. *Brain Research, 767,* 172–5.

Kane, G. (Cox News Service) (1996, November 30). Ritalin puts military careers out of bounds: Rejection of would-be enlistees a problem for recruiters. *Roanoke Times,* p. A1.

Kane, J. M., and Lieberman, J.A. (1992). *Adverse effects of psychotropic drugs.* New York: Guilford.

Kaplan, B.J., McNicol, J., Conte, R.A., and Moghadam, J.K. (1989). Dietary replacement in preschool-aged hyperactive boys. *Pediatrics, 83,* 7–17.

Kaplan, S. (1997, August 14–20). Ritalin info for "Curious Cat" Carter. *Observer* (Charlottesville, Virginia), p. 3.

Karlin, R. (2000, May 7). Ritalin use splits parents, school. *Albany Times Union,* p. 1.

Karon, B., & Vandenbos, G. (1981). *The psychotherapy of schizophrenia: The treatment of choice.* New York: Jason Aronson.

Kauffman, R.E., Smith-Wright, D., Reese, C.A., Simpson, R., and Jones, F. (1981). Medication compliance in hyperactive children. *Pediatric Pharmacology, 1,* 231–237.

Kealey, M. (1997, summer). FDA legislation: A bill to kill. *Public Citizen,* p. 1.

Keane, B. (1997, November 8). Letter

from the psychologist in Lismore, New South Wales, Australia to Peter R. Breggin.

Keirsey, D. (1988). Letter from the psychologist to Peter R. Breggin.

Kennedy, C. (1972, January 31). Medical officer report: Ritalin. Rockville, Maryland: Food and Drug Administration. Obtained through Freedom of Information Act (FOIA).

Kiene, H.E., and Solomon, P. (1937, April). Why people misbehave. *Rhode Island Medical Journal*, 58–62.

Kilborn, P. T. (1996, November 30). Shrinking safety net cradles hearts and hopes of children. *New York Times*, p. 1.

King, A.; Riddle, M. A.; Chappell, P. B.; Hardin, M. T.; Anderson, G. M.; Lombroso, P.; and Scahill, L. (1991, March). Emergence of self-destructive phenomena in children and adolescents during fluoxetine treatment. *Journal of the American Academy of Child and Adolescent Psychiatry* 30:179–186.

Kirk, S., and Kutchins, H. (1992). *The selling of DSM: The rhetoric of science in psychiatry*. New York: Aldine De-Gruyter.

Klein, R.G., Landa, B., Mattes, J.A., and Klein, D.F. (1988). Methylphenidate and growth in hyperactive children. *Archives of General Psychiatry, 45*, 1127–1130.

Klein, R. G. and Mannuzza, S. (1988). Hyperactive boys almost grown up: III. Methylphenidate effects on ultimate height. *Archives of General Psychiatry, 45*, 1131–1134.

Knapp, E. E., Robinson, J.I., and Britt, A. L. (1995). *Annual adverse drug experience report: 1995*. Rockville, Maryland: Surveillance and Data Processing Branch, Division of Pharmacovigilance and Epidemiology, Office of Epidemiology and Biostatistics, Center for Drug Evaluation and Research, Food and Drug Administration.

Koek, W., and Colpaert, F.C. (1993). Inhibition of methylphenidate-induced behaviors in rat: Differences among neuroleptics. *Journal of Pharmacology and Experimental Therapeutics, 267*, 181–191.

Kolata, G. (1996, May 15). Boom in Ritalin sales raises ethical issues. *New York Times*, p. C8.

Kolata, G. (1997, September 16). Companies recall 2 top diet drugs at F.D.A.'s urging. *New York Times*, p. A1.

Koplewicz, H. (1996). *It's nobody's fault.* New York: Times Books.

Koppel, T. (1988, June 10). Nightline: Ritalin/Requiring its use in schoolchildren. Transcript obtained from Journal Graphics, Inc., New York.

Koslow, S. H. (Ed.). (1995). *The neuroscience of mental health, II.* Rockville, Maryland: National Institutes of Health and National Institute of Mental Health. NIH Publication No. 95-4000.

Kosten, T. R. (1990). Neurobiology of abused drugs. *Journal of Nervous and Mental Disease, 178*, 217–227.

Kramer, J.C. (1970). Introduction to amphetamine abuse. In E.H. Ellinwood & S. Cohen (Eds.), *Current concepts on amphetamine abuse: Proceedings of a workshop*, Duke University Medical Center, June 5–6, 1970. Rockville, Maryland: National Institute of Mental Health.

Kramer, J.C., Lipton, M., Ellinwood, Jr., E.H., & Sulser, F. (chairmen). (1970). Discussion of part II. In E.H. Ellinwood & S. Cohen (Eds.), *Current concepts on amphetamine abuse: Proceedings of a workshop*, Duke University Medical Center, June 5–6, 1970. Rockville, Maryland: National Institute of Mental Health.

Kruesi, M., Hibbs, E., Zahn T., Keysor, C., Hamburger, S., Bartko, J., and Rapoport, J. (1992, June). A 2-year prospective follow-up study of children and adolescents with disruptive behavior disorders: Prediction by cerebrospinal fluid 5-hydroxyindoleacetic acid, homovanillic acid, and autonomic measures? *Archives of General Psychiatry* 49:429–435.

Kuczenski, R., and Segal, D.S. (1997). Effects of methylphenidate on extracellular dopamine, serotonin, and norepinephrine: Comparison with amphetamine. *Journal of Neurochemistry*, 68, 2032–2037.

Kuehnel, T.G., & Slama, K.M. (1984). Guidelines for the developmentally disabled. In K.M. Tardiff (Ed.), *The psychiatric uses of seclusion and restraint* (pp. 87–102). Washington, D.C.: American Psychiatric Press.

Kuhl, P.K. (1994). Learning and representation in speech and language. *Current Opinions in Neurobiology, 4*, 812–822.

Kuttner, R. (1997, August 31). Medical firms take scalpel to the FDA. *Los Angeles Times: Science*. www.latimes.com/home/news/science/medicine.

Kwasman, A.K., Tinsley, B.J., and Lepper, H.S. (1991). Pediatricians' knowledge and attitudes concerning diagnosis and treatment of attention deficit and hyperactivity disorders: A national survey approach. *Archives of Pediatric and Adolescent Medicine, 149*, 1211–1216.

Lacroix, D., and Ferron, A. (1988). Electro-physiological effects of methylphenidate on the coeruleo-cortical noradrenergic system of the rat. *European Journal of Pharmacology, 149*, 277–285.

Ladika, S. (1996, February 28). U. N. agency concerned with surge in Ritalin use. Associated Press wire service.

Lake, C.R. and Quirk, R.S. (1984). CNS stimulants and the look-alike drugs. *Pediatric Clinics of North America, 7* (4), 689–701.

Lambert, N. (1998). Stimulant treatment as a risk factor for nicotine use and substance abuse. *Program and Abstracts*, pp. 191–8. NIH Consensus Development Conference Diagnosis and Treatment of Attention Deficit Hyperactivity Disorder. November 16–18, 1998. William H. Natcher Conference Center. National Institutes of Health. Bethesda, Maryland.

Lambert, N., & Hartsough, C.S. (1998). Prospective study of tobacco smoking and substance dependence among samples of ADHD and non-ADHD subjects. *Journal of Learning Disabilities 31*, 533–534.

Lambert, N., Windmiller, M., Sandoval, J., and Moore, B. (1976). Hyperactive children and the efficacy of psychoactive drugs as a treatment intervention. *American Journal of Orthopsychiatry, 46*, 335–352.

Lang, J. (1997, June 9). Generation Rx: Ritalin use booming. *The Journal Gazette* (Fort Wayne, Indiana) (Scripps Howard News Service), p. 1.

Langer, E.J., and Abelson, R. P. (1974). A patient by any other name...: Clinician group difference in labeling bias. *Journal of Consulting and Clinical Psychology, 42*, 4–9.

Lavin, P. (1991). Coordinator for children with attention deficit disorder.

Elementary School Guidance & Counseling, 26, 115–116.

Leary, W. (1993, November 14). Blunder limits supply of crucial drug. *New York Times*, p. 12.

Leber, P. (1985, March 13). Letter to Dr. Barry Sachais, Ciba-Geigy Corporation, from Paul Leber, M.D., Director, Division of Neuropharmacological Drug Products, Office of Drug Research and Review, Center for Drugs and Biologics. Rockville, MD: Food and Drug Administration. Obtained through Freedom of Information Act (FOIA).

Leber, P. (1994, December 22). Letter To Fred A. Baughman, Jr. M.D., from Paul Leber, M.D., Director, Division of Neuropharmacological Drug Products, Office of Drug Evaluation 1, Center for Drug Evaluation and Research. Rockville, MD: Food and Drug Administration. Letter provided by Dr. Baughman.

Lee, J. H. (1981, August 24). Review of Advertising of Ritalin-SR, Ciba-Geigy, NDA 18-029. Rockville, Maryland: Food and Drug Administration. Obtained through Freedom of Information Act (FOIA).

Leff, J., and Berkowitz, R. (1996). Working with families of schizophrenic patients. In P. Breggin, and Stern, E.M. (Eds.). *Psychosocial approaches to deeply disturbed persons*, pp. 185–212. New York: Haworth Press. Also published in (1996) *The Psychotherapy Patient, 9*, 185–212.

Leith, N.J. and Barrett, R.J. (1981). Self-stimulation and amphetamine: Tolerance to *d* and to *l* isomers and cross tolerance to cocaine and methylphenidate. *Psychopharmacology, 74*, 23–28.

Leonard, M. (1997, May 25). Children are the new hot market for antidepressants. *Boston Globe*, p. D1.

Leutwyler, K. (1996, August). In focus: Paying attention. *Scientific American*, pp. 13–14.

Levin, G. M. (1995, November). Attention-deficit/hyperactivity disorder: The pharmacist's role. *American Pharmacy, NS35*, 10–20.

Levin, E. M., Kozak, C., and Shaiova, C.H. (1977). Hyperactivity among white middle-class children. *Child Psychiatry and Human Development, 7*, 156–168.

Levy, F., Hay, D.A., McStephen, M., Wood, C., and Waldman, I. (1997). Attention-deficit hyperactivity disorder: A category or a continuum. Genetic analysis of a large-scale twin study. *Journal of the American Academy of Child and Adolescent Psychiatry, 36*, 737–744.

Lewis, L. (1997, February 2). Each day at every school in Horry County, dozens of children line up at nurses' stations and teachers' desks to take their midday Ritalin pills. *Sun News* (Myrtle Beach, SC), p. 1E.

Lewis-Abney, K. (1993). Correlates of family functioning when a child has attention deficit disorder. *Issues in Comprehensive Pediatric Nursing, 16*, 175–190.

Lewontin, R.C. (1992). *Biology as ideology*. New York: HarperPerennial.

Lewontin, R.C., Rose, S., and Kamin, L. (1984). *Not in our genes: Biology, ideology, and human nature*. New York: Pantheon Books.

Liden, C.B., Zalenski, J.R., and Newman, R.L. (1989). *Pay attention!!!* TRANSACT Health Systems.

Lieberman, J.A., Kane, J.M., and Alivir, J. (1987). Provocative tests with psychostimulant drugs in schizophrenia. *Psychopharmacology, 91,* 415–433.

Eli Lilly. (1997a, February 12, mailing date). Lilly Health Policy Update, Special edition: CAMI campaign news, 1 page. Indianapolis. Eli Lilly and Company.

Eli Lilly and Company. (1997b, July 21). Three-page advertisement for Prozac. *Time,* pp. 18–20.

Lipkin, P.H., Goldstein, I.J., and Adesman, A. R. (1994). Tics and dyskinesias associated with stimulant treatment for attention-deficit hyperactivity disorder. *Archives of Pediatric and Adolescent Medicine, 148,* 859–861.

Livingston, K. (1997, Spring). Ritalin: miracle drug or copout? *Public Interest,* pp. 3–18.

Locy, T. (2000, September 15). Fight over Ritalin is heading to court: Company accused of conspiring to create a diagnosis. *USA Today,* p. 3A.

Long, M., and Barrett, P. (2000, May 15). Lawsuit is filed against Novartis over children's use of Ritalin in Texas. *Wall Street Journal,* p. B19.

Lou, H.C., Henriksen, L., and Bruhn, P. (1984). Focal cerebral hypoperfusion in children with dysphasia and/or attention deficit disorder. *Archives of Neurology, 41,* 825–829.

Lou, H.C., Henriksen, L., Bruhn, P., Børner, H., and Nielsen J. B. (1989). Striatal dysfunction in attention deficit and hyperkinetic disorder. *Archives of Neurology, 46,* 48–52.

Lucas, A., and Weiss, M. (1971). Methylphenidate hallucinosis. *Journal of the American Medical Association, 217,* 1079–1081.

Lucker, J. R. and Molloy, A.T. (1995). Resources for working with children

with attention-deficit/hyperactivity disorder (ADHD). *Elementary School Guidance & Counseling, 29,* 260–267.

Lund, D. S. (1989, May). Tardive dyskinesia suits on increase. *Psychiatric Times,* p. 1.

Maag, J. W., and Reid, R. (1994). Attention-deficit hyperactivity disorders: A functional approach to assessment and treatment. *Behavioral Disorders, 20,* 5–23.

Mach, R.H., Nader, M.A., Ehrenkaufer, R.L.E., Line, S.W., Smith, C.R., Gage, H.D., & Morton, T. E. (1997). Use of positron emission tomography to study the dynamics of psychostimulant-induced dopamine release. *Pharmacology Biochemistry and Behavior, 57,* 477–486.

Mackie, D. (1997, May 29). Crime Watch: Alexandria, Arlington, Falls Church. Thefts/Break-ins. *Washington Post,* p. V07.

Mannuzza, S., Klein, R. G., Bonagura, N., Malloy, P., Giampino, T. L., and Addalli, K.A. (1991). Hyperactive boys almost grown up. *Archives of General Psychiatry, 48,* 77–83.

Markowitz, J., and Patrick, K. (1996). [letter] Polypharmacy side effects. *Journal of the American Academy of Child and Adolescent Psychiatry, 35,* 842.

Marlette, D. (1996, June 25). "Kudzu." Cartoon distributed by Creators Syndicate, Inc.

Marshall, E. (2000, August 4). Duke study faults overuse of stimulants for children. *Science* 289:721.

Martin, W.R., Sloan, J.W., Sapira, J.D., and Jasinksi, D.R. (1971). Physiologic, subjective, and behavioral effects of amphetamine, methamphetamine, ephedrine, phenmetrazine, and methylphenidate in man. *Clinical Pharmacology & Therapeutics, 12* (No. 2, Part I), 245–258.

Mason, Jr., W. (1994a, March 29). Drugs for kids sparks parental concern. *Philadelphia Tribune*, p. PG.

Mason, Jr., W. (1994b, May 27). Ritalin furor rages. *Philadelphia Tribune*, p. PG.

Masson, J. M. (1988). *Against therapy: Emotional tyranny and the myth of psychological healing*. New York: Atheneum.

Mathieu, J-F, Ferron, A., Dewar, K.M., and Reader, T.A. (1989). Acute and chronic effects of methylphenidate on cortical adrenoreceptors in the rat. *European Journal of Pharmacology, 162,* 173–178.

Mattes, J. A. and Gittelman, R. (1983). Growth of hyperactive children on maintenance regimen of methylphenidate. *Archives of General Psychiatry, 40,* 317–321.

Maurer, K. (1996, December). African-American children less likely to get Ritalin. *Clinical Psychiatry News*, p. 1.

Maxmen, J.S., and Ward, N.G. (1995). *Psychotropic drugs fast facts, second edition*. New York: W.W. Norton.

Mayes, S.D., and Bixler, E.O. (1993). Reliability of global impressions for assessing methylphenidate effects in children with attention-deficit hyperactivity disorder. *Perceptual and Motor Skills, 77,* 1215–1218.

Mayes, S.D., Crites, D.L., Bixler, E.O., Humphrey II, F.J., and Mattison, R.E. (1994). Methylphenidate and ADHD: Influence of age, IQ and neurodevelopmental status. *Developmental Medicine and Child Neurology, 36,* 1099–1107.

McCann, U. D., Seiden, L.S., Rubin, L.J., and Ricaurte, G.A. (1997). Brain serotonin neurotoxicity and primary pulmonary hypertension from fenfluramine and dexfenfluramine: A systematic review of evidence. *Journal of the American Medical Association, 278,* 666–672.

McCready, K. (1997). Personal communication from the director of the San Joaquin Psychotherapy Center, Clovis, California to Peter Breggin.

McGinnis, J. (1997, September 18). Attention deficit disaster. *Wall Street Journal*, p. A14.

McGovern, C., and Jenkinson, M. (1996, April 22). "Attention Deficit" made me do it. *Alberta Report/Western Report*, p. 32.

McGuinness, D. (1989). Attention deficit disorder: The emperor's new clothes, animal "pharm," and other fiction. In Fisher, S. and Greenberg, R.P. (Eds.). *The limits of biological treatments for psychological distress*. Hillsdale, NJ: Lawrence Erlbaum Associates, pp. 151–188.

McKinney, J.D., Montague, M., and Hocutt, A. M. (circa 1993). Research synthesis on the assessment and identification of attention deficit disorders. Executive Summary prepared for Division of Innovation and Development, Office of Special Education Programs, Office of Special Education and Rehabilitation Services, U.S. Department of Education, Washington, DC. Prepared by the Chesapeake Institute.

McLeer, S.V., Deblinger, E., &Atkins, M.S. et al. (1988). Post-traumatic stress disorder in sexually abused children. *Journal of American Academy. Child Adolescent Psychiatry, 27,* 650–654.

Medical News. (1979, February 9). Methylphenidate abuse produces retinopathy. *Journal of the American Medical Association, 241,* 546.

Meier, B. (2000, September 14). Suits charge conspiracy by maker and doctors' group to expand Ritalin use. *New York Times,* p. A14.

Medical News Letter (1969, May 30). Methylphenidate (Ritalin), pp. 47–48.

Melega, W.P., Raleigh, M.J., Stout, D.B., Huang, S.C., & Phelps, M.E. (1997a). Ethological and 6-[18F]fluoro-L-DOPA-PET profiles of long-term vulnerability to chronic amphetamine. *Behavioural Brain Research, 84,* 258–268.

Melega, W.P., Raleigh, M.J., Stout, D.B., Lacan, G., Huang, S.C., & Phelps, M.E. (1997b). Recovery of striatal dopamine function after acute amphetamine- and methamphetamine-induced neurotoxicity in the vervet monkey. *Brain Research, 766,* 113–20.

Mendelson, J., Jones, R.T., Upton, R., and Jacob, III, P. (1995). Methamphetamine and ethanol interactions. *Clinical Pharmacology & Therapeutics, 57,* 559–568.

Middleton-Moz, J. (1989). *Children of trauma: Rediscovering your discarded self.* Deerfield Beach, Florida: Health Communications.

Millar, T. P. (1997, August 18). Letter to the editor. *Globe and Mail* (Toronto).

Miller, A. (1983). *For your own good: Hidden cruelty in child rearing and the roots of violence.* New York: Farrar Straus Giroux.

Miller, L.G., and Kraft, I.A. (1994). Application of actigraphy in the clinical setting: Use in children with attention-deficit hyperactivity disorder. *Pharmacotherapy, 14,* 219–223.

Miller, W.G., and Miller, F.D. (1992). Accidental injuries of children. In D.

Templer, Hartlage, L. &Cannon W. (Eds.), *Preventable brain damage,* pp. 41–57. New York:Springer Publishing Company.

Millstein, L. G. (1983, September). The regulation of prescription drug advertising. *American Pharmacy, NS23,* 490–493.

Mintz, J., and Torry, S. (1998, January 15). Internal R.J. Reynolds documents detail cigarette marketing aimed at children. *Washington Post,* p. A1.

Morales, T. (1995, November 26). The Ritalin connection: Criticism of drug maker's funding for CH.A.D.D has local chapter crying foul. *Newsday,* p. A56

Moore, S. D. (1997, August 29). Novartis considers how to make a giant even bigger. *Wall Street Journal,* p. B3.

Moore, T. J. (1995). *Deadly medicine: Why tens of thousands of heart patients died in America's worst drug disaster.* New York: Simon & Schuster.

Morrow, D. J. (1997, September 2). Attention disorder is found in growing number of adults. *New York Times,* p. 1.

Morton, C. T. (1996). Is research in normal and ill children involving radiation exposure ethical? *Archives of General Psychiatry, 53,* 1059.

Mosher, L.R., & Burti, L. (1994). *Community mental health: Principles and practice.* New York: Norton.

Moss, G. (1996, June 5). Comprehensive medication review, 1995–1996, Horry County Schools, submitted to the Horry County Board of Education, South Carolina.

Moss, G. (1997, June 4). Comprehensive medication review, 1996–1997, Horry County Schools, submitted to the Horry County Board of Education, South Carolina.

Mostofsky, S.H., Reiss, A.L., Lockhart, P., and Denckla, M.B. (1998). Evaluation of cerebellar size in attention-deficit hyperactivity disorder. *Journal of Child Neurology 13*, 434–439.

Mother Jones (1993, January/February). Toxic ten: America's truant corporations. 4-page pullout without page numbers.

MTA Cooperative Group. (1999a). A 14-Month randomized clinical trial of treatment strategies for attention-deficit/hyperactivity disorder. *Archives of General Psychiatry*, 56, 1073–1086.

MTA Cooperative Group. (1999b). Moderators and mediators of treatment response for children with attention-deficit/hyperactivity disorder: The multimodal treatment study of children with attention-deficit hyperactivity disorder. *Archives of General Psychiatry*, 56, 1088–1096.

MTA side effects rating scale—parent. (undated). Obtained from http://pioria.cpmc.columbia.edu/mta/SIDE_P.html on March 1, 1999.

MTA side effects rating scale—teacher. (undated). Obtained from http://pioria.cpmc.columbia.edu/mta/SIDE_P.html on March 1, 1999.

Mueller, K. (1993). Locomotor stereotypy is produced by methylphenidate and amfonelic acid and reduced by haloperidol but not clozapine or thioridazine. *Pharmacology Biochemistry and Behavior*, 45, 71–76.

Murphy, K. (1997, August 25). Why Johnny can't sit still. *Business Week*, p. 194E4.

Murray, B. (1996, December). Home schools: How do they affect children? *Monitor*, p. 1.

Murray, B. (1997, June). Parents' role is critical to children's learning. *Monitor*, p. 24.

Nash, M. J. (1997, February 3). Fertile minds. *Time*, pp. 47–56.

Nasrallah, H., Loney, J., Olson., S., Mc-Calley-Whitters, M., Kramer, J., and Jacoby, C. (1986). Cortical atrophy in young adults with a history of hyperactivity in childhood. *Psychiatry Research* 17:241–246.

National Academy of Sciences. (circa 1970). Panel on psychiatric drugs: Ritalin. Washington, D.C.: Author.

National Advisory Mental Health Council. (1988). *Approaching the 21st Century: Opportunities for NIMH Neuroscience Research*. Rockville, Maryland: National Institute of Mental Health.

National Advisory Mental Health Council. (1995). *Basic behavioral science research for mental health*. Rockville, Maryland: National Institute of Mental Health.

National Center for Children in Poverty. (1996–1997, Winter). One in four: America's youngest poor. *News and Issue*, 6, 1. New York: Columbia School of Public Health.

National Information Center for Children and Youth with Attention Deficit Disorder. (1997). Fact sheet number 19: General information about Attention-Deficit/Hyperactivity Disorder. Washington, DC: Author.

National Institute of Mental Health. (undated). Multimodal treatment study for attention-deficit hyperactivity disorder (the MTA study). Obtained from http://pioria.cpmc.columbia.edu/mta/basicq.html on March 1, 1999.

National Institute of Mental Health. (NIMH) (1993). *Learning disabilities: Decade of the brain*. Rockville, Maryland: NIH Publication No. 93-3611.

National Institute of Mental Health.

(NIMH). (1994) *Attention deficit hyperactivity disorder: Decade of the brain.* Rockville, Maryland. NIH publication No. 94-3572.

National Institute of Mental Health and the Food and Drug Administration. (1995, January 24–25). *Psychopharmacology in children and adolescents: Current problems, future prospects.* Conference held in Washington, DC. Complete transcript prepared by Freilicher & Associates, Rockville, Maryland. Obtained through the Freedom of Information Act (FOIA).

National Institutes of Health (1998, November 19). *Consensus statement: Diagnosis and treatment of attention deficit hyperactivity disorder* (draft). Rockville, Maryland: Author. Obtained from the NIH website: http://odp.od.nih.gov/consensus/cons/110/110_statement.

National Institutes of Health. (1998). NIH Consensus Development Conference Diagnosis and Treatment of Attention Deficit Hyperactivity Disorder. November 16–18. William H. Natcher Conference Center. National Institutes of Health. Bethesda, Maryland.

National Institutes of Health (2000). National Institutes of Health Consensus Development Conference Statement: Diagnosis and treatment of attention-deficit/hyperactivity disorder (ADHD). *Journal of the American Academy of Child and Adolescent Psychiatry, 39,* 182–192.

National Toxicology Program. (1995). *NTP technical report on toxicology and carcinogenesis studies of methylphenidate hydrochloride in F344/N rats and B6C3F mice (feed studies).* Rockville, Maryland: National Institutes of Health. NIH Publication No. 95-3355.

Neergaard, L. (Associated Press) (1996, January 13). FDA calls Ritalin safe despite possible cancer signs in mice. *Detroit News.*

Neisworth, J.T., Kurtz, P.D., Jones, R.T., and Madle, R.A. (1974). Biasing of hyperkinetic behavior ratings by diagnostic reports. *Journal of Abnormal Child Psychology, 2,* 323–329.

Nemeroff, C. B. (program chair) (1996, April). *The role of specific neurotransmitter systems in the pathophysiology and treatment of depression.* Atlanta: Emory School of Medicine.

Neurological Drugs Advisory Committee. (NDAC). (1977, February 3). Use of amphetamine in the treatment of MBD, narcolepsy and seizure disorders. Rockville, Maryland: Food and Drug Administration. Obtained through Freedom of Information Act (FOIA).

Neuropharmacology Advisory Committee. (NAC). (1974). Report of the ad hoc panel on Cylert to the NAC. [The report is undated; the NAC met on February 4, 1974. Signing the report were Robert Sprague, Robert Reichler, and Thomas A. Hayes.]. Rockville, Maryland: Food and Drug Administration. Obtained through Freedom of Information Act (FOIA).

Newsweek (1996, March 18). Mother's little helper, p. 51.

New York State Psychiatric Institute and Columbia University Division of Child & Adolescent Psychiatry. (1994). Grand Rounds: The multimodal treatment study of attention deficit hyperactivity disorder (MTA Study)—An NIMH cooperative agreement grant. (unpublished; distributed on March 9, 1994).

Nidecker, A. (1997, September). Spanking predicts later antisocial behavior.

Clinical Psychiatry News, p. 5.

Nies, A.S., and Spielberg, S. P. (1996). Principles of therapeutics. In Hardman, J.G., and L. E. Limbird (Eds.), *Goodman & Gilman's the pharmacological basis of therapeutics, ninth edition*, pp. 43–62. New York: McGraw-Hill.

NIMH MTA Study. (undated, a). Information for parents. Obtained from http://pioria.cpmc.columbia.edu/mta/parent.html. on March 1, 1999.

NIMH MTA Study. (undated, b). Teacher information. Obtained from http://pioria.cpmc.columbia.edu/mta/teacher.html. on March 1, 1999.

Nord, C.W., Brimhall, D., and West, J. (1997, September). *Fathers' involvement in their children's schools: National household education survey*. Washington, DC: National Center for Education Statistics, Office of Educational Research and Improvement, U.S. Department of Education, NCES 98-091.

Novartis. (1996a, March 7). Ciba-Geigy Ltd and Sandoz Ltd announce plans to merge. Basel: Novartis Press Release. http://www.novartis.com.

Novartis. (1996b, August). Strong performance spurred by new products and accelerating growth momentum. Basel: Ciba Press Release. http://www.novartis.com.

Novartis. (1997, August 15—date taken from web site). Pharma—Central Nervous System Disorders. Attention Deficit Hyperactivity Disorder. http://www.novartis.com/healthcare/pharma/add.html.

NYSPI Sponsored Research. (last update, 1998, December 21). Research foundation for Mental Hygiene, Inc., Psychiatric Institute Division. Obtained at http://www.nyspi.cpmc.columbia.educ/nyspi/rfinhgmt.Rf_spon.htm on March 1, 1999.

Oas, P. T. (1997a). Does your child have ADD? Unpublished manuscript by the psychologist who practices in Niceville, Florida.

Oas, P. T. (1997b). Personal communication to Peter and Ginger Breggin.

Office of the Inspector General, Richard P. Kusserow, Inspector General. (1992, June). *Prescription Drug Advertisements in Medical Journals*. Rockville, Maryland: Department of Health and Human Services. OEI-01-90-00482.

Office of Special Education and Rehabilitative Services (OSERS) (1997, February 19). Mission statement. Washington, DC: U. S. Department of Education.

Offir, C. W. (1974, December). A slavish reliance on drugs: Are we pushers for our own children. *Psychology Today*, p. 49.

Ojito, M. (1997, December 14). Ritual use of mercury prompts testing of children for poisoning. *New York Times*, p. 53.

Oprah Winfrey Show. (1987a, April 2). *Mental hospital horror stories* with Peter R. Breggin, Huey Freeman, Rae Unzicker, Leonard Roy Frank, and Dennis Clarke. Journal Graphics, Inc., New York, New York.

Oprah Winfrey Show. (1987b, August 17). *Psychiatric debate* with Peter R. Breggin, Judi Chamberlin, Joseph Rogers, and Paul Fink. Journal Graphics, Inc., New York, N.Y.

OSHERS News in Print (1992, Winter). A clarification of state and local responsibility under federal law to address the needs of children with attention deficit disorders. U.S. Department of Education, Washington, DC, pp. 27–31.

Ostow, M. (1997, December 27).

When mental illness disqualifies candidates. *New York Times*, p. A32.

Ounce of Prevention Fund. (1996). *Starting smart: How early experiences affect brain development*. Chicago, Illinois: Author.

Panksepp, J. (1998). Attention deficit hyperactivity disorders, psychostimulants, and intolerance of childhood playfulness: A tragedy in the making. *Current Directions in Psychological Science, 7*, 91–98.

Parry, M. (1997, January 29). On reading, writing, Ritalin and institutionalized drug use. *Mercer Island Reporter* (Washington State).

Pavlov, I. P. (1957). *Experimental psychology and other essays*. New York: Philosophical Library.

PDR Medical Dictionary. (1995). Montvale, New Jersey: Medical Economics.

Pear, R. (1997, August 13, 1997). President to order drug makers to conduct pediatric studies. *New York Times*, p. A17.

Pear, R. (2000, March 20). White House seeks to curb pills used to calm the young. *New York Times*, p. A1.

Pearson, J., Halliday, G., Sakamoto, N., and Michel, J-P. (1990). Catecholaminergic neurons. In G. Paxinos (Ed.), *The human nervous system* (pp. 1023–1049). New York: Academic Press.

Peck, M.S. (1978). *The road less traveled*. New York: Simon & Schuster.

Pelham, Jr. W.E. (1993). Recent developments in pharmacological treatment for child and adolescent mental health disorders. *School Psychology Review, 22*, 158–161.

Pelliegrino, E.D. (1996). Clinical judgement, scientific data, and ethics: Antidepressant therapy in adolescents and children. *Journal of Nervous and Mental Disease, 184*, 106–108.

Perkins, K. D. (1994, December 5). Some skeptical of surge in attention-disorder diagnoses. *Sacramento Bee*, p. A1.

Perlman, S. E. (1996, March 28). Ritalin caution: Maker urges better control to cure abuse of attention-deficit drug. *Newsday*, p. A05.

Perman, E. S. (1970). Speed in Sweden. *New England Journal of Medicine, 283*, 757–761.

Perry, B. D. (1994). Neurobiological sequelae of childhood trauma: PTSD in children. In M. Murburg (Ed.), *Catecholamine function in posttraumatic stress disorder: Emerging concepts*, pp. 233–255. Washington, DC: American Psychiatric Press.

Perry, B.D., Pollard, R.A., Blakley, T.L., Baker, W. L., and Vigilante, D. (1995). Childhood trauma, the neurobiology of adaptation, and "use-dependent" development of the brain: How "states" become "traits." *Infant Mental Health Journal, 16*, 277–289.

Peterson, R. (1997, July 31). Nurturing may play role in intelligence. *USA Today*, p. 1D.

Physicians' Desk Reference. (1997). Montvale, New Jersey: Medical Economics.

Physicians' Desk Reference. (2000). Montvale, New Jersey: Medical Economics.

Pizzi, W.J., Rode, E.C., and Barnhart, J.E. (1986). Methylphenidate and growth: Demonstration of a growth impairment and a growth-rebound phenomenon. *Developmental Pharmacology and Therapeutics, 9*, 361–368.

Pleak, R.R. (1995). Adverse effects of chewing methylphenidate. *American*

Journal of Psychiatry, 152, 811.

Pollock, G. H. (1986). Report of the Treasurer. *American Journal of Psychiatry, 143,* 1339–1341.

Popper, C.W., and Steingard, R.J. (1994). Disorders usually first diagnosed in infancy, childhood, or adolescence. R. Hales, Yudofsky, S. and Talbott, J. (Eds.), *The American Psychiatric Press textbook of psychiatry,* Second Edition, pp. 729–832. Washington, DC: American Psyciatric Press.

Porrino, L. J., and Lucignani, G. (1987). Different patterns of local brain energy metabolism associated with high and low doses of methylphenidate: Relevance to its action in hyperactive children. *Biological Psychiatry, 22,* 126–128.

Porrino, L. J., Rapoport, J., Behar, D., Ismond, D., and Bunney, W. (1983). A naturalistic assessment of the motor activity of hyperactive boys: Part II. *Archives of General Psychiatry, 40,* 688–693.

Postlewait, G. (1997, July 24). Administrative directive: Improper referral of students for medication. Horry County Schools, South Carolina.

Power, T. J., Hess, L.E., and Bennet, D.S. (1995). The acceptability of interventions for attention-deficit hyperactivity disorder among elementary and middle school teachers. *Journal of Developmental and Behavioral Pediatrics, 16,* 238–243.

Price, J. (1997, May 6). FDA authorization may result in millions of child Prozac users. *Washington Times.*

PR Newswire. (1997, June 6). Transdermal patch formulation of anti-anxiety medication holds promise for treating hyperactive children.

Psychiatric News. (1992, October 2). Media coverage found to influence media prescribing patterns of Ritalin, p. 9.

Psychiatric News. (1996, March 15). APA salutes excellence in residency training, p. 1.

Psychiatric News. (1997a, May 2). NIMH funds nationwide research program to provide data on safe, effective use of psychotropics in youngsters, p. 8.

Psychiatric News. (1997b, August 15). APA racks up good year in advertising revenues, p. 4.

Psychiatric News. (1997c, September 19). Fen-Phen combination said to be neurotoxic, p. 2.

Psychiatric Times. (1993, June). Researchers identify link to attention-deficit disorder, p. 3.

Psychiatric Times. (1995, October). Possible link found between MDMA(Ecstasy), fenfluramine, p. 8.

Psychiatric Services. (1997). Editor's note [letters section]. 48, 601.

PT staff. (1997, September). Indictments impact drug approval process; FDA inspection reveals irregularities. *Psychiatric Times,* p. 19.

Putnam, F.W. (1990). Foreword. In Donovan, D.M. and McIntyre, D. *Healing the hurt child.* New York: W.W. Norton.

Quinn, P. O., and Stern, J.M. (1991). *Putting on the brakes: Young people's guide to understanding attention deficit hyperactivity disorder (ADHD).* New York: Magination Press.

Quinn, P. O. (1997). *Attention deficit disorder: Diagnosis and treatment from infancy to adulthood.* New York: Brunner/Mazel.

Randrup, A., & Munkvad, I. (1970). Correlation between specific effects of amphetamines on the brain and on behavior. In E.H. Ellinwood & S. Cohen (Eds.), *Current concepts on amphetamine abuse: Proceedings of a workshop, Duke University Medical Center, June 5–6, 1970*. Rockville, Maryland: National Institutes of Mental Health.

Rapoport, J.L., Buchsbaum, M., Weingartner, H., Zahn, T.P., Ludlow, C., and Mikkelsen, E. (1980). Dextroamphetamine: Cognitive and behavioral effects in normal and hyperactive boys and men. *Archives of General Psychiatry, 37*, 933–943.

Rapoport, J.L., Buchsbaum, M., Zahn, T.P., Weingartner, H., Ludlow, C., and Mikkelsen, E. (1978). Dextroampheta-mine: Cognitive and behavior effects in normal prepubertal boys. *Science, 199*, 560–563.

Rapoport, J.L., Lott, I., Alexander, D., and Abramson, A. (1970). Urinary noradrenaline and playroom behavior in hyperactive boys. *Lancet, 2*, 1141.

Rappley, M.D., Gardiner, J.C., Jetton, J.R., and Houang, R.T. (1995). The use of methylphenidate in Michigan. *Archives of Pediatric and Adolescent Medicine, 149*, 675–679.

Ready, T. (1997, July 10). The religion of Ritalin. *The Stranger* (Seattle), pp. 12–14.

Regier, D. A. and Leshner, A.I. (1992, February). Request for applications: Cooperative agreement for a multisite, multimodel treatment study of attention-deficit hyperactivity disorder (ADHD)/attention-deficit disorder (ADD). MH-92-03. Washington, D.C.: Department of Health and Human Services; Public Health Service; Alcohol, Drug Abuse and Mental Health Administration; and NIMH.

Resnick, M.D., Bearman, P.S., Blum, R.W., Bauman, K.E., Harris, K.M., Jones, J., Tabor, J., Beuhring, T., Sieving, R.E., Shew, M., Ireland, M., Bearinger, L. H., and Udry, J.R. (1997). Protecting adolescents from harm: Findings from the National Longitudinal Study on Adolescent Health. *Journal of the American Medical Association, 278*, 823–832.

Reuters News Agency. (1997a, April 2). Ky. judge bows out of Lilly Prozac case. Wire service story.

Reuters News Agency. (1997b, August 23). In upset, ulcer drug Prilosec is No. 1 in prescription sales. *Los Angeles Times*, p. D1.

Reuters News Agency. (1997c, August 22). Top 10 US drug sales: Jan–June 1997 vs Jan–June 1996. Obtained from web site of Infoseek.

Reuters News Agency. (1997d, October 20). Lilly profits jump, Prozac sales up on ad push. Obtained from web site of Infoseek.

Richard, M. M. (1996, February 28). Letter from the National President of CHADD to Oscar Schroeder, President, International Narcotics Control Board, Vienna, Austria. http://www.chadd.org/incbresp.htm.

Richards, M.F. (1995). Placebo methylphenidate tablets. *Military Medicine, 160* (5), p. A6.

Richters, J.E., Arnold, L.E., Jensen, P.S., Abikoff, H., Conners, C.K., Greenhill, L.L., Hechtman, L, Hinshaw, S.P., Pelham, W.E., and Swanson, J.M. (1995). NIMH collaborative multisite multimodal treatment study of children with ADHD: I. Background and rationale. *Journal of the American Academy of Child and Adolescent Psychiatry, 34*, 987–1000.

Riddle, Mark A.; King, Robert A.; Hardin, Maureen T.; Scahill, Lawrence; Ort, Sharon I.; Chappell, Phillip; Rasmusson, Ann; and Leckman James F. (1990/1991). Behavioral side efects of fluoxetine in children and adolescents. *Journal of Child and Adolescent Psychopharmacology* 1:193–198.

Rie, H.E., Rie, E.D., Stewart, S., and Ambuel, J.P. (1976a). Effects of methylphenidate on underachieving children. *Journal of Consulting and Clinical Psychology, 44,* 250–260.

Rie, H.E., Rie, E.D., Steward, S., and Ambuel, J.P. (1976b). Effects of Ritalin on underachieving children: A replication. *American Journal of Orthopsychiatry, 46,* 313–322.

Riordan, R. M., and Matyas, D.E. (1994, October 11). Letter from legal counsel for CHADD to Thomas A. Constantine, Administrator, Drug Enforcement Administration, U.S. Department of Justice. With attachments. Obtained through Freedom of Information Act (FOIA).

Robinson, T.E. & Kolb, B. (1997). Persistent structural modifications in the nucleus accumbens and prefrontal cortex neurons produced by previous experience with amphetamine. *Journal of Neuroscience, 17,* 8491–7.

Rosenfeld, A. A. (1979). Depression and psychotic regression following prolonged methylphenidate use and withdrawal: A case report. *American Journal of Psychiatry, 136,* 226–227.

Rosenthal, R., and Jacobson, L. (1968). *Pygmalion in the classroom.* New York: Holt, Rinehart & Winston.

Ross, C.A., and Pam, A. (1995). *Psychoscience in biological psychiatry: Blaming the body.* New York: John Wiley.

Rosse, R.B., and Licamele, W.L. (1984). Slow-release methylphenidate: Problems when children chew tablets. *Journal of Clinical Psychiatry, 45,* 525.

Rowe, K. S., and Rowe, K. J. (1994). Synthetic food coloring and behavior: A dose response effect in a double-blind, placebo-controlled, repeated-measures study. *Pediatrics, 125,* 691–698.

Russell, J. (1997, December). The pill that teachers push. *Good Housekeeping,* p. 110.

Rutter, M. (1997). Child psychiatric disorder (commentary). *Archives of General Psychiatry, 54,* 785–789.

Sabshin, M. (1992, March 10). To aid understanding of mental disorders. *New York Times,* p. A24.

Sackeim, H., Prudic, J., Devanand, D., Kiersky, J., Fitzsimons, L., Moody, B., McElhiney, M., Coleman, E. & Settembrino, J. (1993). Effects of stimulus intensity and electrode placement on the efficacy and cognitive effects of electroconvulsive therapy. *New England Journal of Medicine, 328,* 839–846.

Safer, D. J. (1988). A survey of medication treatment for hyperactive/inattentive students. *Journal of the American Medical Association, 260,* 2256–2258.

Safer, D. J., and Allen, R. P. (1989). Absence of tolerance to the behavioral effects of methylphenidate in hyperactive and inattentive children. *Journal of Pediatrics, 115,* 1003–1008.

Safer, D. J., Allen, R. P., and Barr, E. (1975). Growth rebound after termination of stimulation drugs. *Journal of Pediatrics, 86,* 113–116.

Safer, D.J., and Krager, J.M. (1992). Effect of a media blitz and a threatened lawsuit on stimulant treatment. *Journal of the American Medical Association, 268*, 1004–1007.

Safer, D. J., Zito, J M., and Fine, E. M. (1996). Increased methylphenidate usage for attention deficit disorder in the 1990s. *Pediatrics, 98*, 1084–1088.

Salyer, K. (1991). Learning disabilities as a childhood manifestation of severe psychopathology. *American Journal of Orthopsychiatry, 61*, 230–240.

Sams-Dodd, F., and Newman, J. D. (1997). Effects of administration regimenon the psychomimetic properties of d-amphetamine in the squirrel monkey (*Saimiri sciureus*). *Pharmacology Biochemistry and Behavior, 56*, 471–480.

Sandoval, J., Lambert, N., and Yandell, W. (1976). Current medical practice and hyperactive children. *American Journal of Orthopsychiatry, 46*, 323–332.

Scahill, L., and Lynch, K. A. (1994, October–December). Use of methylphenidate in children with attention-deficit hyperactivity disorder. *Journal of Child and Adolescent Psychiatric Nursing, 7*, 44–46.

Scarnati, R. (1986). An outline of hazardous side effects of Ritalin (methylphenidate). *The International Journal of Addictions, 21*, 837–841.

Schachar, R.J., Tannock, R., Cunningham, C., & Corkum, P.V. (1997). Behavioral, situational, and temporal effects of treatment of ADHD with methylphenidate. *Journal of the American Academy of Child and Adolescent Psychiatry, 36*, 754–763.

Schaepe, H. (1995, June 27). Letter from the Secretary of the Board of the United Nations International Narcotics Control Board to The Counselor for Narcotic Affairs, Permanent Mission of the United States of America to the United Nations.

Schary, W. L. (1980, December 22). Review of a bioequivalency study. Ritalin-SR, NDA # 18-029, Ciba-Geigy Corporation.

Scheflin, A.W., and Opton, Jr., E.M. (1978). *The mind manipulators*. New York: Paddington.

Scher, J. (1966, November). Patterns and profiles of addiction and drug abuse. *Archives of General Psychiatry, 15*, 539–551.

Scherbel, Matt. (1995, January 18). "Ritalin ain't da answer." *Bethesda Almanac*.

Schiller, E., and Hauser, J. (1992a, fall). OSEP's initiatives for meeting the needs of children with attention deficit disorder. *Beyond behavior, 4*: No. 1, p. 17.

Schiller, E., and Hauser, J. (1992b, winter). OSEP's initiatives for meeting the needs of children with attention deficit disorder. *OSERS News in Print*. U.S. Department of Education, Washington, DC, pp. 30–31.

Schiller, E., Jensen, P., and Swanson, J. (1996, November/December). Education of children with attention deficit disorder. *Our Children*, pp. 32–33.

Schiørring, E. (1979). Social isolation and other behavior changes in groups of adult verret monkeys (*Cercopitecus aethiops*) Produced by low, nonchronic doses of d-amphetamine. *Psychopharmacology, 64*, 297–302.

Schiørring, E. (1981). Psychopathology induced by "speed drugs." *Pharmacology Biochemistry & Behavior, 14*, Suppl. 1, 109–122.

Schleifer, M., Weiss, G., Cohen, N., Elman, M., Crejic, H., and Kruger, E.

(1975). Hyperactivity in preschoolers and the effect of methylphenidate. *American Journal of Orthopsychiatry*, 45, 33–50.

Schmidt, W. (1987, May 5). Sales of drug are soaring for treatment of hyperactivity. *New York Times*.

Schmidt, M., Kruesi, M., Elia, J., Borcherding B., Elin, R., Hosseini, J., McFarlin, K., and Hamburger, S. (1994). Effect of dextroamphetamine and methylphenidate on calcium and magnesium concentrations in hyperactive boys. *Psychiatric Research*, 54, 199–210.

Schmidt, W. E. (1987, May 7). Sales of drug are soaring: For treatment of hyperactivity. *New York Times*, p. 1.

Schmitt, R. (2000, September 14). Maker of Ritalin, psychiatric group sued. *Wall Street Journal*, p. B19.

Schmued, L.C., & Bowyer, J.F. (1997). Methamphetamine exposure can produce neuronal degeneration in mouse hippocampal remnants. *Brain Research*, 759, 135–140.

Schrag, P. and Divoky, D. (1975). *The myth of the hyperactive child*. New York: Pantheon.

Schwartz, J. (1997, August 9). FDA relaxes rules for on-air drug ads. *Washington Post*, p. A1.

Schwarz, E.D., and Perry, B.D. (1994). The post-traumatic stress response in children and adolescents. *Psychiatric Clinics of North America*, 17, 311–326.

Schwiebert, V.L., Sealander, K.A., and Tollerud, T. R. (1995). Attention-deficit hyperactivity disorder: An overview for school counselors. *Elementary School Guidance & Counseling*, 29, 249–259.

Scoville, B. (1970, February 27). Review of Reports and Supplements. Ritalin

NDA 10-187; 10-899. Rockville, Maryland: Food and Drug Administration. Obtained through Freedom of Information Act (FOIA).

Scoville, B. (1970, February 27). Review of [corporate] reports and supplements for Ritalin. Rockville, Maryland: Food and Drug Administration. Obtained through Freedom of Information Act (FOIA).

Seattle Clinical Research Center, Inc. (1997, August 13). Advertisement: Attention-Deficit Hyperactivity Disorder Research. *Seattle Times*.

Seppa, N. (1997, June). Parenting programs more popular than ever. *Monitor*, p. 20.

Sexton, J., and Swarns, R. L. (1997, November 15). A slide into peril, with no one to catch her. *New York Times*, p. A1.

Shapiro, L. (1991, August 16). APA and drug companies: Too close for comfort. *Psychiatric News*, p. 20.

Shapiro, N. (1996, December 11). Is Johnny a cash cow? *Eastside Week* (Seattle), p. 7.

Shaywitz, S.E., Hunt, R.D., Jatlow, P., Cohen, D.J., Young, J.G., Pierce, R.N., Anderson, G.M., and Shaywitz, B.A. (1985). Psychopharmacology of attention deficit disorder: Pharmacokinetic, neuroendocrine, and behavioral measures following acute and chronic treatment with methylphenidate. *Pediatrics*, 69, 688–694.

Sheng, P., Ladenheim, B., Moran, T.H., Wang X.-B., & Cadet, J.L. (1996). Methamphetamine-induced neurotoxicity is associated with increased striatal AP-1 DNA-binding activity in mice. *Molecular Brain Research*, 42, 171–174.

Sherman, C. (1995, July). Prozac for kids: "Landmark" study affirms drug's use. *Clinical Psychiatry News*, p. 1.

Shih, T-M, Khachaturian, Z.S., Barry, III, H., and Reisler, K. L. (1975). Differential effects of methylphenidate on reticular formation and thalamic nuclei activity. *Psychopharmacologia*, *44*, 11–15.

Shore, M. (1997, June). Reaching the hard-to-reach. *Readings*, *12*, 4–7.

Silver, L. (1989). *ADHD: Attention deficit-hyperactivity disorder, booklet for parents*. Summit, NJ: Ciba-Geigy.

Silver, L. (1990). *ADHD: Attention deficit-hyperactivity disorder and learning disabilities, Booklet for the Classroom Teacher*. Summit, NJ: Ciba-Geigy.

Silver, L. (1993, January 12). Do doctors too often medicate 'hyper' children? No. *Washington Post Health*, p. 10.

Skinner, B.F. (1971). *Beyond freedom and dignity*. New York: Bantam

Skrzycki, C. (1996, February 18). Slowing the flow of federal rules: New conservative climate chills agencies' activism. *Washington Post*, p. A1.

Sleator, E.K., Ullmann, R.K., and von Neumann, A. (1982). How do hyperactive children feel about taking stimulants and will they tell the doctor? *Clinical Pediatrics*, *21*, 475–479.

Sleek, S. (1997, June). Can "emotional intelligence" be taught in today's schools? *Monitor*, p. 25.

Smith, B.D. (1993, August 1). Relaxed, firm dads save school events. *New York Times: Education life supplement* p.5.

Smith, T.A., and Kronick, R.F. (1979). The policy culture of drugs: Ritalin, methadone, and the control of deviant behavior. *International Journal of Addictions*, *14*, 933–946.

Snyder, J. (1996, November 18). Targeting problems while in cradle may avert later therapy. *Arizona Republic*, B1.

Solanto, M.V., and Wender, E.H. (1989). Does methylphenidate constrict cognitive functioning? *Journal of the American Academy of Child and Adolescent Psychiatry*, *28*, 897–902.

Sommers-Flanagan, J., Sommers-Flanagan, R. (1996). Efficacy of antidepressant medication with depressed youth: What psychologists should know. *Professional Psychology: Research and Practice*, *27*, 145–153.

Sonsalla, P.K., Jochnowitz, N.D., Zeevalk, G.D., Oostveen, J.A., & Hall, E.D. (1996). Treatment of mice with methamphetamine produces cell loss in the substantia nigra. *Brain Research*, *738*, 172–5.

Southam New Media News Service. (1996, June 1). Frustrated parents embrace Ritalin as a panacea for disruptive kids. http.://ww.southam.com/nmc/waves/depth/health/ritalin0601a.html.

Speech, T. J., Rao, S. M., Osmon, D.C., and Sperry, L. T. (1993). A double-blind controlled study of methylphenidate treatment in closed head injury. *Brain Injury*, *7*, 333–338.

Spencer, T.J., Biederman, J., Harding, M., O'Donnell D., Faraone, S., & Wilens, T.E. (1996). Growth deficits in ADHD children revisited: Evidence for disorder-associated growth delays? *Journal of the American Academy Child and Adolescent Psychiatry*, *35*, 1460–69.

Spensley, J. , and Rockwell, D.A. (1972, April 20). Psychosis during methylphenidate abuse. *New England Journal of Medicine*, *286*, 880–881.

Spotts, J.V. and Spotts, C.A. (Eds.) (1980). *Use and abuse of amphetamine and its substitutes.* Rockville Maryland: National Institute on Drug Abuse. DHEW Publication No. (ADM) 80-941.

Squires, S. (1990, November 15). Brain function yields clues to hyperactivity. *Washington Post*, p. A1.

Sroufe, L.A., and Stewart, M.A. (1973). Treating problem children with stimulant drugs. *New England Journal of Medicine, 289*, 407–413.

Stableford, W., Butz, R., Hasazi, J., Leitenberg, H., and Peyser, J. (1976). Sequential withdrawal of stimulant drugs and use of behavior therapy with two hyperactive boys. *American Journal of Orthopsychiatry, 46*, 302–312.

St. Dennis, C., and Synoground, G. (1996). Pharmacology update: Methylphenidate. *Journal of School Nursing, 12*, 5–11.

Stecklow, S., and Johannes, L. (1997a, August 15). Drug makers rely on clinical researchers who now await trial. *Wall Street Journal*, p. A1.

Stecklow, S., and Johannes, L., (1997b, August 15). What became of the drugs tested. *Wall Street Journal*, p. A6.

Stepp, L. S. (1996, February 5). A wonder drug's worst side effect: Kids turning on to easy-to-get Ritalin for a quick—and sometimes deadly—high. *Washington Post*, p. A1.

Still, G.F. (1902). The Coulstonian lectures on some abnormal physical conditions in children. *Lancet, 1*, 1008–1168.

Stout, D. (1996, April 18). 2 wells are closed in area with concern over cancer. *New York Times*, B4.

Stout, D. (1997, August 9). Drug makers get leeway on TV ads. *New York Times*, p. 27.

Strauch, B. (1997, August 10). Use of antidepressant medication for young patients has soared: To bolster market, makers seek F.D.A. sanction. *New York Times*, p. 1.

Strayhorn, J. M. and Weidman, C.S. (1989). Reduction of attention deficit and internalizing symptoms in preschools through parent-child interaction training. *Journal of the American Academy of Child and Adolescent Psychiatry, 28*, 888–896.

Struzzi, D. (1995, April 24). Teens learn dangers of Ritalin use: 19-year-old man dies after snorting stimulant at party. *Roanoke Times*, C1.

Subcommittee of the Committee on Government Operations (1970, September 29). *Federal involvement in the use of behavior modifying drugs on grammar school children.* House of Representatives, 91st Congress, Second Session. Washington, DC: U. S. Government Printing Office.

Suplee, C. (1997, August 30). FDA seeks ban on laxative ingredient. A *Washington Post* story obtained off the web site of the *Los Angeles Times*.

Suro, R. (1997, June 25). Other drugs supplanting cocaine use: Methamphetamine, heroin on the rise, White House reports. *Washington Post*, p. A1.

Susman, E. (1996, May 1). Alternatives sought for Ritalin. *Psychopharmacology Update, 7*, 1.

Swanson, J. (1998). Biological bases of ADHD: Neuroanatomy, genetics, and pathology. *Program and Abstracts*, pp. 37–42. NIH Consensus Development Conference Diagnosis and Treatment of Attention Deficit Hyperactivity Disorder. November 16–18, 1998. William H. Natcher Conference Center. National Institutes of Health. Bethesda, Maryland.

Swanson, J.M. (circa 1993). Research synthesis of the effects of stimulant medication on children with attention deficit disorder: A review of reviews. Executive Summary prepared for Division of Innovation and Development, Office of Special Education Programs, Office of Special Education and Rehabilitation Services, U.S. Department of Education, Washington, DC. Prepared by the Chesapeake Institute.

Swanson, J.M. (1993, January 27–29). Medical intervention for children with attention deficit disorder. *Proceedings of the Forum on the Education of Children with Attention Deficit Disorder*, pp. 27–34. Washington, DC: U.S. Department of Education, Office of Special Education and Rehabilitation Services and Office of Special Education Programs, Division of Innovation and Development.

Swanson, J.M., Cantwell, D., Lerner, M., McBurnett, K., Pfiffner, L. and Kotkin, R. (1992, fall). Treatment of ADHD: Beyond medication. *Beyond behavior* 4:No. 1, pp. 13–16 and 18–22.

Swanson, J.M., Lerner, M., and Williams, L. (1995). More frequent diagnosis of attention deficit-hyperactivity disorder. *New England Journal of Medicine, 333*, 944.

Tanouye, E. (1997, April 4). Pharmaceuticals: Antidepressant makers study kids' market. *Wall Street Journal*, p. 1.

Taylor, E. (1994). Syndromes with attention deficit and hyperactivity. M. Rutter, Taylor, E., and Hersov, L. (Eds.). *Child and adolescent psychiatry:Modern approaches*, pp. 285–307. Oxford:Blackwell.

Teicher, MH, Andersen, S.L., Glod, C.A., Navalta, C.P., and Gelbard, H. A. (1997). Neuropsychiatric disorders of childhood and adolescence. In Yudofsky, S., and Hales, R.E. (Eds.), *The American Psychiatric Press textbook of neuropsychiatry*, pp. 903–942. Washington, DC: American Psychiatric Press.

Thadani, P. V. (1995). Biological mechanisms and perinatal exposure to abused drugs. *Synapse, 19, 228–232.*

The White House. (1999, June 7). Remarks by the President, the First Lady, the Vice President, and Mrs. Gore at the White House Conference on Mental Health, Blackburn Auditorium, Howard University, Washington, D.C. Provided to the media by the White House Office of the Press Secretary.

Thomas, S.F. (1990, October 24). Give attention deficit disorders their due. *Education Week*, p. 1.

Thomas, K. (1995, November 16). Ritalin maker's ties to advocates probed. *USA Today*.

Thomas, K. (2000, August 8). Parents pressured to put kids on drugs. Courts, schools force Ritalin use. *USA Today*, p. 1.

Thomson, C. (1997, June 5). Woke up this morning feeling so blue. Took an antidepressant. But what'll it do? *The Bulletin* [European, English-language], p. 2531.

Thurow, L. C. (1997, January 27). Changes in capitalism render one-earner families extinct. *USA Today*, p. 17A.

Tienari, P., Sorri, A., Lahti, L., Naarala, M., Wahlberg, E., Moring, J., Pohjola, J., and Wynn, L.C. (1987). Genetic and psychosocial factors in schizophrenia: The Finnish adoptive family study. *Schizophrenia Bulletin, 13,* 477–484.

Tork, I., and Hornung, J-P. (1990). Raphe nuclei and the serotonergic system. In G. Paxinos (Ed.). *The Human Nervous System,* pp. 1001–1022. New York: Academic Press.

Tousignant, M. (1995, April 11). Children's cure or adults' crutch. *Washington Post,* p. B1.

Treadwell, D. (1987, December 28). A "Miracle Drug" gets closer look. *Los Angeles Times,* p. 1.

Tucker, M. E. (1997, March). 'Dear Doctor' a reminder of potential Cylert risk. *Clinical Psychiatry News,* p. 4.

Turner, J. (1996, May 16). Ritalin sharer expelled: Friend who sold drug also booted. *Roanoke Times,* p. A1.

Twin studies unravel relationship between genes and environment. (1992, December) *Psychiatric Times,* p. 20.

Ubell, E. (1997, October 12). Are our children overmedicated? *Parade Magazine,* p. 4.

Unis, A.S., Dawson, T.M., Gehlert, D.R., and Wamsley, J.K. (1985). Autoradiographic localization of [^{3}H]methyl-phenidate binding sites in rat brain. *European Journal of Pharmacology, 113,* 155–157.

United Nations Information Service (1995, February 28). Dramatic increase in methylphenidate consumption in U.S.: Marketing methods questioned. Vienna: Author.

United Nations Information Service (1997a, March 4). INCB sees continuing risk in stimulant prescribed for children. Vienna: Author.

United Nations Information Service (1997b, March 4). Drugs of abuse: INCB annual report, background note no. 8. Vienna: Author.

Up from Prozac. (1996, June 13). *Sacramento News & Review.*

USA Today. (2000, August 15). Editorial: Reading, writing and Ritalin.

U.S. Department of Education (undated). *Attention deficit disorder: What teachers should know.* Washington, DC: Division of Innovation and Development, Office of Special Education Programs, Office of Special Education and Rehabilitation Services.

U.S. Department of Education (undated). *Attention deficit disorder: Beyond the myths.* Washington, DC: Division of Innovation and Development, Office of Special Education Programs, Office of Special Education and Rehabilitation Services.

U.S. Department of Education (circa 1993). Executive summaries of research syntheses and promising practices on the education of children with attention deficit disorder. Prepared for Division of Innovation and Development, Office of Special Education Programs, Office of Special Education and Rehabilitation Services, U.S. Department of Education, Washington, DC. Prepared by the Chesapeake Institute.

U.S. Department of Health and Human Services. (1999). *Mental health: A report of the Surgeon General.* Rockville, MD: U.S. Department of Health and Human Services, Substance Abuse and Mental Health Services Administration, Center for Mental Health Services, National Institutes of Health, National Institute of Mental Health.

U.S. House of Representatives (2000, September 29). Behavioral drug use in schools: Questions and concerns. Hearings before the Committee on

Education and the Workforce, Subcommittee on Oversight and Investigations, Washington, DC. The entire hearing was filmed by C-Span and can be purchased from www.viewer@c-span.org. The title for purchasing is Behavioral Drug Use, ID: 159514-09/29/2000.

Valentine, M.R. (1987). *How to deal with discipline problems in the schools: A practical guide for educators.* Dubuque, Iowa: Kendall/Hunt Publishing Company.

Valentine, M.R. (1988). *How to deal with difficult discipline problems: A family-systems approach.* Dubuque, Iowa: Kendall/Hunt Publishing Company.

Valentine, M. R. (1997). ADHD: A growing educational, social and legal problem. Summary of a workshop presentation. Dr. Valentine can be contacted at 23565 Via Paloma, Coto de Caza, CA 92679.

van Meerendonk, F. (1997, July 30). Interview with Peter Breggin.

Van Pelt, J. C. (1997, September 15). Ritalin column distorts the truth. *Bangor Daily News.*

Vatz, R.E. (1994, July 27). Attention deficit delirium. *Wall Street Journal*, p. A10.

Vatz, R.E., and Weinberg, L.S. (1993). Treatment of attention-deficit hyperactivity disorder. *Journal of the American Medical Association, 269,* 2368.

Vatz, R.E., and Weinberg, L.S. (1995, January 1). Overreacting to attention deficit disorder. *USA Today Magazine,* p. 84.

Vigue, D. I. (2000, January 1). Ritalin use challenged: Lawrence parents say children pressed to use drug. *Boston Globe,* p. B4.

Vitiello, B., and Jensen, P. S. (1997).

Medication development and testing in children and adolescents. *Archives of General Psychiatry, 54,* 871–876.

Vobejda, B. (1997, September 10). Love conquers what ails teen, study finds. *Washington Post,* p. A1.

Volkow, N.D., Ding, Y-S., Fowler, J.S., Wang, G-J., Logan, J., Gatley, J.S., Dewey, S., Ashby, C., Lieberman, J., Hitzemann, R., & Wolf, A.P. (1995, June). Is methylphenidate like cocaine? *Archives of General Psychiatry, 52,* 456–463.

Volkow, N.D., Wang, G.-J., Fowler, J.S., Logan, J., Gatley, S.J., Hitzemann, R., Chen, A.D., Dewey, S.L., and Pappas, N. (1997). Decreased striatal dopaminergic responsiveness in detoxified cocaine-dependent subjects. *Nature, 386,* 830–833.

Vorhees, C.V. (1994). Developmental neurotoxicity induced by therapeutic and illicit drugs. *Environmental Health Perspectives, 102* (supple. 2), 145–153.

Wagner, G.C., Ricaurte, G.A., Johanson, C.E., Schuster, C.R., and Seiden, L.S. (1980). Amphetamine induces depletion of dopamine and loss of dopamine uptake sites in caudate. *Neurology, 30,* 547–550.

Walker, III, S. (1974, December) Drugging the American child: We're too cavalier about hyperactivity. *Psychology Today,* pp. 43–48.

Wallander, J.L., Schroeder, S.R., Michelli, J.A., and Gualtieri, C.T. (1987). Classroom social interactions of attention deficit disorder with hyperactivity children as a function of stimulant medication. *Journal of Pediatric Psychology, 12,* 61–76.

Wang, G-J, Volkow, N., Fowler, J., Ferrieri, R., Schlyer, D., Alexoff, D., Pappas, N., Lieberman, J., King, P.

Warner, D., Wong, C., Hitzemann, R., and Wolf, A. (1994). Methylphenidate decreases regional cerebral blood flow in normal human subjects. *Life Sciences, 54,* 143–146.

Weiler, I.J., Hawrylak, N., and Greenough, W.T. (1995). Morphogenesis in memory formation: Synaptic and cellular mechanisms. *Behavioral Brain Research, 66,* 1–6.

Weiss, G. (1981). Controversial issues of the pharmacotherapy of the hyperactive child. *Canadian Journal of Psychiatry, 26,* 385–392.

Weiss, F., Imperato, A., Casu, M.A., Mascia, M.S., & Gessa G.L. (1997). Opposite effects of stress on dopamine release in the limbic system of drug-naive and chronically amphetamine-treated rats. *European Journal of Pharmacology, 337,* 219–222.

Weithorn, C. J., and Ross, R. (1976). Stimulant drugs for hyperactivity: Some additional disturbing questions. *American Journal of Orthopsychiatry, 46,* 168–173.

Welke, R. (1990, Spring). Litigation involving Ritalin and the hyperactive child. *Detroit College of Law Review, (1),* 125–176.

Welsh, P. (1995, June 11). The case for going public. *Washington Post,* p. C1.

Wender, P.H. (1971). *Minimal brain dysfunction in children.* New York: John Wiley.

Wender, P.H. (1973). *The hyperactive child: A handbook for parents.* New York: Crown Publishers.

Wender, P.H. (1987). *The hyperactive child, adolescent,and adult.* New York: Oxford University Press.

Wender, P.H. (1995). *Attention-deficit hyperactivity disorder in adults.* New York:Oxford University Press.

Wender, P.H. (1997). Attention deficit hyperactivity disorder in adults: A wide view of a widespread condition. *Psychiatric Annals, 27,* 556–562.

Whalen, C. and Henker, B. (1991). Social impact of stimulant treatment for hyperactive children. *Journal of Learning Disabilities, 248,* 231–241.

Whalen, C. and Henker, B. (1997). Stimulant pharmacotherapy for attention-deficit/hyperactivity disorders: An analysis of progress, problems, and prospects. In S. Fisher, and R. Greenberg, R. (Eds.) *From placebo to panacea: Putting psychotherapeutic drugs to the test,* pp. 323–356. New York: J. Wiley & Sons.

Whalen, C., Henker, B., Collins, B., Finck, D., &Dotemoto, S. (1979). A social ecology of hyperactive boys: Medication effects in structured classroom environments. *Journal of Applied Behavior Analysis, 12,* 65–81.

Wilens, T.E. and Biederman, J. (1992). The stimulants. *Pediatric Psychopharmacology, 15,* 191–222.

Wiley, R. F. (1971). Abuse of methylphenidate (Ritalin). (letter). *New England Journal of Medicine, 285,* 464.

Williams, L. (1988, January 15). Parents and doctors fear growing misuse of drug used to treat hyperactive kids. *Wall Street Journal,* p. 25.

Williamson, P. (1990). *Good kids, bad behavior.* New York: Simon & Schuster.

Williamson, S., Gossop, M., Powis, B., Griffiths, P., Fountain, J., and Strang, J. (1997). Adverse effects of stimulant drugs in a community sample of users. *Drug and Alcohol Dependence, 44,* 87–94.

Wilson, J.M., Kalasinsky, K.S., Levey,

A.I., Bergeron, C., Reiber, G., Anthony, R.M., Schmunk, G.A., Shannak, K., Haycock, J.W., and Kish. S.J. (1996). Striatal dopamine nerve terminal markers in human, chronic methamphetamine users. *Nature Medicine, 2,* 699–702.

Wolraich, M. L. (Ed.). (1996). *The classification of child and adolescent mental diagnoses in primary care.* Elk Grove Village, Illinois: American Academy of Pediatrics.

Woodward, B., and Weiser, B. (1994, February 4). Costs soar for children's disability program. *Washington Post,* p. A1.

Wren, C. (1996, February 14). Sharp rise in use of methamphetamines generates concern. *New York Times,* p. A16.

Wulf, S. (1997, May 26). A new lesson plan. *Time,* p. 75.

Wyeth-Ayerst Laboratories. (1997, August 19). Press release: Multisite clinical study will evaluate possible behavioral and cognitive effects of Redux. Obtained from the web site of the *Los Angeles Times* Bizwire.

Young, J. G. (1981). Methylphenidate-induced hallucinosis: Case histories and possible mechanisms of action. *Developmental and Behavioral Pediatrics, 2,* 35–38.

Younger, D. (1995). Pollutants and industrial hazards. In L. Rowland (Ed.), *Merritt's textbook of neurology,* ninth edition, pp. 987–995. Baltimore:Williams &Wilkins.

Yuan, J., McCann, U., & Ricaurte, G. (1997). Methylphenidate and brain dopamine neurotoxicity. *Brain Research, 767,* 172–175.

Yudofsky, S., Hales, R.E., and Ferguson, T. (1991). *What you need to know about psychiatric drugs.* New York: Grove Weidenfeld.

Zachary, G. P. (1997, May 2). Boys used to be boys, but do some now see boyhood as a malady. *Wall Street Journal,* p.1.

Zaczek, R., Battaglia, G., Contrera, J.F., Culp, S., & De Souza, E.B. (1989). Methylphenidate and pemoline do not cause depletion of rat brain monoamine markers similar to that observed with methamphetamine. *Toxicology and Applied Pharmacology, 100,* 227–233.

Zametkin, A.J. (1991, Spring/Summer). The neurobiology of attention-deficit hyperactivity disorder. *Chadder,* pp. 10–11.

Zametkin, A.J. (1992, August 28). Deposition testimony in the case of Laverne Miller v. Lehman Lindsey et al. Superior Court for the County of Gwinnett, State of Georgia, Civil Action No. 89-A-0261-5.

Zametkin, A.J., Liebenauer, L.L., Fitzgerald, G.A., King, A.C., Minkunas, D.V., Herscovitch, P., Yamada, E.M. and Cohen, R.M.. (1993). Brain metabolism in teenagers with attention-deficit hyperactivity disorder. *Archives of General Psychiatry, 50,* 333–340.

Zametkin, A.J., Nordahl, T.E., Gross, M., King, A. C., Semple, W.E., Rumsey, J., Hamburger, S. and Cohen, R.M. (1990). Cerebral glucose metabolism in adults with hyperactivity of childhood onset. *New England Journal of Medicine, 323,* 1361–1366.

Zito, J.M., Safer, D.J., dosReis, S., Magder, L.S., Riddle, M.A. (1997). Methylphenidate patterns among

Medicaid youths. *Psychopharmacology Bulletin*, *33*, 143–147.

Zito, J.M., Safer, D .J., dosReis, S., Gardner, J.F., Boles, J., and Lynch, F. (2000). Trends in the prescribing of psychotropic medications to preschoolers. *Journal of the American Medical Association*, *283*, 1025–1030.

INDEX

ABOUT THE AUTHOR

Peter R. Breggin, M.D., is a psychiatrist in full-time private practice in Bethesda, Maryland, where he has treated adults, children, and families since 1968.

Dr. Breggin is one of the world's foremost critics of biological psychiatry, including medication, and is a strong advocate for psychological and social human services. He is the founder and director of the International Center for the Study of Psychiatry and Psychology, a reform-oriented research and educational network. He is also the founder and co-editor of Ethical Human Sciences and Services. Dr. Breggin has been on the faculty of the counseling departments of the University of Maryland and Johns Hopkins University, and has also taught at George Mason University and the Washington School of Psychiatry.

Dr. Breggin was trained at Harvard College and Case Western Reserve Medical School. His three years of residency in psychiatry were at the Massachusetts Mental Health Center where he was a teaching fellow at the Harvard Medical School and also at the State University of New York, Upstate Medical Center. He is a former officer in the U. S. Public Health Service and a former full-time consultant with the National Institute of Mental Health (NIMH).

Dr. Breggin gives workshops and seminars throughout North America and Europe, and frequently appears in the media as an expert on national programs such as "60 Minutes," "20/20," and "Nightline." He participates as a medical expert in a variety of forensic activities, including malpractice and product liability lawsuits, and helped to formulate the original class action lawsuit against Novartis, the manufacturer of Ritalin.

Dr. Breggin is an editor on several journals. He has published many professional articles and books, including Toxic Psychiatry (1991), Talking Back to Prozac (1994, with Ginger Breggin), Brain-Disabling Treatments in Psychiatry (1997), The Heart of Being Helpful (1997), The War Against Children of Color (1998, with Ginger Breggin), Your Drug May Be Your Problem: How and Why to Stop Taking Psychiatric Medication (1999, with David Cohen), Reclaiming Our Children (2000), and The Antidepressant Fact Book (2001).

More information about Dr. Breggin's work can be found on his web site, www.breggin.com.